Neurology and Neurobiology

EDITORS

Victoria Chan-Palay
University Hospital, Zurich

Sanford L. Palay
The Harvard Medical School

ADVISORY BOARD

Albert J. Aguayo
McGill University

Günter Baumgartner
University Hospital, Zurich

Masao Ito
Tokyo University

Tong H. Joh
Cornell University Medical
College, New York

Gösta Jonsson
Karolinska Institute

Bruce McEwen
Rockefeller University

William D. Willis, Jr.
The University of Texas, Galveston

ORGANIZATION OF THE AUTONOMIC NERVOUS SYSTEM
Central and Peripheral Mechanisms

ORGANIZATION OF THE AUTONOMIC NERVOUS SYSTEM
Central and Peripheral Mechanisms

Proceedings of a Satellite Symposium of the XXX Congress
of the International Union of Physiological Sciences
Held in Montreal, July 8–10, 1986

Editors

John Ciriello
Department of Physiology
Health Sciences Centre
University of Western Ontario
London, Ontario

Franco R. Calaresu
Department of Physiology
Health Sciences Centre
University of Western Ontario
London, Ontario

Leo P. Renaud
Neurosciences Unit
Montreal General Hospital and
McGill University
Montreal, Quebec

Canio Polosa
Department of Physiology
McGill University
Montreal, Quebec

ALAN R. LISS, INC., NEW YORK

Address all Inquiries to the Publisher
Alan R. Liss, Inc., 41 East 11th Street, New York, NY 10003

Copyright © 1987 Alan R. Liss, Inc.

Printed in the United States of America

Library of Congress Cataloging-in-Publication Data
Organization of the autonomic nervous system.

(Neurology and neurobiology ; v. 31)
Contains papers presented at the satellite
symposium of the 30th Congress of the International
Union of Physiological Sciences, held in Montreal,
Canada, July 8–10, 1986.
Includes bibliographies and index.
1. Nervous system, Autonomic—Congresses.
I. Calaresu, Franco R., 1931–   . II. International
Union of Physiological Sciences. Congress (30th : 1986 :
Vancouver, B.C.) III. Series: [DNLM: 1. Autonomic
Nervous System—physiology—congresses. 2. Central
Nervous System—physiology—congresses. 3. Peripheral
Nerves—physiology—congresses.   W1 NE337B v.31 /
WL 600 068 1986]
QP368.O74 1987   599′.0188   87-3970
ISBN 0-8451-2733-0

Contents

I. FUNCTIONAL PROPERTIES OF SYMPATHETIC PREGANGLIONIC AND POST-GANGLIONIC NEURONS

II. SPINAL MECHANISMS

III. SYMPATHETIC TONE AND PERIODICITIES

IV. VENTROLATERAL MEDULLA AND CARDIOVASCULAR REGULATION

V. SUPRASPINAL MECHANISMS IN THE CONTROL OF THE CIRCULATION

VI. CELLULAR MECHANISMS FOR HYPOTHALAMIC REGULATION: THE MAGNOCELLULAR NEUROSECRETORY NEURON

Contributors

H.-H. Abel, Institute of Physiology, Free University of Berlin, D-1000 Berlin 33, Federal Republic of Germany [179]

W. Steve Ammons, Department of Physiology, Thomas Jefferson University, Philadelphia, PA [91]

J. A. Armour, Department of Physiology and Biophysics, Dalhousie University, Halifax, Nova Scotia, B3H 4H7, Canada [67]

Manjit Bachoo, Department of Physiology, McGill University, Montreal, Quebec, H3G 1Y6 Canada [189]

D. Banks, Department of Physiology, The Medical School, University of Birmingham, Birmingham, England B15 2TJ [337]

Susan M. Barman, Departments of Pharmacology/Toxicology and of Physiology, Michigan State University, East Lansing, MI 48824 [203, 239]

Robert W. Blair, Department of Physiology and Biophysics, The University of Oklahoma Health Sciences Center, Oklahoma City, OK 73190 [91]

Charles W. Bourque, M.R.C. Neuropharmacology Research Group, Department of Pharmacology, School of Pharmacy, University of London, London, WC1N 1AX, England [387]

Chandler McCuskey Brooks, Department of Physiology #31, SUNY, Health Science Center at Brooklyn, Brooklyn, NY 11203, [459]

D. Les Brown, Department of Pharmacology, University of Virginia, Charlottesville, VA 22908; present address: Department of Pediatrics, University of North Carolina, Chapel Hill, NC 27514 [215]

Franco Calaresu, Department of Physiology, Health Sciences Centre, University of Western Ontario, London, Ontario, N6A 5C1 Canada [363]

Monica M. Caverson, Department of Physiology, Health Sciences Centre, University of Western Ontario, London, Ontario, N6A 5C1 Canada [227]

John Ciriello, Department of Physiology, Health Sciences Centre, University of Western Ontario, London, Ontario, N6A 5C1 Canada [227]

Howard L. Cohen, Department of Physiology, State University of New York, Health Science Center at Brooklyn, Brooklyn, NY 11203 [133]

Morton I. Cohen, Department of Physiology and Biophysics, Albert Einstein College of Medicine, Bronx, NY 10461 [133]

The numbers in brackets are the opening page numbers of the contributors' articles.

C.A. Connelly, Rehabilitation Research and Development Center, Hines VA Center, Hines, IL 60141 [169]

E.T. Cunningham, Jr., Department of Neuroscience, University of California at San Diego, La Jolla, CA 92037 [267]

Jürgen Czachurski, I. Physiologisches Institut, Universität Heidelberg, D-6900 Heidelberg, Federal Republic of Germany [3]

Maria F. Czyzyk, Department of Human Physiology, Medical Academy, Warsaw 00927, Poland [143]

R.A.L. Dampney, University of Sydney, Sydney, N.S.W. 2006, Australia [251]

Trevor A. Day, Department of Physiology and Centre for Neuroscience, University of Otago Medical School, Dunedin, New Zealand [425]

William C. de Groat, Department of Pharmacology and Center for Neuroscience, University of Pittsburgh, Pittsburgh, PA 15261 [81]

Klaus Dembowsky, I. Physiologisches Institut, Universität Heidelberg, D-6900 Heidelberg, Federal Republic of Germany [3]

Steven M. DiRusso, Department of Immunology, Emory University School of Medicine, Atlanta, GA [133]

F. Edward Dudek, Department of Physiology, Tulane University School of Medicine, New Orleans, LA [377]

Richard E.J. Dyball, Department of Anatomy, University of Cambridge, Cambridge, CB2 3DY England and Department of Physiology, University of Occupational and Environmental Health, School of Medicine, Kitakyushu 807, Japan [417,447]

Larry P. Eberle, Department of Physiology, State University of New York Health Science Center at Brooklyn, Brooklyn, NY 11203 [133]

András Erdélyi, Department of Physiology, National Institute of Occupational Health, Budapest, Hungary 1450 [295]

Susan Erdman, Department of Pharmacology and Center for Neuroscience, University of Pittsburgh, Pittsburgh, PA 15261 [81]

Ludwik Fedorko, Department of Human Physiology, Medical Academy, Warsaw 00927, Poland [143]

Alastair V. Ferguson, Department of Physiology, Queen's University, Kingston, Ontario, K7L 3N6 Canada [435]

Robert D. Foreman, Department of Physiology and Biophysics, The University of Oklahoma Health Sciences Center, Oklahoma City, OK 73190 [91]

Donald N. Franz, Department of Pharmacology, University of Utah, Salt Lake City, UT 84132 [121]

Gerard L. Gebber, Departments of Pharmacology/Toxicology and of Physiology, Michigan State University, East Lansing, MI 48824 [203]

A.K. Goodchild, University of Sydney, Sydney, N.S.W. 2006, Australia [251]

Norman Gootman, Department of Pediatric Cardiology, Schneider Children's Hospital, Long Island Jewish Medical Center, New Hyde Park, NY 11042 [133]

Phyllis M. Gootman, Department of Physiology, State University of New York, Health Science Center at Brooklyn, Brooklyn, NY 11203 [133]

Valentin K. Gribkoff, Department of Physiology, Tulane University School of Medicine, New Orleans, LA **[377]**

Patrice G. Guyenet, Department of Pharmacology, University of Virginia, Charlottesville, VA 22908 **[215]**

M.C. Harris, Department of Physiology, The Medical School, University of Birmingham, Birmingham, England B15 2TJ **[337]**

S.M. Hilton, Department of Physiology, The Medical School, University of Birmingham, Birmingham B15 2TJ, England **[315]**

Mary B. Houston, Department of Pharmacology and Center for Neuroscience, University of Pittsburgh, Pittsburgh, PA 15261 **[81]**

Zhong-Sun Huang, Departments of Pharmacology/Toxicology and of Physiology, Michigan State University, East Lansing, MI 48824 **[203]**

Kiyotoshi Inenaga, Department of Physiology, University of Occupational and Environmental Health, School of Medicine, Kitakyushu 807, Japan **[417]**

A.Y. Ivanov, Department of Autonomic Nervous System Physiology, Bogomoletz Institute of Physiology, Kiev-24, USSR **[37]**

S. Jamieson, Department of Physiology, The Medical School, University of Birmingham, Birmingham, England, B15 2TJ **[337]**

Wilfrid Jänig, Physiologisches Institut, Universität Kiel, 2300 Kiel, Federal Republic of Germany **[57]**

Jack H. Jhamandas, Neurosciences Unit, Montreal General Hospital and McGill University, Montreal, Quebec, H3G 1A4 Canada **[397]**

Hiroshi Kannan, Department of Physiology, University of Occupational and Environmental Health, School of Medicine, Kitakyushu 807, Japan **[417]**

Masahito Kawatani, Department of Pharmacology and Center for Neuroscience, University of Pittsburgh, Pittsburgh, PA 15261 **[81]**

D. Klüßendorf, Institute of Physiology, Free University Berlin, D-1000 Berlin 33, Federal Republic of Germany **[179]**

H. P. Koepchen, Institute of Physiology, Free University Berlin, D-1000 Berlin 33, Federal Republic of Germany **[179]**

Kiyomi Koizumi, Department of Physiology, State University of New York, Health Science Center at Brooklyn, Brooklyn, NY 11203 **[153]**

Mark Kollai, Department of Physiology, State University of New York, Health Science Center at Brooklyn, Brooklyn, NY 11203 **[153]**

M. Lambertz, Institute of Physiology, The Free University of Berlin, D-1000 Berlin 33, Federal Republic of Germany **[347]**

P. Langhorst, Institute of Physiology, The Free University of Berlin, D-1000 Berlin 33, Federal Republic of Germany **[347]**

Gareth Leng, Department of Neuroendocrinology, AFRC Institute of Animal Physiology and Genetics Research, Cambridge, England CB2 4AT **[447]**

M.C. Levin, The Salk Institute for Biological Studies, San Diego, CA 92138 **[267]**

Renea Livingstone, Department of Biomedical Engineering, The Johns Hopkins University School of Medicine, Baltimore, MD 21205 [111]

Sheilagh M. Martin, Department of Biology, Mount Saint Vincent University, Halifax, N.S., B3M 2J6 Canada [327]

R.M. McAllen, Department of Physiology, University of Bristol, Bristol BS8 1TD, U.K. [251]

Robert B. McCall, Cardiovascular Diseases Research, The Upjohn Company, Kalamazoo, MI 49001 [283]

Elspeth M. McLachlan, Baker Medical Research Institute, Prahran, Victoria 3181, Australia [47]

Robert L. Meckler, Department of Physiology, Michigan State University, East Lansing, MI 48824-1101 [101]

Steven W. Mifflin, Department of Physiology, Royal Free Hospital School of Medicine, London NW3 2PF, England [307]

Lewis C. Miner, Department of Pharmacology, University of Utah, Salt Lake City, UT 84312 [121]

S. Nishi, Department of Physiology, Kurume University School of Medicine, Kurume-Shi 830 Japan [15]

Nobukuni Ogata, Department of Pharmacology, Faculty of Medicine, Kyushu University, Japan [407]

Quentin J. Pittman, Department of Medical Physiology and Neuroscience Research Group, Faculty Medicine, University of Calgary, Calgary, Alberta, T2N 4N1 Canada [327]

Canio Polosa, Department of Physiology, McGill University, Montreal, Quebec, H3G 1Y6 Canada [15,189]

John C. R. Randle, Neurosciences Unit, Montreal General Hospital and McGill University, Montreal, Quebec, H3G 1A4, Canada [397]

W.S. Redfern, Department of Physiology, The Medical School, University of Birmingham, Birmingham B15 2TJ, England [315]

Leo P. Renaud, Neurosciences Unit, Montreal General Hospital and McGill University, Montreal, Quebec, H3G 1A4 Canada [397]

Colleen L. Riphagen, Department of Medical Physiology and Neuroscience Research Group, Faculty Medicine, University of Calgary, Calgary, Alberta, T2N 4N1 Canada [327]

Alan P. Rudell, Department of Physiology, State University of New York, Health Science Center at Brooklyn, Brooklyn, NY 11203 [133]

Michael Rutigliano, Department of Pharmacology and Center for Neuroscience, University of Pittsburgh, Pittsburgh, PA 15261 [81]

Chaichan Sangdee, Department of Pharmacology, University of Utah, Salt Lake City, UT 84132 [121]

Akio Sato, Department of Physiology, Tokyo Metropolitan Institute of Gerontology, Itabashiku, Tokyo 173, Japan [27]

Yuko Sato, Department of Physiology, Tokyo Metropolitan Institute of Gerontology, Itabashiku, Tokyo 173, Japan [27]

P.E. Sawchenko, The Salk Institute for Biological Studies, San Diego, CA 92138 [267]

Lawrence P. Schramm, Department of Biomedical Engineering, The Johns Hopkins University School of Medicine, Baltimore, MD 21205 [111]

G. Schulz, Schering AG, D-1000 Berlin 65, Federal Republic of Germany **[347]**

Horst Seller, I. Physiologisches Institut, Universität Heidelberg, D-6900 Heidelberg, Federal Republic of Germany **[3]**

Anthony L. Sica, Department of Pulmonary Division, Schneider Children's Hospital, Long Island Jewish Medical Center, New Hyde Park, NY 11042 **[133]**

László Simon, First Institute of Anatomy, Semmelweis University Medical School, Budapest, Hungary 1094 **[295]**

V.I. Skok, Department of Autonomic Nervous System Physiology, Bogomoletz Institute of Physiology, Kiev-24, USSR **[37]**

K. Michael Spyer, Department of Physiology, Royal Free Hospital School of Medicine, London NW3 2PF, England **[307]**

Scott C. Steffensen, Department of Pharmacology, University of Utah, Salt Lake City, UT 84132 **[121]**

Reuben D. Stein, Department of Physiology, Michigan State University, East Lansing, MI 48824-1101 **[101]**

G. Stock, Schering AG, D-1000 Berlin 65, Federal Republic of Germany **[347]**

W.N. Stokes, Department of Physics, University of Birmingham, Birmingham, England, B15 2TT **[337]**

Miao-Kun Sun, Department of Pharmacology, University of Virginia, Charlottesville, VA 22908 **[215]**

Harue Suzuki, Department of Physiology, Tokyo Metropolitan Institute of Gerontology, Itabashiku, Tokyo 173, Japan **[27]**

Tibor Tóth, Department of Physiology, National Institute of Occupational Health, Budapest, Hungary 1450 **[295]**

Andrzej Trzebski, Department of Human Physiology, Medical Academy, Warsaw 00927, Poland **[143]**

Kurt J. Varner, Departments of Pharmacology/Toxicology and of Physiology, Michigan State University, East Lansing, MI 48824 **[203]**

Lynne C. Weaver, Department of Physiology, Michigan State University, East Lansing, MI 48824-1101; present address: J.P. Robarts Institute, London, Ontario, N6A 5K8 Canada **[101]**

Deborah J. Withington-Wray, Department of Physiology, Royal Free Hospital School of Medicine, London NW3 2PF, England **[307]**

R.D. Wurster, Department of Physiology, Loyola University Medical Center, Maywood, IL 60153; and: Rehabilitation Research and Development Center, Hines Veterans Administration Medical Center, Hines, IL 60141 **[169]**

Hiroshi Yamashita, Department of Physiology, University of Occupational and Environmental Health, School of Medicine, Kitakyushu 807, Japan **[417]**

M. Yoshimura, Department of Physiology, Kurume University School of Medicine, Kurume-Shi 830 Japan **[15]**

Preface

This volume contains the papers presented at the satellite symposium of the XXX Congress of the International Union of Physiological Sciences entitled "Organization of the Autonomic Nervous System: Central and Peripheral Mechanisms", held in Montreal, Canada, July 8–10, 1986.

In light of the surge of new information regarding many aspects of the structure and function of the autonomic nervous system, the objective of the symposium was to bring together investigators whose current work in various areas of the autonomic nervous system was considered significant and provocative. It is hoped that this volume as a summary of present scientific accomplishments will serve as a benchmark against which future progress can be measured. The purpose of this volume is therefore twofold, to make available to the scientific community an up-to-date body of data and concepts on the autonomic nervous system, and to serve as a stimulus for an expanded research effort in the field.

The organizing committee would like to thank all the contributors for making the symposium successful and Alan R. Liss, Inc. for kindly agreeing to publish the results of this effort as a volume. The organizing committee also acknowledges the following for their financial contributions to the symposium: the Medical Research Council of Canada, the Fonds de la Recherche en Santé du Quèbec, the Faculty of Medicine and the Faculty of Graduate Studies of McGill University.

SECTION I: Functional Properties of Sympathetic Preganglionic and Post-Ganglionic Neurons

This section is devoted to the properties of pre- and post-ganglionic neurons. The characteristics of these output neurons are of considerable interest because they can markedly influence the information generated in the central nevous system or in sensory systems before it reaches the effector organs of the autonomic nervous system. The papers presented here show some of the most interesting trends of present research in this area.

The paper by Dembowsky, Czachurski and Seller describes membrane properties of sympathetic preganglionic neurons identified by "in vivo" intracellular recording. Indirect evidence is presented for the existence of several membrane currents. Some of these currents are of potential importance in determining the response of the neuron to synaptic inputs, and in accounting for the presence or absence of spontaneous activity.

The paper by Nishi, Yoshimura and Polosa presents an analysis of synaptic potentials recorded in sympathetic preganglionic neurons "in vitro" in response to focal stimulation. In addition, the paper compares properties of these potentials and of the potentials evoked by application of putative transmitters, as a step towards identifying the chemicals mediating synaptic transmission to this neuron. An important contribution of this paper is the first demonstration of slow synaptic potentials in this neuron.

The paper by Sato, Sato and Suzuki presents a study, the first of this kind, of the spontaneous activity of sympathetic preganglionic neurons as a function of age. The neurons studied are those which innervate the adrenal medulla.

The functional meaning of the pattern of innervation of sympathetic ganglion cells by preganglionic axons is investigated in the paper by Skok and Ivanov. The question of the heterogeneity of the sympathetic ganglion cell population is taken up in the paper by McLachlan. In addition to the already known chemical heterogeneity of these cells, shown, for instance, by differences in neuropeptide content, heterogeneity of membrane properties relevant to the control of repetitive firing is demonstrated. Cells firing with phasic or tonic patterns are described, and evidence is presented for differences in the tonic patterns are described, and evidence is presented for differences in the distribution of various types of K^+ channels among different neurons.

The heterogeneity of preganglionic and postganglionic neurons is also the topic of the paper by Jänig, which describes the topographical distribution within the spinal cord of the somata of preganglionic neurons which project to pelvic organs and colon through the lumbar splanchnic and hypogastric nerves as well as through the lumbar sympathetic trunk. In addition, this paper suggests a further classification of the preganglionic and postganglionic neurons innervating pelvic organs and colon on the basis of their response to various physiological stimuli.

Finally, the paper by Armour is concerned with the anatomical heterogeneity of sympathetic ganglia. These authors propose the hypothesis that sensory neurons and interneurons are present in thoracic sympathetic ganglia. This would result in the ability of the ganglia to mediate reflex response.

Organization of the Autonomic Nervous System:
Central and Peripheral Mechanisms, pages 3–14
© **1987 Alan R. Liss, Inc.**

ELECTROPHYSIOLOGICAL PROPERTIES OF SYMPATHETIC
PREGANGLIONIC NEURONES IN VIVO

Klaus Dembowsky, Jürgen Czachurski, Horst Seller
I. Physiologisches Institut, Univ. Heidelberg
Im Neuenheimer Feld 326, D-6900 Heidelberg,
F. R. G.

INTRODUCTION

The existence of a spontaneous or background activity
in sympathetic nerves has first been postulated by Bernard
(1852) to account for the increase in blood flow and skin
temperature after section of the cervical sympathetic trunk.
Later on, its existence has been verified by Adrian and co-
workers (1932) with the first recordings of the electrical
activity of sympathetic nerves. Studies with extracellular
recordings of individual sympathetic preganglionic neurones
(SPNs) have revealed that only a minority of these neurones
(20-30%) show this background activity (Polosa, 1968). The
vast majority, however, are not spontaneously active. It is
a generally accepted view that the spontaneously active SPNs
are mainly involved in the control of the cardiovascular
system (Jänig, 1985).

The background activity of single SPNs is characterized
by the irregular discharge of action potentials at low rates
between 0.1 and 5 spikes/s (Polosa, 1968; Seller, 1973). In
studies with intracellular recordings of SPNs the importance
of the on-going, mostly subthreshold synaptic activity has
been emphasized for the generation of this spontaneous activity (Coote and Westbury, 1979; Dembowsky et al., 1985a; Mc-
Lachlan and Hirst, 1980). This on-going synaptic activity in
SPNs mainly consists of excitatory post-synaptic potentials
(EPSPs) from which intermittently action potentials are initiated.

In addition to these extrinsic, synaptic factors intrinsic membrane properties might also be important for the generation and maintenance of this sympathetic background activity. In this report some active and passive electrophysiological properties of SPNs will be considered that have been obtained from intracellular recordings of these neurones by conventional techniques.

METHODS

Experiments were performed on cats that had been anaesthetized with alpha-chloralose (70 mg/kg i.v.). A femoral artery and vein were catheterized and a tracheotomy was performed. The animals were paralyzed with hexacarbacholine and artificially ventilated. A bilateral pneumothorax was performed to reduce the respiratory movements of the spinal cord. The left white ramus of the third thoracic segment (WR-T3) was exposed retropleurally and placed on bipolar electrodes for antidromic stimulation of preganglionic axons. A laminectomy was performed between the spinal segments C8 and T6 after fixing the animal rigidly by clamps on adjacent spinous processes. The left dorsal rootlets were partly removed. Intracellular recordings of SPNs were obtained by conventional techniques. Glass microelectrodes were drawn from filament glass tubing and backfilled with a solution of 3 M KCl, 2 M K-citrate or 4 M K-acetate. Intracellular potentials were recorded with a preamplifier with capacity compensation and bridge circuitry for current injection. Data were stored on magnetic tape and were analyzed off-line with a digital oscilloscope and an x/y pen recorder.

RESULTS

Intracellular recordings were obtained from SPNs which were identified by recording the antidromic action potential in response to WR-T3 stimulation (Fig.1). The resting membrane potential (MP) of SPNs was estimated in most neurones after sudden loss of the recording. In some neurones showing a continuous deterioration of the recording it was determined at the very beginning of the recording just after penetration of the electrode. Values of the resting MP in SPNs ranged from -48 to -86 mV.

Antidromic action potentials had peak amplitudes from 70 to 107 mV with an overshooting component of 12-50 mV.

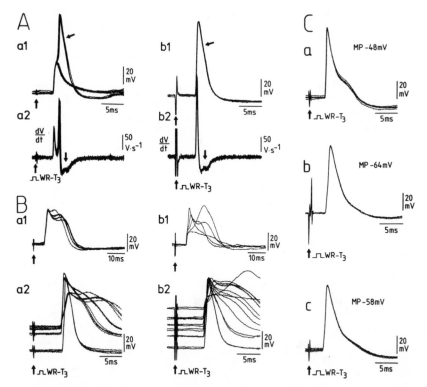

Figure 1. Antidromic action potentials and their first derivatives (dV/dt). A: The pronounced shoulder is indicated by arrows; two different SPNs (a, b). B: In damaged SPNs, this shoulder attained a plateau depolarization (a1, b1) which is reduced by hyperpolarization with negative current (a2, b2). C: Antidromic action potentials showing an afterdepolarization in three different SPNs (a, b and c). (Modified from Dembowsky et al., 1986; reproduced with permission of the Springer Verlag.)

Their duration was measured from the beginning of the upstroke to the point at which the declining phase had returned to prespike levels and ranged from 2.9 to 7.7 ms (4.7±1.1 ms, mean±S.D.). In neurones showing a depolarizing afterpotential (Fig. 1C) this duration was significantly longer (8.2 ±1.2 ms). The action potential rising phase showed an inflection which commonly is believed to indicate the IS and SD components of the action potential (Brock et al., 1953).

With increasing membrane hyperpolarization this inflection was accentuated before a blockade of the large SD component occurred (Fig. 1A). The remaining IS component had an amplitude between 20 and 35 mV and mostly a longer, but occasionally also a shorter duration than the full spike (Fig. 1A). Action potentials of all SPNs showed a more or less pronounced shoulder in the early action potential falling phase which was caused by a short-lasting slowing of the rate of repolarization (Fig. 1). In damaged SPNs, this shoulder took the form of a plateau depolarization with a duration up to 30 ms (Fig. 1B). This plateau could be shortened by membrane hyperpolarization with negative current (Fig. 1B). Not only in these recordings of apparently and seriously damaged SPNs, but also in good and stable recordings it was consistently noted that the spike repolarization was very sensitive to changes in the MP. Thus, the rate of repolarization was always decreased by depolarization and increased by hyperpolarization.

A portion of SPNs showed an afterdepolarization of the action potential (Fig. 1C). This afterdepolarization was independent of the way by which the action potential was evoked, i.e. either by antidromic, orthodromic or direct current stimulation. The afterdepolarization was smoothly continuous with the action potential falling phase and the subsequent afterhyperpolarization; it showed no notch-like inflections. The duration of this afterpotential was 5-12 ms. It was never evoked in the absence of a preceding full spike. The afterdepolarization could be abolished by two means: (1) By steady state membrane hyperpolarization to values between -55 and -65 mV and a duration of at least 30-50 ms; (2) during repetitive discharges that were evoked by antidromic, orthodromic or direct stimulation. In this case the second and all following action potentials missed this afterdepolarization. On the other hand, an afterdepolarization was never observed in SPNs with a high resting MP when they were depolarized beyond -50 mV with current injection.

The neuronal input resistance (R_N) was determined by passing short (50-200 ms), de- and hyperpolarizing current pulses through the recording electrode into cells. Values of R_N ranged from 10 to 47 MΩ (Fig. 2). Many SPNs had a quite linear current-voltage relation over a wide range of injected current intensities (Fig. 2A). Some neurones, however, displayed a prominent inward rectification with hyperpolarizing pulses that caused a voltage deflection of at least

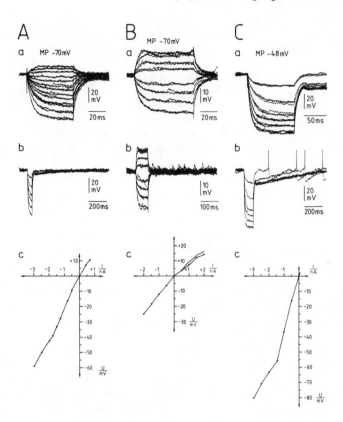

Figure 2. Current-voltage curves in three different SPNs (A, B and C). Voltage deflections during the current pulses are shwon on a fast (a) and a slow (b) time base. B: I-V curves were determined at 13 ms after the onset (open circles) and at the end of depolarizing current pulses (solid circles).

30 to 50 mV negative to MP (Fig. 2C). Other neurones showed a marked outward rectification with depolarizing pulses after a short latency (Fig. 2B): The voltage trajectory of these depolarizing pulses showed an early depolarization which rapidly within 10-20 ms fell back towards a steady state level. This short latency rectification was seen in cells with a high resting MP (Fig. 2B) or after hyperpolarization with negative current. The possibility of an additional out-ward rectification after a longer latency which is charac-

teristic of the M-current (Adams et al., 1982a) was not investigated. In many neurones it was observed that the voltage
trajectory at the termination of hyperpolarizing pulses only
slowly returned to control levels (Fig. 2A, C). In some neurones (Fig. 2C) this voltage trajectory was preceded by a
small and short depolarizing notch. This slow return to control levels was only observed with hyperpolarizing pulses
causing a voltage deflection of at least 10 mV negative to
MP and having a duration of at least 50 ms. The latency of
spontaneously occurring or anodal break action potentials
was delayed by this slow return of the MP (Fig. 2C). This
voltage trajectory is typical of the A-current (I_A), a transient outward current which is activated by depolarization
after a preceding hyperpolarization (Adams et al., 1982a).

Action potentials of SPNs were followed by a prominent
afterhyperpolarization (AHP) (Fig. 3). In most neurones this
AHP had a duration from 50 to 500 ms and an amplitude from
3 to 17 mV. Two different time courses of this AHP were observed: (1) After rapidly reaching the peak, the MP returned
curvilinearly to resting values; (2) in other neurones the
decay of the AHP was almost completely linear (Fig. 3).

In several neurones showing an AHP with a curvilinear
decay the underlying conductance change and the reversal potential could be determined. By injecting short hyperpolarizing current pulses at various times during the AHP it was
found that at its peak R_N is reduced to values between 50
and 70% of control. The amplitude of this type of AHP was
readily reduced by membrane hyperpolarization with negative
current. Occasionally, when no SD blockade occurred by
hyperpolarizing the MP, it actually could be reversed. In a
few neurones a linear relation was found between the MP and
the amplitude of the AHP which allowed an estimation of its
reversal potential: In these neurones it ranged from -77 to
-98 mV.

The second type of AHP with a linear decay phase was
only observed in neurones with a resting MP of at least -60
mV, although it was not necessarily recorded in all neurones
with a high resting MP. The linear decay of the AHP started
either directly at or 10-20 ms after the peak had been
reached (Fig. 3); this onset was shifted towards the peak by
membrane hyperpolarization that either occurred naturally or
was evoked by current injection. This earlier onset resulted
in a prolongation of the AHP and in lower discharge rates of

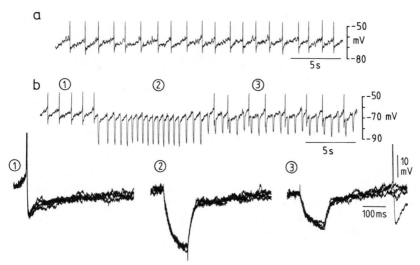

Figure 3. Comparison of the time course of the AHP (b1) with the voltage trajectory at the termination of hyperpolarizing current pulses (b2: -1nA, b3: -0.5nA) indicates that the A-current might be activated during the AHP and causes this linear decay.

spontaneously active SPNs. The time course of this AHP great-ly resembled the voltage trajectory that has been described at the termination of hyperpolarizing pulses (Fig. 2 and 3) and which is caused by the activation of I_A. Furthermore, in some SPNs with this linearly decaying AHP this rather typi-cal voltage trajectory was already observed at the termina-tion of hyperpolarizing pulses causing a voltage deflection similar to that seen during the peak of the AHP (Fig. 3b).

In a few SPNs action potentials were followed by an AHP with a much longer duration from 1200 to 4250 ms. In two SPNs the AHP showed a long-lasting (1-2 s) plateau before decaying curvilinearly. Mostly, however, this very long AHP was composed of an early and late component: The early com-ponent closely resembled the above described AHP with a curvilinear decay. It was followed by a much longer, slowly decaying component. Occasionally, this slow AHP had a second peak which, however, was always smaller than the peak of the early AHP. During repetitive discharges a summation of this late component was observed which resulted in a steady mem-brane hyperpolarization. The early AHP was little affected by this summation. Neurones showing this long-lasting AHP appeared to have a slightly broader action potential.

According to differences in some of the described properties thoracic SPNs fell into three groups: Not spontaneously active SPNs had a significantly higher resting MP (-60 to -86 mV) and low values of R_N (12-23 MΩ); their action potentials showed a prominent IS-SD inflection and a marked shoulder in the falling phase. On the other hand, spontaneously active SPNs had a lower resting MP (-48 to -68 mV) and a high R_N (21-47 MΩ). Both the IS-SD inflection and the shoulder of action potentials of these SPNs were not as prominent as in silent SPNs. Spontaneously active SPNs could further be subdivided with respect to the presence or absence of an afterdepolarization of the action potential. No differences existed in the amplitude and duration of the AHP and the axonal conduction velocity.

DISCUSSION

Using conventional intracellular recording techniques indirect evidence has been obtained for the existence of several membrane currents in SPNs that might play a role in the generation and maintenace of the sympathetic background activity.

The broad action potential with its prominent shoulder is suggestive of a major calcium component of the action potential (Dunlap and Fischbach, 1981; North, 1973). A similar plateau of the action potential as shown in the present study has been observed in many other neurones after blocking delayed potassium currents and has been shown to present a calcium influx (Dunlap and Fischbach, 1981). More direct evidence for this calcium component has been obtained in a recent in vitro study of cat SPNs (Yoshimura et al., 1986). The short depolarizing notch at the termination of hyperpolarizing pulses may represent the activation of a low threshold calcium current after a prior hyperpolarization (Carbone and Lux, 1984). The increase in the rate of spike repolarization by membrane hyperpolarization might involve this current which is activated by hyperpolarization and may trigger a fast, calcium sensitive potassium current (Adams et al., 1982b; MacDermott and Weight, 1982). Similar effects on repolarization, however have also been attributed to I_A (Belluzzi et al., 1985).

A characteristic feature of SPNs ist their prolonged AHP. The present findings suggest that at least three different mechnisms are involved in the generation of this AHP. The most frequently observed AHP had a curvilinear decay phase. The observed conductance increase and the estimated reversal potential suggest that it is due to increased potassium conductance. Although its time course is considerably slower it shows many similarities with a fast, transient component of the AHP that has been attributed to activation of a voltage-dependent delayed potassium current (Barrett and Barrett, 1976; Thompson, 1977).

The most reasonable explanation for the long-lasting AHP of SPNs with a duration up to 5 s is at present the assumption of a slow, calcium-dependent potassium current (I_K (Ca)) (Barrett and Barrett, 1976; Thompson, 1977). A similar long-lasting AHP has been reported in myenteric AH neurones (Hirst et al., 1974) where this AHP is attributed to a pronounced I_K (Ca)) (Grafe et al., 1980; North, 1973). The finding that this long-lasting AHP is only rarely recorded in the present in vivo study, but can easily be observed by in vitro recordings (Yoshimura et al., 1986) can be explained by a variety of factors. Thus, in vivo recordings are more likely to result in cell injury, whereas in vitro recordings are performed in a rather artificial situation. Furthermore, the length of the dendritic tree of SPNs in the longitudinal direction is four times as long as the thickness of the spinal cord transverse slices that were used in this in vitro study (Dembowsky et al., 1985b; Yoshimura et al., 1986). Thus, in vitro recordings of SPNs are likely to be performed in the absence of a great part of their dendrites.

Some neurones showed a linear decay phase of the AHP which is proposed to represent activation of I_A. The existence of this transient outward current in SPNs is indicated by the present current clamp recordings (Adams et al., 1982a; Belluzzi et al., 1985). The assumption that I_A plays a role in the AHP of SPNs is based on the finding that the linear AHP decay closely resembles the voltage trajectory that is seen at the termination of hyperpolarizing current impulses. Additionally, this typical voltage trajectory is already evident with hyperpolarizing current pulses which cause a membrane deflection to similar values also achieved during the peak of the AHP. It is concluded that I_A is activated in some SPNs during the peak of the AHP and leads to its prolongation and consequently, to a limitation of discharge rates to rather low rates. In line with this assumption is the observation that 4-aminopyridine, a substance known to block I_A (Belluzzi et al., 1985) causes an increase in the discharge rate of SPNs (Laskey et al., 1984).

Some SPNs displayed a depolarizing afterpotential which is similar to that seen in motoneurones (MN) (Granit et al., 1963; Nelson and Burke, 1967). Interestingly, this afterdepolarization was never observed in in vitro recordings of SPNs (Yoshimura et al., 1986). Although some properties of this afterdepolarization are different in SPNs and MNs, e.g. abolition by hyperpolarization in SPNs, but enhancement in MNs, it can yet be interpreted as the equivalent of some active dendritic processes (Pongrácz, 1985; Traub and Llinás, 1977). It seems reasonable to assume that in SPNs this process is either turned off or in case of dendritic action potentials does not reach threshold for their activation by membrane hyperpolarization.

The importance of some of these membrane currents in the determination of the discharge rates of spontaneously active SPNs is obvious. Quantitative and qualitative differences in these various currents in subpopulations of SPNs are already evident and must be the subject of future research. Likewise, at present it can only be speculated about the origin of the difference in resting MP and R_N between spontaneously active and silent SPNs. Since SPNs of these subgroups have similar axonal conduction velocities, these differences are probably unrelated to cell size. The observed differences in the shape of the action potential most probably are secondary to differences in the level of the resting MP.

REFERENCES

Adams PR, Brown DA, Constanti A (1982a). M-currents and other potassium currents in bullfrog sympathetic neurones. J Physiol (Lond) 330: 537-572.
Adams PR, Constanti A, Brown DA, Clark RB (1982b). Intracellular Ca^{2+} activates a fast voltage sensitive K^+ current in vertebrate sympathetic neurones. Nature 296: 746-749.
Adrian ED, Bronk DW, Phillips G (1932). Discharges in mammalian sympathetic nerves. J Physiol (Lond) 74: 115-133.
Barrett EF, Barret JN (1976). Separation of two voltage-sensitive potassium currents, and demonstration of a

tetrodotaxin-resistant calcium current in frog motoneurones. J. Physiol (Lond) 255: 737-774.

Belluzzi, O, Sacchi O, Wanke E (1985). A fast transient outward current in rat sympathetic neurone studied under voltage-clamp conditions. J Physiol (Lond) 358: 91-108.

Bernard C (1852). Influence du grand sympathique sur la sensibilité et sur la calorification. Comp rend Soc biol 3: 163.

Brock LG, Coombs JS, Eccles JC (1953). Intracellular recording from antidromically activated motoneurones. J Physiol (Lond) 122: 429-461.

Carbone E, Lux HD (1984). A low voltage-activated, fully inactivated Ca channel in vertebrate sensory neurones. Nature 310: 501-503.

Coote JH, Westbury DR (1979). Intracellular recordings from sympathetic preganglionic neurones. Neurosci Lett 15: 171-175.

Dembowsky K, Czachurski J, Seller H (1985a). An intracellular study of the synaptic input to sympathetic preganglionic neurones of the third thoracic segment of the cat. J Autonom Nerv Syst 13: 201-244.

Dembowsky K, Czachurski J, Seller H (1985b). Morphology of sympathetic preganglionic neurons in the thoracic spinal cord of the cat: An intracellular horseradish peroxidase study. J comp Neurol 238: 453-465.

Dunlap K, Fischbach GD (1981). Neurotransmitters decrease the calcium conductance activated by depolarization of embryonic chick sensory neurones. J Physiol (Lond) 317: 519-535.

Grafe P, Mayer CJ, Wood JD (1980). Synaptic modulation of calcium dependent potassium conductance in myenteric neurones in the guinea-pig. J Physiol (Lond) 305: 235-248.

Granit R, Kernell D, Smith RS (1963). Delayed depolarization and the repetitive response to intracellular stimulation of mammalian motoneurones. J Physiol (Lond) 168: 890-910.

Hirst GDS, Holman ME, Spence I (1974). Two types of neurones in the myenteric plexus of duodenum in the guinea-pig. J Physiol (Lond) 236: 303-326.

Jänig W (1985). Organization of the lumbar sympathetic outflow to skeletal muscle and skin of the cat hindlimb and tail. Rev Physiol Biochem Pharmacol 102: 119-213.

Laskey W, Schondorf R, Polosa C (1984). Effects of 4-aminopyridine on sympathetic preganglionic neuron activity. J Autonom Nerv Syst 11: 201-206.

MacDermott AB, Weight FF (1982). Action potential repolarization may involve a transient, Ca^{2+}-sensitive outward current in a vertebrate neurone. Nature 300: 185–188.

McLachlan EM, Hirst GDS (1980). Some properties of preganglionic neurons in upper thoracic spinal cord of the cat. J Neurophysiol 43: 1251–1265.

Nelson PG, Burke RE (1967). Delayed depolarization in cat spinal motoneurons. Exp Neurol 17: 16–26.

North RA (1973). The calcium–dependent slow, after–hyperpolarization in myenteric plexus neurones with tetrodotoxin-resistant action potentials. Brit J Pharmacol 49: 709–711.

Polosa C(1968). Spontaneous activity of sympathetic preganglionic neurons. Can J Physiol Pharmacol 46: 887–896.

Pongrácz F (1985). The function of dendritic spines: A theoretical study. Neuroscience 15: 933–946.

Seller H (1973). The discharge pattern of single units in thoracic and lumbar white rami in relation to cardiovascular events. Pflügers Arch 343: 317–330.

Thompson SH (1977). Three pharmacologically distinct potassium channels in molluscan neurones. J Physiol (Lond) 265: 465–488.

Traub RD, Llinás R (1977). The spatial distribution of ionic conductances in normal and axotomized motoneurons. Neuroscience 2: 829–849.

Yoshimura M, Polosa C, Nishi S (1986). Electrophysiological properties of sympathetic preganglionic neurons in the cat spinal cord in vitro. Pflügers Arch 406: 91–98.

Organization of the Autonomic Nervous System:
Central and Peripheral Mechanisms, pages 15–26
© 1987 Alan R. Liss, Inc.

SYNAPTIC POTENTIALS AND PUTATIVE TRANSMITTER ACTIONS IN
SYMPATHETIC PREGANGLIONIC NEURONS

S. Nishi, M. Yoshimura and C. Polosa
Department of Physiology, Kurume University School
of Medicine, Kurume, 830 Japan (S.N., M.Y.) and
Department of Physiology, McGill University
Montreal, Quebec, Canada H3G 1Y6

Synaptic input from sensory systems and from central
nervous system sites converges on the membrane of the
sympathetic preganglionic neuron (SPN, Polosa et al., 1979)
where it contributes to generating synaptic responses that
mediate appropriate output to its target cells, the
ganglion neurons, and the related effector cells. The
present study was undertaken to analyze the properties of
postsynaptic potentials of the SPN and the mechanism of
action of several putative transmitters.

The experiments were performed on transverse slices of
upper thoracic spinal cord (Yoshimura and Nishi, 1982). In
cats anaesthetized with chloralose and pentobarbital (60
and 10 mg/kg, respectively, I.P.), the second and third
thoracic spinal cord segments were excised and cut into 500
μm thick slices. These were transferred to a recording
chamber and superfused with Krebs solution, equilibrated
with 95% O_2 and 5% CO_2, containing (in mM): NaCl 117; KCl
3.6; NaH_2PO_4 1.2; $CaCl_2$ 2.5; $MgCl_2$ 1.2; glucose 11.0;
$NaHCO_3$ 25.0. Temperature was maintained at 37°C. Cells
were impaled using glass micropipettes filled with 3 M KCl
or 2 M K citrate. In some experiments 1 M CsCl-filled
micropipettes were used in order to block the K
conductances of the SPN membrane that contribute to its
rectifying characteristics. Electrode resistance varied
between 40 and 110 MΩ. Intracellular recordings were
obtained using a high input impedance amplifier with an
active bridge circuit, enabling simultaneous measurement of
membrane potential and intracellular current injection.
The amplifier output was monitored on a digital

oscilloscope. A DC pen recorder was used to record
membrane potential continuously. The neurons were
identified as SPNs by antidromic stimulation, as described
previously (Yoshimura et al., 1986). This study is based
on a sample of 85 antidromically identified SPNs. Drugs
were applied by superfusion, except for N-methyl-d-
aspartate (NMDA) which was applied by pressure pulses.
Pressure pipettes which contained 10 mM NMDA had tip
diameters of 2-5 μm and typically pressure pulses of 20 psi
for 250-350 ms were used. Focal stimulation was performed
with a monopolar, 50 μm diameter electrode, insulated
except at the tip.

In response to focal stimulation, the SPN showed four
types of synaptic response, a fast excitatory postsynaptic
potential (EPSP), a fast inhibitory postsynaptic potential
(IPSP), a slow EPSP and a slow IPSP, as seen in Fig. 1.

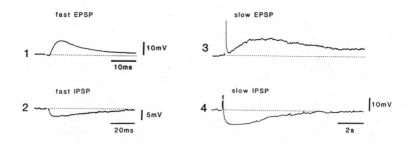

Fig. 1. Four types of postsynaptic potentials recorded
intracellularly from sympathetic preganglionic neurons.

Below is a description of the properties of these PSPs and
of responses to putative transmitters which closely
resemble the former.

The Fast EPSP

Fast EPSPs were evoked in most of these neurons. They ranged in amplitude from 5 to 20 mV and often reached firing threshold. The rise time varied from 2 to 8 ms, and the total duration from 40 to 100 ms. Hyperpolarization of the cell membrane caused an increase in the fast EPSP amplitude, and depolarization caused a decrease. However, because of the rectifying properties of the cell membrane, mostly due to the voltage dependence of K ion channels, the relationship of the EPSP amplitude to membrane potential was non-linear, and it was difficult to obtain the EPSP equilibrium potential (E_{epsp}) by extrapolation of this relationship. Moreover, because of the presence of depolarization- induced outward K current, extremely large cathodal currents were required to reverse the fast EPSP and an accurate measurement of E_{epsp} was technically difficult. In order to block such outward K currents, Cs ions were injected intracellularly from a recording electrode filled with 1 M CsCl (Johnston and Hablitz, 1980). During the first 10-20 min after impalement with a CsCl electrode, the membrane progressively depolarized, presumably due to block of rectifying K channels by Cs ions leaking from the electrode tip. In these conditions, membrane potential could be shifted to any desired level up to + 30 mV. Spontaneous firing only occurred when the

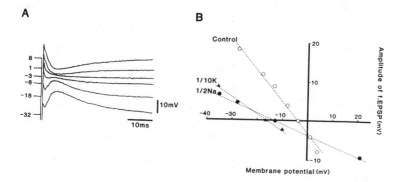

Fig. 2. Reversal of fast EPSP. A: Fast EPSP of a
Cs-loaded SPN (CsCl-electrode) at different levels of
cathodal depolarization. Note the reversal of EPSP at -3
mV. B: Fast EPSP amplitude - membrane potential
relationship obtained from the same neuron shown in A in
normal Krebs (open circles), 1/10 K Krebs (triangles) and
1/2 Na Krebs (filled circles) solutions.

membrane potential was more negative than - 30 mV.

Fig. 2A illustrates a typical reversal of the fast
EPSP, recorded with a Cs-filled electrode, at an
approximate potential of -3 mV. The average reversal
potential estimated with the same method in seven neurons
was -2.2 ± 0.8 mV (mean ± S.E.). Decreasing external Na to
1/2 by replacing the appropriate amount of Na with Tris
shifted the E_{epsp} toward resting membrane potential (-12.5
± 1.3 mV, n = 4, Fig. 2B). Decreasing external K by
replacing 9/10 of KCl with NaCl shifted the E_{epsp} in the
same direction as in the low Na medium (-22.3 ± 2.7 mV, n =
4, Fig. 2B). Increasing internal chloride by ionophoresis
with a CsCl-filled electrode did not significantly shift
the E_{epsp}. These findings imply that the fast EPSP is
generated by an increased Na and K conductance of the
subsynaptic membrane. From the E_{epsp} value in normal Krebs
solution, the ratio of the increased Na conductance to the
increased K conductance would be approximately 1.9.

The fast EPSP was not significantly affected by
superfusion with d-tubocurarine (50 µM), atropine (10 µM),
phentolamine (1 µM) or propranolol (1 µM).

Responses To Putative Neurotransmitters

Noradrenaline (NA, 10-50 µM) caused a long-lasting
depolarization in 30% of the neurons, a short-lasting
hyperpolarization followed by a long-lasting depolarization
in 14% of the neurons, a long-lasting hyperpolarization in
40% of the neurons, and no response in the remaining 16% of
the neurons. The NA-induced depolarization was associated
with an increased input resistance (R_N), while the

NA-induced hyperpolarization was associated with a decreased R_N. 5-Hydroxytryptamine (5-HT, 10-30 μM) induced a long-lasting depolarization with an increased R_N in 42% of the neurons and was without effect in the remainder of the neurons. The 5-HT-elicited depolarization was also observed in neurons which were either depolarized or hyperpolarized by NA. Tetrodotoxin (TTX, 1 μM) did not eliminate the NA- or 5-HT induced responses.

Eighty percent of the neurons were depolarized by glutamate (0.5 mM), and 52% of the neurons were depolarized by aspartate (0.5 mM). The glutamate depolarizations were associated with a decreased R_N (84%) or an increased R_n (16%), while the aspartate-induced depolarizations were accompanied by an increased R_N (73%) or a decreased R_N (27%). Glutamate and aspartate responses were not affected by TTX (1 μM).

Acetylcholine (ACh, 0.5-1 mM) depolarized 57% of the neurons. The ACh depolarization was associated with a decreased R_N in 80% of the neurons and was almost completely eliminated by d-tubocurarine (50 μM).

Despite the abundance of NA- and 5-HT-containing nerve fibers in the lateral horn of the thoracic spinal cord (Carlsson et al., 1964; Dahlström and Fuxe, 1965), the association of the NA- and 5-HT-induced depolarizations with an increased R_N rules out the possibility of their synaptic mediation of the fast EPSP. The same applies to aspartate which in many neurons caused an R_N- increasing depolarization. ACh depolarized the neurons and decreased R_N. Yet it is probably not the neurotransmitter of the fast EPSP because the EPSP was insensitive to nicotinic and muscarinic blocking drugs. Among the candidate substances examined, glutamate appeared to be a relatively promising transmitter candidate for the fast EPSP based on its R_N-decreasing depolarizing action on the majority of neurons.

The fast EPSP was markedly depressed during the glutamate-induced depolarization. EPSP depression was observed even during the decay of the glutamate-evoked depolarization and when, during glutamate superfusion, the membrane potential was prevented from depolarizing by injection of hyperpolarizing current into the cell. The

EPSP amplitude recovered completely after washing the preparation for about 10 min. D-glutamylglycine (DGG, 1 mM), a glutamate antagonist (Davies and Watkins, 1981), reversibly depressed the fast EPSP.

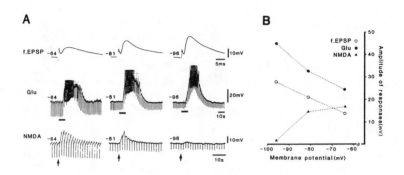

Fig. 3.   Effect of changing membrane potential on fast EPSP and on responses to glutamate (Glu. 2 mM, applied by superfusion) and NMDA (applied by pressure pulse from a micropipette filled with 10 mM NMDA). A: Responses recorded with a KCl-filled electrode from the same neuron at the membrane potentials indicated. B: Graphic presentation of records in A.

As seen in Fig. 3, the effect of anodal hyper-polarization on the fast EPSP and the glutamate induced depolarization were similar in that both responses were increased, while the response to N-methyl-d-aspartate (NMDA), one of the three types of glutamate agonists, was decreased and almost nullified. 2-Amino-phosphonovalerate (250 µM), a glutamate antagonist that blocks NMDA receptors (Davies et al., 1981), eliminated the NMDA-induced depolarization but did not affect the fast EPSP and the glutamate depolarization (but cf. Dun et al., 1986). It is known that the suppression of the NMDA-type response by

anodal hyperpolarization is reversed by removal of Mg ions
from the superfusing medium (Nowak et al., 1984; Mayer et
al., 1984). Comparison, in the present experiment, of the
EPSP amplitude at different levels of anodal hyperpolarization in normal Krebs and in Mg-free Krebs solution
did not yield any significant differences. These results
suggest that if the fast EPSP were mediated by glutamate,
the glutamate receptor would be of the quisqualate or
kainate type but not of the NMDA type.

The Slow EPSP

The fast EPSP was often followed by a slow
depolarization (slow EPSP, Fig. 4A1). Increasing the

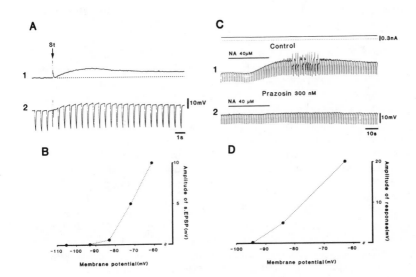

Fig. 4   The slow EPSP.   A: Slow EPSP of the same
neuron with (2) or without (1) superimposed anodal pulses.
Note increased R_N in record 2.   B: Reduction of slow EPSP
amplitude by hyperpolarization.   C: Elimination of the
NA-induced depolarization by prazosin.   Notice in C1
increased R_N during the depolarization.   D: Reduction of
the NA-induced depolarization by membrane
hyperpolarization.

strength or number of the stimulating pulses enhanced the amplitude and duration of the slow EPSP, the maximum values of which were 25 mV and 20 s, respectively. The slow EPSP was associated with an increase in R_N (Fig. 4A2). Anodal hyperpolarization decreased the amplitude of the slow EPSP, which was nullified when membrane potential reached approximately -90 mV (Fig. 4B). No reversal of the slow EPSP was observed by hyperpolarizing the membrane beyond -90 mV. Thus the slow EPSP does not behave like a postsynaptic depolarization generated by an increased ion conductance. Ionophoretic injection of Cl from the intracellular KCl-electrode or reduction of the external Cl to 1/5 by replacing Cl with isethionate did not appreciably alter the amplitude or duration of the slow EPSP. Reduction of external K to 1/10 augmented and elevation of K to 10 mM (2.8 times) decreased the slow EPSP amplitude. These observations suggest that the slow EPSP is caused by synaptic inactivation of a K conductance (G_K) of the cell membrane.

Since NA produced an R_N-increasing depolarization, as mentioned above, the effect of a NA antagonist was tested on the slow EPSP and NA-depolarization, to examine comparatively if the slow EPSP were catecholaminergic in nature. Prazosin, an alpha-1 adrenoceptor blocking drug, at 0.1-0.5 µM blocked both the slow EPSP and the NA (40 µM)-induced depolarization. Moreover, the behaviour of the NA-induced depolarization at different levels of membrane potential and in various ionic environments was essentially similar to that of the slow EPSP as partially illustrated in Fig. 4A-D. Based on these results and on the finding of abundance of NA-containing fibers in the lateral horn (Carlsson et al., 1964; Dahlström and Fuxe, 1965) NA is a likely candidate as the transmitter that mediates the slow EPSP. Similar analogies between properties of slow EPSP and of NA-evoked depolarization, including sensitivity to prazosin, were found in a previous study of raphe neurons (Yoshimura et al., 1985).

The Fast IPSP

Fast IPSPs were rarely produced by focal stimulation. In cells showing fast IPSPs, it was generally difficult to induce the IPSP without also inducing a fast EPSP or an

action potential. The fast IPSP ranged in amplitude from 2
to 8 mV. The rise time varied from 2 to 5 ms, and the
total duration from 50 to 90 ms. The IPSP decreased in
amplitude with anodal hyperpolarization, and was nullified
at approximately -70 mV. Hyperpolarization beyond this
level reversed the polarity of the fast IPSP. Because of
the limited numbers of cells which showed an IPSP, its
ionic requirement and the transmitter candidates have not
yet been explored.

The Slow IPSP

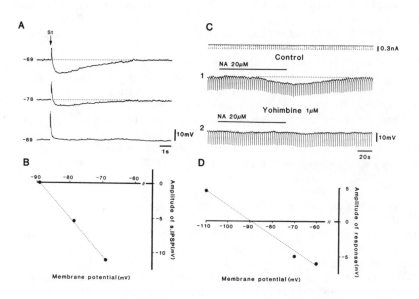

Fig. 5   Slow IPSP. A: Changes in slow IPSP amplitude
with hyperpolarization of cell membrane. B: relationship
of IPSP amplitude to membrane potential obtained from A.
C: Elimination of NA-induced hyperpolarization by
yohimbine. D: relationship of NA-hyperpolarization
amplitude to membrane potential.

In some cells the fast EPSP was followed by a slow hyperpolarizing response (slow IPSP) (Fig. 5A, uppermost record). Increasing the number of stimuli applied at 10 to 20 Hz enhanced and prolonged the slow IPSP. The slow IPSP reached its peak (5-15 mV) in 0.3 to 1.0 s and lasted 4 to 12 s. The slow IPSP was always associated with a decrease in R_N. Anodal hyperpolarization reduced the amplitude of the slow IPSP and in most cases the IPSP was nullified or reversed in polarity at approximately -90 mV (Fig. 5A and B). All these characteristics of the slow IPSP differ from those of the slow EPSP. Interestingly, NA, which mimicked the slow EPSP was also able to mimick the slow IPSP. Namely, in the cells which showed a slow IPSP in response to focal stimulation, NA (10-30 µM) applied by superfusion produced a slow hyperpolarization (Fig. 5 C1). The NA-induced hyperpolarization was always accompanied by a decrease in R_N (Fig. 5 C1), as the slow IPSP. Moreover, both the slow IPSP and the NA-induced hyperpolarization (Fig. 5 C2) were completely and reversibly blocked by the same concentration (0.1-1.0 µM) of yohimbine, an alpha-2 adrenoceptor blocker. The behaviour of the NA-induced hyperpolarization during anodal hyperpolarization was also similar to that of the slow IPSP; it was nullified at about -90 mV and reversed its polarity beyond -90 mV (Fig. 5D). These results suggest that the slow IPSP is mediated by NA.

It seems remarkable that NA produces a hyperpolarization in one cell and a depolarization in another. In 14% of neurons NA produced a biphasic response consisting of an early hyperpolarization followed by a depolarization. Occasionally it was observed that after elimination of the slow EPSP by prazosin a slow IPSP was unmasked. The variability of the responses to NA might be due to differences in the density of distribution of alpha-1 and alpha-2 adrenoceptors in individual neurons.

SUMMARY

In response to focal stimulation, the sympathetic preganglionic neurons in the lateral horn of cat spinal cord slices produced four distinctly different synaptic responses: fast and slow EPSP, fast and slow IPSP. The fast EPSP, although not conclusively established yet, might be mediated by glutamate acting on non-NMDA-type subsynaptic receptors and increasing G_{Na} and G_K. The slow EPSP is likely to be mediated by NA via alpha-1 receptors, activation of which produces a decrease in G_K. Because of the infrequent occurrence of the fast IPSP, the possible transmitter and the ionic conductance involved have not been studied. The slow IPSP is characteristically different in electrogenesis from the slow EPSP, but like the slow EPSP, is likely to be mediated by NA. The receptor appears to be of the alpha-2 type.

Supported by grants to S.N. from the Ministry of Education, Science and Culture of Japan and to C.P. from the Medical Research Council of Canada.

REFERENCES

Carlsson A, Falck B, Fuxe K, Hillarp NA (1964). Cellular localization of monoamines in the spinal cord. Acta Physiol Scand 60: 112-119.

Dahlström A, Fuxe K (1965). Evidence for the existence of monoamine neurons in the central nervous system. II. Experimentally induced changes in the intraneuronal amine levels of bulbospinal neuron systems. Acta Physiol Scand Suppl 247, 64:1-36.

Davies J, Francis AA, Jones AW, Watkins JC (1981). 2-amino-phosphonovalerate (2APV), a potent and selective antagonist of amino acid-induced and synaptic excitation. Neurosci Lett 21: 77-81.

Davies J, Watkins JC (1981). Differentiation of kainate and quisqualate receptors in the cat spinal cord by selective antagonism with γ-D (and L)-glutamylglycine. Brain Res 206: 172-177.

Dun NJ, Mo N, Jiang ZG (1986). Excitatory synaptic potentials evoked in rat lateral horn neurons and possible involvement of amino acids. Fed Proc 45: 158.

Johnston D, Hablitz JJ (1980). Voltage clamp discloses slow inward current in hippocampal burst-firing neurones. Nature 286: 391-393.

Mayer ML, Westbrook GL, Guthrie PB (1984). Voltage-dependent block by Mg^{2+} of NMDA responses in spinal cord neurones. Nature 309: 261-263.

Nowak L, Bregestovski P, Ascher P (1984). Magnesium gates glutamate-activated channels in mouse central neurones. Nature 307: 462–465.

Yoshimura M, Higashi H, Nishi S (1985). Noradrenaline mediates slow excitatory synaptic potentials in rat dorsal raphe neurons in vitro. Neurosci Lett 61: 305–310.

Yoshimura M, Nishi S (1982). Intracellular recordings from lateral horn cells of the spinal cord in vitro. J Auton Nerv Syst 6: 5–11.

Yoshimura M, Polosa C, Nishi S (1986). Electrophysiological properties of sympathetic preganglionic neurons in the in vitro spinal cord of the cat. Pflügers Arch 406: 91–98.

Organization of the Autonomic Nervous System:
Central and Peripheral Mechanisms, pages 27–36
© 1987 Alan R. Liss, Inc.

CHANGES IN SYMPATHO-ADRENAL MEDULLARY FUNCTIONS DURING AGING.

Akio Sato, Yuko Sato and Harue Suzuki

Department of Physiology, Tokyo Metropolitan Institute of Gerontology, 35-2 Sakaecho, Itabashiku, Tokyo 173, Japan.

Recently, the population of aged people has rapidly increased in many countries, and therefore interest in the physiological study of the aged has also increased. In particular, the autonomic nervous functions of the aged are an important area of investigation. Furthermore, the aged often have diseases which give us an erroneous impression of disturbed or decreased functions. Thus, it is important to study these functions during aging in order to distinguish normal change from diseases.

First of all, the most important summary of aging research to date seems to have been delivered by Dr. Shock, whose fundamental work (1960) indicated that various physiological functions gradually decrease with age with different declining degrees. For example, when various physiological functions at 30 years old are presented as 100%, various functions all show a tendency to decline. For example, fasting blood glucose level is quite stable, still almost 100% at 80 years old. Nerve conduction velocity is also maintained at a high level only about 15% decrease at 80 years old, though the data on nerve conduction velocity was gathered only from thick myelinated fibers of somatic nerves. However, other functions such as renal blood flow, maximum breathing capacity, maximum oxygen uptake and etc. decrease markedly. In particular, the maximum oxygen uptake decreases almost 70%.

When we first read about these characteristics, we were impressed with the preservation of nerve functions. Therefore, our laboratory began our aging research by examining the conduction velocity of autonomic nerves. For this purpose we used male Wistar rats of various ages from 28 days to 900 days for our experiments. In our institute, 50% of male animals survive to 750 days but only 16% survive to 900 days. The maximum conduction velocities for both myelinated and unmyelinated fibers of autonomic vagus nerves were measured. For comparison, the conduction velocities of somatic cutaneous sural (SU) and muscle gastrocnemius-soleus (GS) nerves were also measured (Fig. 1). The conduction velocities of myelinated fibers in these 3 different nerves gradually increased up to 300 days due to thickening of their myelin sheaths. Between 700 and 800 days the maximum conduction velocity of the muscle GS nerve declined about 15%. Thus, the GS conduction velocity is compatible with the data presented by Dr. Shock. It is noticeable, however, that the conduction velocities of the other two nerves, the cutaneous sural and autonomic vagal nerves, were well maintained up to 900 days. Even more interestingly, the conduction velocities of the unmyelinated fibers in all three nerves remained quite stable up to 900 days.

After the foregoing, we became interested in sympathetic preganglionic neuronal function and especially age-dependent changes in their spontaneous activity. To determine whether there are any changes, we used urethane-chloralose anesthetized Wistar rats, and dissected a single

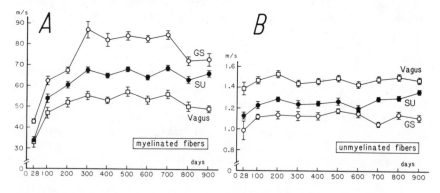

Figure 1. Changes in the maximum conduction velocity of the myelinated (A) and unmyelinated (B) fibers of peripheral nerves in rats during aging. GS: gastrocnemius and soleus muscle nerves. SU: cutaneous sural nerve (from Sato A, Sato Y and Suzuki H, 1985).

nerve unit from the preganglionic sympathetic nerves innervating the adrenal gland. As shown in Fig. 2 we recorded
their unitary spontaneous discharge activities in the
resting state. The adrenal gland is a unique organ which
is innervated by preganglionic sympathetic neurones. Two
typical examples of unitary discharge activities in young
adult and aged rats are shown in Fig. 2A. The nerve
activity was counted and averaged over a 1-5 min period.
In Fig. 2B, the results from all 102 units dissected are
plotted. The abscissa is rat age in days, and the ordinate
is the rates of unitary spontaneous discharge.

At ages from 100 through 300 days, the means of
spontaneous discharge rates of the preganglionic adrenal
sympathetic neurones were about 1.4 impulses/second. At
400 days the spontaneous discharge rate increased to 3.2
imp/s. This increase was maintained up to 900 days, but
after 400 days there was a significant increase in the
variation. Then, the variations of spontaneous nerve
activities in young adults of 100 to 200 days and aged rats
of 800 to 900 days were compared (Fig. 3). The discharge
frequencies are plotted in abscissae, and numbers of the
filaments in percentage in ordinates. For young adult rats
the discharge rates were between 0.1 and 2.5 imp/s. In

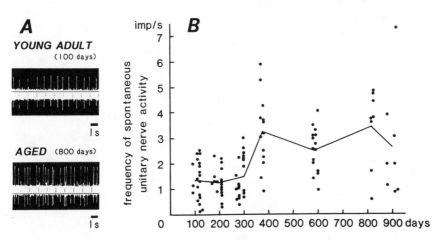

Figure 2. Spontaneous adrenal sympathetic unitary nerve
activities in urethane-chloralose anesthetized rats at
different ages (100-900 days). The mid-line inside the
graph (B) represents mean values for nerve activities
(modified from Ito K, Sato A, Sato Y and Suzuki H, 1986).

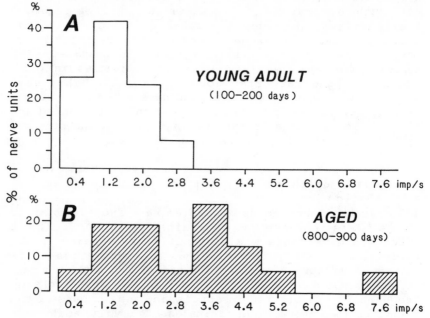

Figure 3. Ranges of spontaneous adrenal sympathetic unitary nerve activities in young adult(A) and aged (B) rats and % of numbers of adrenal nerve units corresponding to the frequencies indicated on abscissae.

aged rats the discharge rates were spread from 0.6 to 7.3 imp/s.

After looking at these results, we began to wonder if the increased adrenal sympathetic nerve activity during aging would influence adrenal catecholamine (CA) secretion. Catecholamines in the systemic blood of young and aged rats have been repeatedly measured, with inconsistent results (Avakian et al., 1984, Chiueh et al., 1980, McCarty, 1981). In human beings, it is well established that noradrenaline in systemic blood increases during aging (Wallin et al., 1981, Ziegler et al., 1976). However, CA concentrations in systemic blood are not an accurate reflection of adrenal medullary functions because of metabolic alterations in systemic blood circulation and large doses of noradrenaline secreted from the nerve terminals of the general sympathetic nervous system. Therefore, the secretion rates of both CAs from the adrenal gland were directly measured. For this purpose, a thin polyethylene tube was inserted

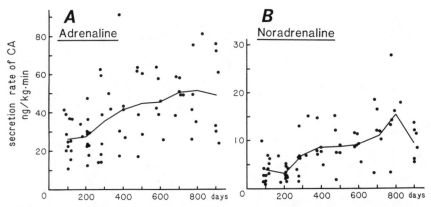

Figure 4. Secretion rate of adrenaline and noradrenaline from the adrenal gland in urethane-chloralose anesthetized rats with different ages (100-900 days). Mid-lines in A and B shows means of secretion rates in each age group (modified from Ito K, et al., 1986).

into an adrenal vein and a small amount of adrenal blood was collected. Adrenaline and noradrenaline in this adrenal venous blood plasma were separated by high performance liquid chromatography, and then measured by an electro-chemical detector. Concentrations of adrenaline and noradrenaline in the adrenal venous blood were almost 50 to 1000 times higher than those in systemic blood. From the concentrations of CAs in the adrenal venous blood and the rate of adrenal venous flow, the secretion rates of CAs from the adrenal gland were calculated. Figure 4 shows the secretion of adrenaline and noradrenaline for all animals from 100 to 900 days. The secretion rates of both adrenaline and noradrenaline increased almost proportional-ly with age after 300 days up to 800 days. These increases in CA secretion rates coincided with the increases in adrenal sympathetic nerve activity. The present results suggest that the increased adrenal CA secretions were in fact produced by the increased adrenal sympathetic nerve activity.

Again, variations in secretion rates also increased with age as did nerve activities. Figure 5 shows the differences in the CA secretion rates for young adult rats of 100 to 200 days and aged rats of 700 to 900 days; in the young adult rats the ranges were quite narrow while in the aged rats the ranges were widely spread.

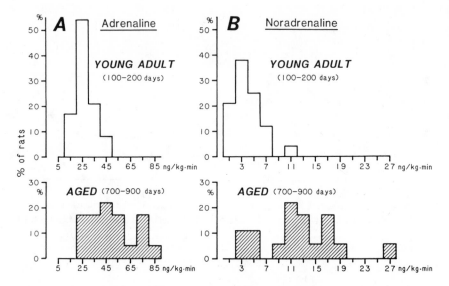

Figure 5. Ranges of spontaneous adrenal secretions of adrenaline (A) and noradrenaline (B) in young adult (upper traces) and aged (lower traces) rats and % of numbers of rats corresponding to the secretion rates indicated on abscissae.

Our next step was to determine whether this increased adrenal CA secretion in aged rats would be reflected in the CA concentration of systemic peripheral blood. In systemic blood, the adrenaline and noradrenaline concentrations were found to be almost twice as high in aged animals as in the young (Fig. 6A,B). These increases in adrenaline and noradrenaline would appear to be produced by the increased secretion rates from the adrenal gland. On the other hand, increased noradrenaline in systemic peripheral blood can be produced also by increases in sympathetic nerve activities of the more generalized sympathetic nervous systems. Furthermore, the physiological significance of these increased CAs in the systemic peripheral blood will be our next study. As a first approach, we have recorded systemic arterial blood pressure in both young and aged rats anesthetized with urethane and chloralose, and noted that both systolic and diastolic pressures did not change significantly in the aged group (Fig. 6C). Thus it is evident that increases in CA in systemic peripheral blood are not directly related to changes in systemic blood pressure.

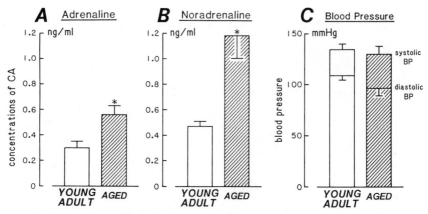

Figure 6. Concentrations of adrenaline (A), noradrenaline (B) in peripheral blood plasma and systemic arterial blood pressure (C) in young adult (100-200 days) and aged (800-900 days) rats anesthetized with urethane-chloralose. The means ± S.E. for adrenaline in 9 young adult and 7 aged rats were 0.30 ± 0.05 and 0.56 ± 0.07 ng/ml, respectively, while those for noradrenaline in young adult and aged rats were 0.47 ± 0.04 and 1.18 ± 0.18 ng/ml, respectively. The means ± S.E. of systolic and diastolic blood pressure in 22 young adult rats were 135 ± 5 and 109 ± 4 mmHg, respectively, while those in 19 aged rats were 130 ± 8 and 96 ± 7 mmHg, respectively. *:p<0.01 by Student t test.

To summarize, our present experiments indicate that the increases in CAs in peripheral blood in the aged were produced by increases in CA secretion rates from the adrenal gland, and these increases were probably due to increased adrenal sympathetic nerve activities. The most important question is the mechanism by which aging produces such increases in adrenal sympathetic nerve activities. Decreases in baroreceptor sensitivity, decreases in central inhibitory mechanisms, or increases in central excitatory mechanisms might be causative factors. At this moment we do not have any answers.

With this question in mind, it is interesting to note that the sympathetic neural mechanisms of hypertension in genetically controlled spontaneously hypertensive rats (SHR) are being analyzed by other investigators. Schramm and Chornoboy (1982) have been studying the effect of

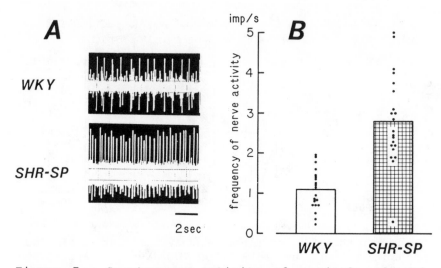

Figure 7. Spontaneous activity of a single adrenal sympathetic nerve fibers in normotensive WKY and SHR-SP (15-20 weeks in age) anesthetized with halothane. A: an example of single nerve recordings. B: dots represent the frequency of individual single nerve fiber activities and columns show mean frequencies of all fibers dissected (from Sato A, Sato Y, Shimamura K and Suzuki H, 1986).

excitatory and inhibitory descending systems originating at the brainstem on spinal sympathetic neurones in the SHR and have found that adrenal sympathetic nerves in SHR exhibited much larger responses after stimulation of the descending sympathoexcitatory pathways. Loewy and his colleagues found that the amount of substance P (SP) and the numbers of the SP receptor in the region of intermediolateral cell column at the spinal cord were increased in SHR and suggested that the activity of the excitatory descending pathway containing SP on the preganglionic sympathetic neurones at the spinal level was increased in SHR (Takano et al., 1985). Fukuda et al.(1986) have reported an increased sensitivity of the carotid chemoreceptor activity in SHR, while Coote and Sato (1977) emphasized a decreased sensitivity of baroreceptor activity in SHR. Such changes in the chemo- and baroreceptors sensitivities seem to produce an increase in sympathetic nerve activity. We hope the experimental approaches used with SHR by these investigators can be applied to our present aging research on adrenal sympathetic preganglionic neurones.

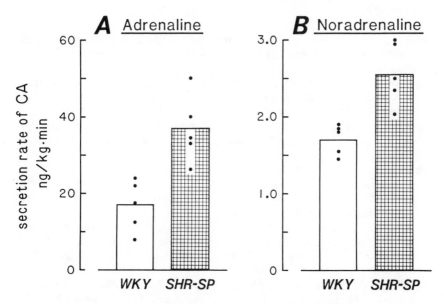

Figure 8. Spontaneous secretion rates of adrenaline (A) and noradrenaline (B) from the adrenal gland in WKY and SHR-SP (15-20 weeks in age) anesthetized with halothane. Dots represent the secretion rate of CA of an individual animal and columns show mean secretion rates of all animals (from Sato A, et al., 1986).

Finally, we would like to briefly introduce some of our results on the stroke-prone SHR (SHR-SP). Using the usual techniques employed in aging studies, we investigated sympatho-adrenal medullary functions in young normotensive Wistar Kyoto rats (WKY) and in young hypertensive SHR-SP rats aged 15-20 weeks and anesthetized with halothane. Adrenal sympathetic preganglionic neuronal activities in SHR-SP were above twice those in WKY (Fig. 7). Adrenaline secretion from the adrenal gland was about doubled and noradrenaline secretion was about 50% greater in SHR-SP (Fig. 8). From this we can see that there are similarities between the increased sympatho-adrenal medullary functions in normotensive normal aged rats and in young hypertensive SHR-SP rats. Therefore, studies of the sympatho-adrenal medullary functions of young SHR (or SHR-SP) rats may give us valuable insights into the mechanisms involved in both hypertension and aging.

REFERENCES

Avakian EV, Horvath SM, Colburn RW (1984). Influence of age and cold stress on plasma catecholamine levels in rats. J Auton Nerv Syst 10: 127-133.

Chiueh CC, Nespor SM, Rapoport S (1980). Cardiovascular, sympathetic and adrenal cortical responsiveness of aged Fischer-344 rats to stress, Neurobiol Aging 1: 157-163.

Coote JH, Sato Y (1977). Reflex regulation of sympathetic activity in the spontaneously hypertensive rat, Circ Res 40: 571-577.

Fukuda Y, Sato A, Trzebski A (1986). Carotid chemoreceptor discharge responses to hypoxia and hypercapnia in the normotensive and spontaneously hypertensive rats. J Auton Nerv Syst (in press).

Ito K, Sato A, Sato Y, Suzuki H (1986). Increases in adrenal catecholamine secretion and adrenal sympathetic nerve unitary activities with aging in rats. Neurosci Lett 69: 263-268.

McCarty R (1981). Aged rats: Diminished sympathetic-adrenal medullary responses to acute stress. Behav Neural Biol 33: 204-212.

Sato A, Sato Y, Shimamura K, Suzuki H (1986). An increase in the sympatho-adrenal medullary function in stroke-prone spontaneously hypertensive rats under anesthetized and resting conditions. Neurosci Lett (in press).

Sato A, Sato Y, Suzuki H (1985). Aging effects on conduction velocities of myelinated and unmyelinated fibers of peripheral nerves. Neurosci Lett 53: 15-20.

Schramm LP, Chornoboy ES (1982). Sympathetic activity in spotaneously hypertensive rats after spinal transection. Am J Physiol 243: R506-R511.

Shock NW (1960). In Strehler BL, Ebert JD, Glass HB, Shock NW (eds.) "The Biology of Aging." Washington, D.C.: American Institute of Biological Sciences.

Takano Y, Sawyer WB, Loewy AD (1985). Substance P mechanisms of the spinal cord related to vasomotor tone in the spontaneously hypertensive rat. Brain Res 334: 105-116.

Wallin BG, Sundlof G, Eriksson BM, Dominiak P, Grobecker H, Lindblad LE (1981). Plasma noradrenaline correlates to sympathetic muscle nerve activity in normotensive man. Acta Physiol Scand 111: 69-73.

Ziegler MC, Lake CR, Kopin IJ (1976). Plasma noradrenaline increases with age. Nature 261: 333-335.

**Organization of the Autonomic Nervous System:
Central and Peripheral Mechanisms, pages 37–46
© 1987 Alan R. Liss, Inc.**

ORGANIZATION OF PRESYNAPTIC INPUT TO NEURONES OF A
SYMPATHETIC GANGLION

V.I. Skok and A.Y. Ivanov
Department of Autonomic Nervous System
Physiology, Bogomoletz Institute of
Physiology, Kiev-24, USSR.

INTRODUCTION

It has long been known that some neurones in autonomic
ganglia are singly innervated by preganglionic fibres
(Martin and Pilar, 1963; Nishi et al., 1965), while others
receive multiple preganglionic innervation (Skok, 1973;
Gabella, 1976). There is usually one fibre among those
converging on the same neurone in a mammalian sympathetic
ganglion with an excitatory action strong enough to trigger
a postsynaptic discharge. Other converging fibres can
trigger a postsynaptic discharge only if two to eight
fibres (Blackman and Purves, 1969; Sacchi and Perri, 1971)
fire simultaneously. These two types of presynaptic inputs
were called dominant and accessory, respectively (Skok and
Ivanov, 1983). The postsynaptic spikes evoked through
these inputs differ markedly in their characteristics. In
particular, accessory spikes have one or more notches on
their rising phase which is not observed in dominant
spikes. The dominant input is apparently analogous to
presynaptic input in singly innervated cells.

An intriguing question is what is the physiological
significance of the multiple innervation of ganglion cells
compared with their single innervation. One possibility is
that multiple innervation provides an additional mechanism
that may regulate the number of discharging neurones by
changing the combinations of simultaneously firing
preganglionic fibres that converge on common neurones.
According to this "key-lock" hypothesis (Skok, 1974, 1986),
the group of neurones stimulated through a part of the

combination would respond with excitatory postsynaptic potentials (EPSP) while those stimulated through the full combination would respond with spikes. One would thus expect that more neurones discharge synchronously with a discharging neurone than with a neurone responding with an EPSP. The first purpose of this work was to check whether such difference is observed. The second purpose of the work was to investigate whether dominant and accessory presynaptic inputs differ in their functions. The responses of tonically active neurones to stimulation of arterial chemoreceptors were used for their functional identification. It is known that tonic activity in cat vasoconstrictor neurones supplying skeletal muscles is modulated by cardiac rhythm and increases in response to arterial hypercapnia in contrast to that in the neurones supplying hairy skin (see Janig, 1985).

METHODS

The experiments were performed on rabbits (1.5 - 2.5 kg) anaesthetized with urethane (1 g/kg i.v.), tracheotomized and spontaneously breathing. The superior cervical ganglion with its preganglionic input left intact was fixed in situ between two horizontal perspex rings. Conventional intracellular electrodes filled with 0.5 M potassium acetate or with 3 M potassium chloride and connected to a DC amplifier (upper frequency 30 kHz) were inserted through the upper ring. The external carotid nerve which contains postganglionic fibres was drawn into a suction recording electrode connected to an AC amplifier (bandwidth 3 Hz - 3 kHz). The ECG was recorded with needle electrodes inserted under the skin in forepaw and hindlimb. The respiratory movements of the chest were recorded using a tensiometric circuit.

The paired records of tonic activity obtained simultaneously from a single neurone and from the postganglionic nerve were stored on magnetic tape in analog form for subsequent analysis with an SM-3 computer. To improve the signal-to-noise ratio in postganglionic nerve activity correlated to intracellular spikes or EPSPs the postganglionic records were triggered either by intracellular spikes or by EPSPs; 100 to 600 records were stored and averaged for each spike or EPSP.

Arterial chemoreceptors were stimulated by ventilating the animal with CO_2-enriched air through the tracheal cannula for a period of 15-20 s (see Gregor and Janig, 1977).

RESULTS

Number of Cells Discharged by a Single Tonic Preganglionic Volley

Attempts to obtain a postganglionic response correlated with an intracellular spike or with an EPSP were made for 22 neurones. For 16 of these neurones responses correlated with the intracellular spike were recorded.

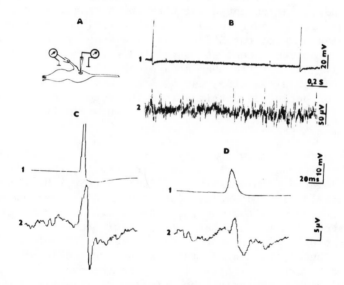

Figure 1. Separation of nerve action potential correlated with intracellular spike and EPSP from whole-nerve recordings. A. A scheme of the experimental arrangement. B. Synchronous records of intracellular tonic activity (1) and of the activity of the whole external carotid nerve (2). C. Average tonic intracellular spike (1) correlated with average nerve tonic action potential (2). D. Average tonic EPSP (1) correlated with average nerve tonic action

potential (2). Records C and D were obtained from the same cell at 100 summations each.

Fig. 1, A illustrates the experimental arrangement. In Fig. 1,B, a pair of original records obtained from a single cell and from the postganglionic nerve is shown. The average intracellular spike used to trigger the nerve records and the average nerve action potential obtained from 100 records are shown in Fig. 1, C, 1 and 2, respectively. Mean amplitude of the nerve action potential obtained from pooled results was 43.0 ± 2.1 µV, and mean area covered by the first (upward) phase of the action potential was 313 ± 94 µV • ms (n=9).

Only in 9 of these 16 neurones showing a correlation of the nerve action potential with the intracellular spike there was also a correlation with the EPSP. No cell showed a correlation with the EPSP only. The mean amplitude of the nerve action potential correlated with the EPSP was 30.0 ± 1.7 µV, and the mean area of the first phase of the action potential was 183 ± 46 µV • ms (n=9). Examples of the action potential obtained from 100 records and of the averaged EPSP used for triggering are shown in Fig. 1,D,2 and 1,D,1, respectively.

In order to know how many neurones sending their axons into the external carotid nerve correlate their discharge with the intracellular spike or with the EPSP, the areas of both nerve action potentials obtained as described above were compared with that of the nerve action potential correlated with the discharge of a single neurone. A discharge of a single neurone was evoked by direct stimulation of the neurone through the intracellular electrode, with parallel monitoring of the evoked intracellular spike using the bridge circuit. Six neurones chosen for direct stimulation were preliminarily tested by antidromic stimulation to be sure they sent their axons to the external carotid nerve. The experimental procedure is illustrated by Fig. 2, A. The nerve action potential correlated with the single cell discharge is shown in Fig. 2, B. Its mean amplitude and mean area of the first phase were 1.1 ± 0.1 µV and 1.2 ± 0.3 µV • ms (n=6), respectively. The areas of the nerve action potentials correlated with the tonic intracellular spike and with the

A   **B**

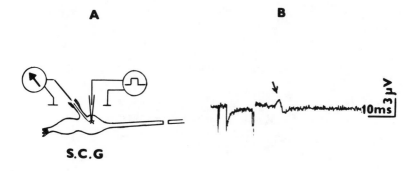

Figure 2. Separation of nerve action potential correlated
with intracellular spike evoked by direct cell stimulation
from whole-nerve recordings. A. A scheme of experimental
arrangement. B. Average action potential recorded from
external carotid nerve (300 summations coherent with
intracellular spike evoked by direct cell stimulation).
The action potential (indicated by arrow) is preceded by
stimulus artifacts.

EPSP are 261 and 153 times larger than that of the nerve
action potential correlated with the single cell discharge,
respectively. On the assumption of linear summation
(Bigland et al. 1955) this result suggests that at least
261 neurones correlate their discharges with the tonic
intracellular spike while at least in 153 neurones the
discharges correlate with the tonic EPSP.

Functional Identification of Tonically Active Neurones

Tonic activity was studied in 98 neurones. In 67
neurones single spikes and EPSPs appeared at regular or
irregular intervals. The remainder of the neurones
exhibited regular burst-like activity. The frequency of
single spikes appearance increased (first group, 30
neurones), decreased (second group, 15 neurones) or did not
change (22 neurones) in response to inhalation of
CO_2-enriched air (Fig. 3); in the neurones exhibiting
regular burst-like activity (third group, 31 neurones) the
responses to CO_2 were not studied.

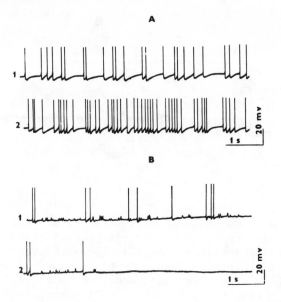

Figure 3. Tonic activity recorded from the neurones of the first (A) and second (B) groups in control conditions (1) and during inhalation of CO_2-enriched air (2).

The interspike interval power spectrum analysis showed that in the first group 33% of neurones had cardiac rhythm, 17% had respiratory rhythm, 40% showed both and in 10% of neurones the spectrum was noise-like, i.e. contained neither cardiac nor respiratory frequencies.

In the second group of neurones, no cardiac rhythm was found, 19% of neurones showed respiratory rhythm, 62% had noise-like spectrum and in 19% a new frequency component at 1.5 - 2.5 Hz was found. One can suggest from these results that the neurones of the first group are vasoconstrictors to skeletal muscle while those of the second group are vasoconstrictors to skin (see Gregor and Janig, 1977; Janig, 1985).

Mean frequency of spike appearance was higher in the first group (3.6 ± 0.5 spikes per second) than in the second group (2.3 ± 0.2 spikes per second). The most striking feature of the third group was that both spikes and EPSPs appeared in the same burst-like manner indicating that all converging fibres possess similar pattern in their tonic activity.

The neurones whose tonic activity contains only dominant spikes, only accessory spikes or both types of spikes constituted 23%, 31% and 46% in the first group, 23%, 54% and 23% in the second group, and 14%, 18% and 68% in the third group, respectively. Thus, although the contribution of dominant and accessory presynaptic inputs differs somewhat among the three groups, each group possesses both synaptic inputs.

DISCUSSION

The results obtained in this work indicate that each spike in the tonic activity of a single neurone in the ganglion correlates with spikes in at least 261 other neurones, while each EPSP correlates with spikes in at least 153 neurones, as an average. These estimates are the lowest limits because only the neurones sending their axons into the external carotid nerve are considered. Both estimates can be called functional neural units in contrast to structural neural unit which is the number of cells innervated by one preganglionic fibre. According to different authors, the structural nerve unit in mammalian sympathetic ganglion contains 50 to 200 neurones (Purves, 1975; Gabella, 1976; Purves and Wigston, 1983), i.e. about 120 neurones, as an average.

Thus, at least 2.4 structural nerve units correlate their discharges with each discharge of one tonically active neurone, while only 1.3 structural nerve units correlate thir discharge with the EPSP. This means that two or more preganglionic neurones may fire synchronously during their tonic activity, and their number varies markedly in each volley. The actual number of synchronously firing preganglionic neurones is probably much higher because only about half of a structural neural unit usually responds with a discharge to a stimulus applied to a single preganglionic fibre in the rabbit parasympathetic ganglion (Hume and Purves, 1983).

One more result of this work is that the failure to

discharge in response to tonic preganglionic volley in one neurone of the ganglion correlates with the failure in many other neurones. This result follows from the difference between the numbers of neurones correlating their discharges with tonic intracellular spike and EPSP. Thus, tonic preganglionic volleys are not equal in their ability to evoke postganglionic discharge. It is evident that the central nervous system may regulate the number of discharging cells in the ganglion simply by changing the number of the combination of preganglionic fibres that fire synchronously. Assuming that the amount of transmitter released by a single preganglionic fibre is limited (see Fonnum et al., 1984), this mechanism might have the advantage that one additional preganglionic fibre in the combination may markedly increase the number of discharging cells by adding a small EPSP to a subthreshold one evoked by other converging fibres, thus triggering a discharge in a much more numerous cell population than if the cells were singly innervated. This suggestion is consistent with the "key-lock" hypothesis (Skok, 1974, 1986). One more recent observation is consistent with this hypothesis: each neurone tends to be preferentially innervated by presynaptic fibres of similar conduction velocity (Wigston, 1983) which fire synchronously (see Johnson and Purves, 1983).

The fact that ganglion cells defined as muscle or skin vasoconstrictor neurones do not differ essentially in contribution of dominant and accessory presynaptic inputs indicates that neither of these two inputs has functional specificity. This is in agreement with the observation that dominant and accessory spikes may occur in the same cell and that dominant and accessory inputs do not differ in their preganglionic fibre conduction velocities (Skok and Ivanov, 1983).

REFERENCES

Bigland B, Hutter OF, Lippold OCJ (1953). Action potentials and tension in mammalian nerve-muscle preparations. J Physiol 121:55P.
Blackman JG, Purves RD (1969). Intracellular recordings from ganglia of the thoracic sympathetic chain of the guinea-pig. J Physiol 203:173-198.
Fonnum F, Malhlen J, Nja A (1984). Functional, structural

and chemical correlates of sprouting of intact preganglionic sympathetic axons in the guinea-pig. J Physiol 347:741-749.

Gabella G (1976). "Structure of the Autonomic Nervous System". London: Chapman and Hall, p. 8, 40.

Gregor M, Janig W (1977). Cardiac and respiratory rhythmicities in cutaneous and muscle vasoconstrictor neurones to the cat's hindlimb. Pflugers Arch 370:299-302.

Hume RI, Purves D (1981). Geometry of neonatal neurones and the regulation of synapse elimination. Nature 293:469-471.

Janig W (1985). Organization of the lumbar sympathetic outflow to skeletal muscle and skin of the cat hindlimb and tail. Rev Physiol Biochem Pharmacol 102:119-213.

Johnson DA, Purves D (1981). Post-natal reduction of neural unit size in the rabbit ciliary ganglion. J Physiol 318:143-159.

Martin AR, Pilar G (1963). Dual mode of synaptic transmission in the avian ciliary ganglion. J Physiol 168:443-463.

Nishi S, Soeda H, Koketsu K (1965). Studies on sympathetic B and C neurons and patterns of preganglionic innervation. J Cell Comp Physiol 66:19-32

Purves D (1975). Functional and structural changes in mammalian sympathetic neurones following interruption of their axons. J Physiol 252:429-463.

Purves D, Wigston DJ (1983). Neural units in the superior cervical ganglion of the guinea-pig. J Physiol 334:169-178.

Sacchi O, Perri V (1971). Quantal release of acetylcholine from the nerve endings of the guinea-pig superior cervical ganglion. Pflugers Arch 329:207-219.

Skok VI (1973). "Physiology of Autonomic Ganglia". Tokyo: Igaku Shoin Ytd., p 101-104.

Skok VI (1974). Convergence of preganglionic fibres in autonomic ganglia. In "Mechanisms of Neuronal Integration in Nervous Center" (Ed. Kostyuk PG) Leningrad: Nauka, p 27-24 (in Russian).

Skok VI (1986). Spontaneous and reflex activities: general characteristics. In "Autonomic and Enteric Ganglia. Transmission and its Pharmacology" (Ed. Karcmar AG, Koketsu K, Nishi S). New York, London: Plenum Press, p 425-438.

Skok VI, Ivanov AY (1983). What is the ongoing activity of sympathetic neurones? J Auton Nerv Syst 7:263-270.

Wigston DJ (1983). Innervation of individual guinea-pig superior cervical ganglion cells by axons with similar conduction velocities. J Physiol 334:179-187.

**Organization of the Autonomic Nervous System:
Central and Peripheral Mechanisms, pages 47–56
© 1987 Alan R. Liss, Inc.**

FUNCTIONAL SPECIALIZATION OF MEMBRANE PROPERTIES OF
SYMPATHETIC POSTGANGLIONIC NEURONES

Elspeth M. McLachlan

Baker Medical Research Institute, Prahran,
Victoria 3181, Australia

Postganglionic neurones of the sympathetic nervous
system are usually thought of as a uniform population that
relays signals originating within the central nervous
system to the vascular and visceral affector organs. The
noradrenaline (NAd) is released to excite or inhibit
effector function; many consider the actions of NAd to
resemble those of hormones. This generalized concept of
uniformity of the sympathetic neuronal population, like
all generalizations, has exceptions. For example,
cholinergic neurones in sympathetic ganglia perform
sudomotor function in skin (Sjöqvist, 1963); cholinergic
secretomotor or vasodilator responses in salivary glands
(see Emmelin et al., 1968) and some pelvic organs (e.g.
Dail et al., 1985; Hammarström, 1985) can be activated via
the sympathetic outflow. These cholinergic neurones
apparently develop from noradrenergic neurones (Landis and
Keefe, 1983).

Recently, because of the current interest in neuropeptides, subtypes of noradrenergic neurones have been
revealed. Different noradrenergic neurones have been shown
to possess immunoreactivity for Neuropeptide Y (NPY)
(Lundberg et al., 1982), somatostatin (SS) (Hökfelt et al.,
1977), and enkephalins (Shimosegawa et al., 1985), while
others lack immunoreactivity to any of the antibodies so
far tested. Cholinergic sympathetic postganglionic
neurones are also immunoreactive for vasoactive intestinal
polypeptide (VIP) (Lundberg et al., 1979). By correlating
cell body populations with terminals of extrinsic origin
within the wall of the small intestine in the guinea pig,

three neurone types have been distinguished on broad
'functional' grounds (Costa and Furness, 1984):-
(i) NAd/NPY neurones to blood vessels (vasoconstriction),
(ii) NAd/- neurones to the myenteric plexus (motility
regulation), and (iii) NAd/SS neurones to the submucous
plexus and circular muscle (regulation of secretion and
motility).
This kind of methodology undoubtedly will yield further
and more discrete identification of functional sympathetic
sub-types.

Two major sub-types of sympathetic neurones can be
distinguished in the lumbar region by their projections
from (a) the caudal lumbar sympathetic chain (LSC) via the
lumbosacral plexus to the vasculature in skeletal muscle
and skin of the hindlimb (McLachlan and Jänig, 1983;
McLachlan et al., 1985), and (b) the distal lobe(s) of the
inferior mesenteric ganglion (IMG) via the hypogastric
nerves to the pelvic organs (bladder, rectum, internal
reproductive organs) (McLachlan, 1985; Baron et al., 1985a).

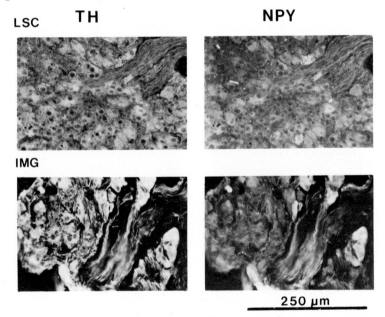

Figure 1. Immunofluorescent double staining with antibodies
to TH and NPY in the same 10 µm sections of LSC and IMG of
guinea pig (for details of methods see McLachlan and
Llewellyn-Smith, 1986).

Most of the vascular innervation in the pelvic organs
arises from the sacral sympathetic chain (Costa and
Furness, 1973), so that most IMG neurones are likely to be
concerned with motility (relaxation or contraction),
secretory neurones(i.e. ACh/VIP) to these organs being
located predominantly in the pelvic ganglia. Thus vascular
and motility regulating sympathetic neurones are located
separately.

The LSC and IMG neurones in the guinea pig have
immunohistochemical properties consistent with this
functional distinction. After colchicine treatment, 90%
of neurones in the LSC contain NPY, compared with only 22%
of neurones in the IMG (McLachlan and Llewellyn-Smith,
1986). Double staining for tyrosine hydroxylase (TH) and
NPY using two fluorescent second antibodies shows both
substances are present in LSC neurones (Fig. 1), but only in
17% of IMG neurones, in agreement with the functional
pathways described above.

Electrophysiological experiments on these two ganglia
isolated in vitro have revealed major differences between
the membrane properties of the vascular neurones and those

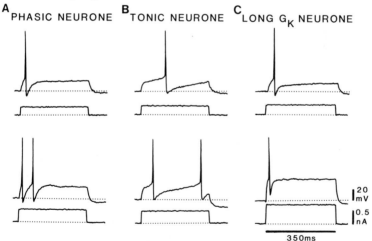

$$\text{A}_{\text{PHASIC NEURONE}} \quad \text{B}_{\text{TONIC NEURONE}} \quad \text{C}_{\text{LONG } G_K \text{ NEURONE}}$$

20 mV

0.5 nA

350ms

Figure 2. Responses of guinea pig sympathetic neurones in
vitro to just threshold (above) and suprathreshold (below)
depolarizing current. Membrane potential (upper records),
current passed through the recording microelectrode (lower
records). Neurones in (A) L5 paravertebral ganglion, (B)
distal lobe of IMG, (C) ventral lobe of the coeliac ganglion.

of the diverse (but mainly non-vascular) IMG population
(Cassell et al., 1986). While the number and kind of
synaptic inputs to the ganglion cells differ (Cassell and
McLachlan, 1986), the major distinction between neurones
from these two sites is in their response to depolarization.
When small depolarizing currents are passed via an intracellular microelectrode, nearly all neurones in the LSC
discharge at the onset of the current step. When the
current is increased, several action potentials occur in a
burst which terminates (Fig. 2A). Only about 15% of
neurones in the IMG behave in this way. Instead, the
majority depolarize slowly, and a just threshold action
potential is initiated after a delay of about 100 ms (Fig.
2B). Increased current produces low frequency rhythmic
discharge that persists if current is maintained. Such
phasic and tonic discharge patterns have been reported
previously in some sympathetic (e.g. Weems and Szurszewski,
1978; Decktor and Weems, 1983) and other (Connor and
Stevens, 1971; Madison and Nicoll, 1984) neurones.
Although mixed populations with differing proportions of
these discharge characteristics have been noted in
different sympathetic ganglia, their significance and the
underlying mechanisms were unknown.

By using a single microelectrode to voltage clamp the
soma (Finkel and Redman, 1984), the conductance changes
underlying the discharge patterns have been defined. In
such studies, the dendrites of the neurones may not always
be controlled by the somatic voltage clamp. However, the
electrotonic length of the dendrites of sympathetic
neurones is only about 0.5λ, and control of dendritic
voltage can usually be achieved within a few ms of a large
conductance change. The conventional addition of tetrodotoxin and tetraethylammonium (to prevent the fast Na^+ and
K^+ conductances associated with the action potential) need
not be employed. Instead, uncontrolled brief 'action
currents' occur, but the ensuing slower conductance changes
during and after various command steps can be examined
under good voltage control. This approach permits a
description of neuronal membrane behaviour in the voltage
range over which phasic and tonic firing normally occur.

Under voltage clamp, when the membrane is stepped
from resting membrane potential (RMP) to 15 to 25 mV more
positive, the bases for the early firing of phasic neurones
and the delayed firing of tonic neurones are obvious. In

phasic neurones (Fig. 3A), an early transient inward (Na+)
current is observed when the depolarization is just subthreshold. Larger voltage steps cause one or more 'action
currents' only in the first part of the voltage step. In
tonic neurones (Fig. 3B), the outward membrane current
declines until, after about 100 ms, a small inward
deflection is detected. A slightly larger voltage step
initiates an 'action current' only after the transient
raised conductance has declined. Additional discharges
with larger voltage commands may occur late in the voltage
step. Thus a maintained outward current of relatively
slow onset is present in phasic neurones, preventing
discharge at later times after the onset of depolarization.
In tonic neurones, a transient outward current (with decay
time constant of 25 ms) is initiated by depolarization;
this delays threshold, so that firing is slow and rhythmic.

Potassium currents with these properties have been
described in other neurones. The M current (Brown et al.,
1982) is slow in onset and maintained; the A current
(Connor and Stevens, 1971) is a fast transient current.
In sympathetic neurones, these currents are also carried
by K+ ions as they are reversed in direction at RMP >-90mV

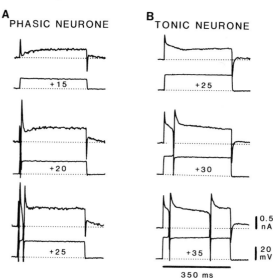

Figure 3. Current responses (upper records) to voltage
clamp steps (lower records) from resting membrane potential
(-60 mV) in an LSC neurone (A) and an IMG neurone (B).

(in 5 mM K^+), they are abolished and then reversed by raising the K^+ concentration by 10-15 mM, and they are abolished in the presence of Ba^{++} ions.

As predicted, the discharge of phasic neurones becomes 'tonic' when a muscarinic agonist (which blocks M channels) is added to the bathing solution (Cassell et al., 1986). On the other hand, the A channels in tonic neurones are unusual. In most neurones, even though A channels are present, their participation in normal activity seems doubtful because their activation/inactivation character- istics are such that few will ever be open at physiological membrane potentials. In tonic neurones, the voltage range over which the A channels become inactivated is 10-15 mV more positive than in other neurones (Fig. 4). This means that some A channels are open at rest (-60 mV) (RMP is 3-4 mV more negative than in phasic neurones, Cassell et al., 1986). Also, A currents are opened by small depolarizations from RMP, i.e. during excitatory synaptic potentials, so that their amplitude and particularly their duration become markedly attenuated (Cassell and McLachlan, 1986). This unique property makes the A channels dominate the behaviour of tonic neurones.

Both kinds of lumbar sympathetic neurones also have Ca-activated K^+ conductances (McAfee and Yarowsky, 1979) that cause afterhyperpolarizations lasting several hundred ms. After a brief voltage command step that initiates an

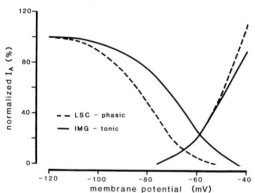

Figure 4. Normalized activation/inactivation curves describing the voltage sensitivity of A channels. Half-inactivation in tonic neurones occurs at -71 mV, compared with -84 mV for phasic neurones.

'action current', exponential tail currents have similar
time constants (120 ms) but they are usually larger in
tonic neurones. These slow K^+ conductances cannot therefore contribute significantly to the cessation of discharge
in phasic neurones (cf. Madison and Nicoll, 1984), but
probably potentiate the effect of the A channels in slowing
firing in tonic neurones by permitting reactivation of A
channels during the afterhyperpolarization.

Thus LSC neurones differ from those of the IMG, not
only in their functional destination and neurochemistry,
but also in terms of the populations of voltage-dependent
K^+ channels present in their membranes. The latter have
two important roles: first, in determining the patterns of
neuronal discharge that can be transmitted at these
ganglionic synapses, and secondly, as potential mechanisms
whereby specific channel block might modify synaptic
transmission.

There are however more than two types of electrical
behaviour. Tonic neurones are more diverse than phasic
neurones in many ways, possibly reflecting the range of
functions performed. In our preliminary studies of the
guinea pig coeliac ganglion, the majority of neurones
discharged phasically and tonic neurones were rare (<5%).
However the phasic population could be subdivided into a
major proportion (at lease 60%) largely indistinguishable
from phasic LSC neurones, while another group (particularly
in the ventral lobes) discharged only once over a wide
range of depolarizing steps (Fig. 2C). In these latter

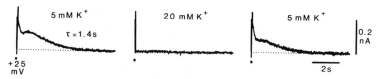

Figure 5. Prolonged K^+ conductance responsible for the long
afterhyperpolarization in a coeliac neurone. Two phases of
outward tail current recorded at -52 mV holding potential
after initiating an 'action current' at the beginning of
each trace. Decay time constants, early phase = 150 ms,
late phase 1.4 s. Both phases are reversibly abolished by
increasing extracellular K^+ to 20 mM (i.e. shifting E_K to
-50 mV).

neurones, two Ca-activated K^+ conductances follow the
action potential (Fig. 5), as in some myenteric neurones
(Hirst et al., 1985) and sensory ganglion cells (Fowler
et al., 1986). This very prolonged gK clearly does
contribute to the prevention of discharge during maintained
depolarization.

In summary, at least three types of sympathetic postganglionic neurones have been identified on electrophysiological grounds in the guinea pig. Similar subgroups
probably exist in the cat (e.g. Decktor and Weems, 1981).
The results of future studies, when correlated with data
from studies of anatomical projection and immunohistochemistry, will clarify whether electrophysiological
properties are specified according to the function of
particular sympathetic neurones.

I am indebted to John Cassell and Ida Llewellyn-Smith
for their collaboration, and to Karen Walls for technical
assistance. This work was supported by the National
Health and Medical Research Council of Australia and the
National Heart Foundation of Australia.

REFERENCES

Baron R, Jänig W, McLachlan EM (1985). The afferent and
    sympathetic components of the lumbar spinal outflow to
    the colon and pelvic organs in the cat: III. The colonic
    nerves, incorporating an analysis of all components of
    the lumbar prevertebral outflow. J Comp Neurol 238:
    158-168.
Brown DA, Adams PR, Constanti A (1982). Voltage-sensitive
    K-currents in sympathetic neurons and their modulation
    by neurotransmitters. J Auton Nerv Syst 6:23-35.
Cassell JF, Clark AL, McLachlan EM (1986). Characteristics
    of phasic and tonic sympathetic ganglion cells of the
    guinea pig. J Physiol 372:457-483.
Cassell JF, McLachlan EM (1986). The effect of a transient
    outward current (I_A) on synaptic potentials in
    sympathetic ganglion cells of the guinea pig. J Physiol
    374:273-288.
Connor JA, Stevens CF (1971). Voltage clamp studies of a
    transient outward membrane current in gastropod neural
    somata. J Physiol 213:21-30.
Costa M, Furness JB (1973). The origins of the adrenergic

fibres which innervate the internal anal sphincter, the rectum, and other tissues of the pelvic region in the guinea pig. Z Anat Entwickl -Gesch 140:129-142.

Costa M, Furness JB (1984). Somatostatin is present in a subpopulation of noradrenergic nerve fibres supplying the intestine. Neurosci 13:911-919.

Dail WG, Minorsky N, Moll MA, Manzanares K (1986). The hypogastric nerve pathway to penile erectile tissue: histochemical evidence supporting a vasodilator role. J Auton Nerv Syst 15:341-349.

Decktor DL, Weems WA (1983). An intracellular characterization of neurones and neural connexions within the left coeliac ganglion of cats. J Physiol 341:197-211.

Emmelin N, Garrett JR, Ohlin P (1968). Neural control of salivary myoepithelial cells. J Physiol 196:381-396.

Finkel AS, Redman SJ (1984). Theory and operation of a single microelectrode voltage clamp. J Neurosci Meth 11:101-127.

Fowler JC, Greene R, Weinreich D (1985). Two calcium-sensitive spike after-hyperpolarizations in visceral sensory neurones of the rabbit. J Physiol 365:59-75.

Hammarström M (1985). Autonomic nervous control of endometrial secretion in the guinea pig. Acta Physiol Scand 125:461-469.

Hirst GDS, Johnson SM, van Helden DF (1985). The slow calcium-dependent potassium current in a myenteric neurone of the guinea pig ileum. J Physiol 361:315-337.

Landis SC, Keefe D (1983). Evidence for neurotransmitter plasticity in vivo: developmental changes in properties of cholinergic sympathetic neurons. Dev Biol 98:349-372.

Lundberg JM, Hokfelt T, Schultzberg M, Uvnas-Wallenstein K, Kohler C, Said SIB (1979). Occurrence of vasoactive intestinal polypeptide (VIP)-like immunoreactivity in certain cholinergic neurons of the cat. Evidence from combined immunohistochemistry and acetylcholinesterase staining. Neuroscience 4:1539-1559.

Lundberg JM, Terenius L, Hökfelt T, Martling CR, Tatemoto K, Mutt V, Polak J, Bloom S, Goldstein M (1982). Neuropeptide Y (NPY)-like immunoreactivity in peripheral noradrenergic neurons and effects of NPY on sympathetic function. Acta Physiol Scand 116:477-480.

Madison DV, Nicoll RA (1984). Control of the repetitive discharge of rat CA1 pyramidal neurones in vitro. J Physiol 354:319-331.

McAfee DA, Yarowsky PJ (1979). Calcium-dependent potentials in the mammalian sympathetic neurone. J Physiol 290:507-523.

McLachlan EM (1985). The components of the hypogastric nerve in male and female guinea pigs. J Auton Nerv Syst 13:327-342.

McLachlan EM, Jänig W (1983). The cell bodies of origin of sympathetic and sensory axons in some skin and muscle nerves of the cat hindlimb. J Comp Neurol 214:115-130.

McLachlan EM, Oldfield BJ, Sittiracha T (1985). Localization of hindlimb vasomotor neurones in the lumbar spinal cord of the guinea pig. Neurosci Lett 54:269-275.

Shimosegawa T, Koizumi M, Toyota A, Goto Y, Kobayashi S, Yanaihara C, Yanaihara N (1985). Methionine- enkephalin-Arg[6]- Gly[7]- Leu[8]- immunoreactive nerve fibers and cell bodies in lumbar paravertebral ganglia and celiac-superior mesenteric ganglion complex of the rat: an immunohistochemical study. Neurosci Lett 57:169-174.

Sjöqvist F (1963). The correlation between the occurence and localization of acetylcholinesterase-rich cell bodies in the stellate ganglion and the outflow of cholinergic sweat secretory fibres to the forepaw of the cat. Acta Physiol Scand 57:339-351.

Weems WA, Szurszewski JH (1978). An intracellular analysis of some intrinsic factors controlling neural output from inferior mesenteric ganglion of guinea pigs. J Neurophysiol 41:305-321.

Organization of the Autonomic Nervous System:
Central and Peripheral Mechanisms, pages 57–66
© **1987 Alan R. Liss, Inc.**

FUNCTIONAL ORGANIZATION OF THE LUMBAR SYMPATHETIC OUTFLOW
TO PELVIC ORGANS AND COLON

Wilfrid Jänig

Physiologisches Institut, Universität Kiel,
Olshausenstr. 40, 2300 Kiel, FRG

INTRODUCTION

In the cat most lumbar sympathetic preganglionic
neurons project to the distal lumbar sympathetic trunk
(LST) or to the lumbar splanchnic nerves (LSN) (Fig. 1A).
Most neurons projecting to the distal LST synapse with
postganglionic neurons which supply target organs in
skeletal muscle and skin (in particular of hindlimb and
tail; see Janig, 1985); few preganglionic neurons synapse
in the sacral sympathetic trunk with postganglionic neurons
which project through the pelvic nerve to the pelvic
viscera (Kuo et al., 1984). The pre- and postganglionic
neurons which are involved in the regulation of target
organs in skeletal muscle and skin exhibit distinct
response patterns to natural stimulation of skin, viscera,
arterial baroreceptors and chemoreceptors as well as to
central stimuli. Six different types of sympathetic
neurons exist; muscle and cutaneous vasoconstrictor neurons
are numerically the largest groups (Janig, 1985).

Do the lumbar sympathetic neurons which innervate
viscera (colon, pelvic organs) also consist of different
types? The target tissues of the visceral sympathetic
neurons are blood vessels, non-vascular smooth muscle of
the visceral organs (lower urinary tract, genital tract,
internal anal sphincter), other neurons (e.g. in the
enteric nervous system of the colon and possibly in the
pelvic ganglia) and possibly secretory epithelia. Thus,
the lumbar sympathetic supply to the colon and pelvic
organs is involved in regulation of vascular resistance and

blood flow, of motility of the organs and possibly of
secretory processes.

This article summarizes the data obtained from three
groups of investigations:
1) Topographical distribution within the spinal cord of
preganglionic neurons which project to the distal LST, the
LSN and the hypogastric nerves (HGN; Baron et al, 1985 a-d;
Janig and McLachlan, 1986 a,b).
2) Functional discrimination of different types of
preganglionic neurons that project to the LSN (Bahr et al,
1986 a-c; Bartel et al, 1986).
3) Functional discrimination of pre- and postganglionic
neurons that project to the HGN (Janig, Schmidt, Schnitzler
and Wesselmann, unpublished observations).

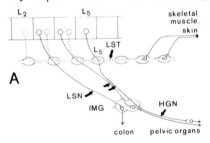

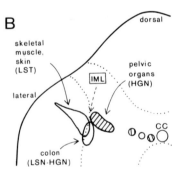

Figure 1. Location of preganglionic neurons in the spinal
segment L4. A. Arrangement of nerves. The arrows indicate
the sites where the horseradish peroxidase solution was
applied to the cut central ends of the nerves. B.
Transverse section. Schematized from Janig and McLachlan
(1986b). LST, lumbar sympathetic trunk; LSN, lumbar
splanchnic nerves; HGN, hypogastric nerves; IML, intermediolateral column; IMG, inferior mesenteric ganglion.

RESULTS

1) Localization in the spinal cord of preganglionic somata with different functions.

Cell bodies of preganglionic neurons that project to the distal LST, the LSN and the HGN have been labeled retrogradely with horseradish peroxidase applied to the central end of their cut axons (application sites indicated by arrows in Fig. 1A). About 4500 preganglionic neurons project to the distal LST and 2300 preganglionic neurons to the LSN on one side, 1700 neurons of the latter group project further to the HGN. The preganglionic neurons are located in the spinal segments T12 - L5 (LST, maximum L3), L1 - L4 (neurons terminating with their axons in the inferior mesenteric ganglion, maximum L3) and L2 - L5 (HGN, maximum L4) (Baron et al, 1985d; Janig and McLachlan, 1986a).

The topographical locations of the preganglionic cell bodies in the spinal cord are as follows (Fig. 1B): Most preganglionic neurons that project to the distal LST are situated in the pars funicularis and pars principalis of the intermediolateral cell column. Most preganglionic neurons that project to the HGN are situated medial to the preganglionic LST somata spreading in small groups towards the central canal (see also Morgan et al, 1986). Preganglionic neurons which synapse with postganglionic neurons in the inferior mesenteric ganglion without projecting to the HGN are probably associated with the postganglionic neurons with destination to the colon. The positions of these preganglionic neurons were evaluated after subtracting hypogastric preganglionic neurons from preganglionic neurons which project to the LSN. The somata of these neurons are located close to the border between white and gray matter, overlapping with the LST neurons in the ILp and lying slightly ventrally and medially to them. Some of these neurons are also located more medially.

This analysis shows that sympathetic preganglionic neurons with different functions are organized in discrete rostro-caudal cell columns in the spinal cord.

2) Reflex patterns of preganglionic neurons that project to the lumbar splanchnic nerves

Most preganglionic neurons that project to the LSN are probably involved in regulation of blood vessels and of motility of colon and pelvic organs. In order to discriminate between different types of preganglionic neurons, reflex responses elicited in the neurons by stimulation of functionally relevant afferent inputs were analyzed. The following types of afferents were stimulated: arterial baro- and chemoreceptors, sacral afferents from the urinary bladder (distension and contraction), sacral afferents from the colon (distension and contraction), sacral afferents from the mucosal skin of the anus (mechanical shearing stimuli) (see Bahns et al, 1985). The activity of the preganglionic neurons was recorded from their axons which were isolated from one of the LSN in cats (anesthetized with chloralose, immobilized, artificially ventilated; for details see Bahr et al, 1986a).

Type of Neurone

	VVC	MR_I	MR_2	MR_A	?
ongoing activity	all	most	most	most	most
arterial barorecept.	↓,CR	$\emptyset^x$	$\emptyset^x$	$\emptyset^x$	$\emptyset$
arterial chemorecept.	↑	$\emptyset$	$\emptyset$	$\emptyset$	$\emptyset$
anal skin	$\emptyset^o$	↑↓	↑↓	↑↓	$\emptyset$
urinary bladder	$\bigcirc^o$	↑	↓	$\bigcirc$	$\emptyset$
colon	$\emptyset^o$	↓	↑	$\emptyset$	$\emptyset$

Figure 2. Reflex patterns. Responses to natural stimulation of different types of afferents. ↑, excitation; ↓, inhibition; φ, no response; CR, cardiac rhythmicity of the activity (see Janig, 1985); VVC, visceral vasoconstrictor neuron; MR, neuron regulating motility (A, responding to anal stimulation only); x, some neurons excited during increase of blood pressure induced by adrenaline i.v.;

o, some VVC neurons excited by visceral stimuli.
Several types of preganglionic neurons were found:
a) Visceral vasoconstrictor (VVC) neurons. These neurons
were inhibited by stimulation of arterial baroreceptors and
excited by stimulation of arterial chemoreceptors. Stimulation of the visceral organs had either no or only weak
effects on most VVC neurons. A few VVC neurons were
excited by one of these visceral stimuli (Fig. 2; see Bahr
et al, 1986b).
b) Neurons regulating motility (MR) of the visceral organs.
These neurons were not influenced by stimulation of the
arterial baro- and chemoreceptors but were excited or
inhibited by the other visceral stimuli used (Fig. 2). The
MR neurons could be further classified into those which
were excited from the urinary bladder and sometimes
inhibited from the colon (MR1 neurons), those which were
inhibited from the urinary bladder and sometimes excited
from the colon (MR2 neurons) and those which were not
influenced from either organ but excited or inhibited from
the anal canal (MRA neurons) (Fig. 2). The details of the
classification of these neurons are described in Bahr et al
(1986a).
c) We identified preganglionic neurons which did not
respond to any of the stimuli used. In fact this group
should be numerically considerably larger than shown in
Fig. 3 since we could not detect silent preganglionic
neurons of this type (see Bahr et al, 1986c).
The upper lines of Fig. 3 list the frequencies of the
different types of preganglionic neurons which we found in
our experiments (see Bahr et al, 1986c).

	VVC	MR$_1$	MR$_2$	MR$_A$	MR$_?$	?
preganglionic:						
all (N = 192)	25.5% --------		68.2%	------	-6.2%	
MR (N = 110)		59.1%	29%	11.8%		
postganglionic:						
all (N = 150)	16% ---------		- 68%	--------	-16%	
MR (N = 84)		60.7%	25%	14.3%		

Figure 3. Percentages of different types of functionally
identified preganglionic neurons (LSN) and postganglionic
neurons (HGN).

There are several other differences between preganglionic VVC and MR neurons which support the functional classification (Bahr et al, 1986c):
a) VVC axons conduct more slowly than MR axons (2.8 versus 8.1 m/s).
b) VVC neurons have higher rates of ongoing activity than MR neurons (1.6 versus 0.8 Hz).
c) Almost all VVC neurons show short and long latency reflexes upon electrical stimulation of lumbar somatic and visceral afferents, whereas only about 50% of the MR neurons show mostly short latency reflexes.
d) VVC axons pass through the white rami L1 to L4 (maximum in L3); MR axons pass through the white rami L3 to L5 (maximum in L4).
e) VVC neurons are silent and display no reflexes after transecting the spinal cord between T8 and T13; ongoing activity and excitatory reflexes in MR neurons are barely affected after spinalization (Bartel et al, 1986).

3) Reflex patterns of pre- and postganglionic neurons that project to the hypogastric nerves

The discharge patterns of pre- and postganglionic neurons which project to the HGN were analyzed using the same approach as in the experiments on the preganglionic neurons which project to the LSN. Since the preganglionic axons in the HGN conduct very slowly (mean 2.4 m/s) and since the percentage of preganglionic axons in one HGN is low (about 9%; see Baron et al, 1986 b,d) it was difficult to isolate single preganglionic axons from the HGN. Only ten such neurons were found and 5 of them were of the MR type (no influence from the arterial baroreceptors and reactions to stimulation of the visceral organs).

The reflex patterns in the postganglionic neurons were similar to those found for the preganglionic neurons which project to the LSN: VVC, MR1, MR2 and MRA neurons. VVC neurons were less frequent at the postganglionic than at the preganglionic site (Fig. 3). The proportions of different types of functionally identified MR neurons were pre- and postganglionically nearly identical (Fig. 3). The percentage of postganglionic neurons which did not react to any of the natural stimuli used was higher at the post-ganglionic than at the preganglionic site. However, this finding is expected since it is impossible to recognize silent preganglionic axons which exhibit no reflexes.

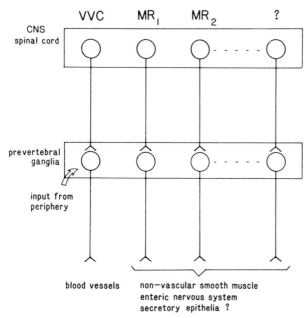

Figure 4. Organization of the visceral pre- and post-ganglionic sympathetic neurons.

CONCLUSION AND SUMMARY

Generally it can be concluded that the populations of visceral sympathetic neurons which project to the LSN (preganglionic) and the HGN (postganglionic) are similar in their compositions of functionally different types (Fig. 3). VVC neurons are functionally similar in their reflex pattern to muscle vasoconstrictor neurons (for details see Bahr et al, 1986c; Janig, 1984). The MR neurons are functionally very different from all other sympathetic neurons. At present it is difficult to relate different types of MR neurons to distinct functions or target organs. Reflexes which occur in MR1, MR2 and MRA neurons are seen in whole nerve recordings made from the lumbar colonic nerve and the HGN. Thus it is possible that these neurons are involved in regulation of the lower urinary tract and the distal bowel (for discussion see Janig, 1986). The functional classification of the MR neurons into different types as proposed by us is at present somewhat tentative; it is possible that other types of MR neurons projecting to the pelvic organs exist. It is unlikely that the internal reproductive organs are innervated by the MR1, MR2 and MRA neurons; we rather believe that the sympathetic neurons to these visceral organs are part of the group of pre- and postganglionic neurons which could not be classified.

Finally, it seems justified to conclude that the centrally generated discharge patterns in the different types of visceral sympathetic neurons are faithfully transmitted from the preganglionic to the postganglionic neurons in the inferior mesenteric ganglion. The preservation of the distinct discharge patterns in the postganglionic neurons argues in favor of the idea that the different visceral sympathetic systems are functionally separate (Fig. 4). This separation does not preclude integration of preganglionic and peripheral inputs in the inferior mesenteric ganglion (see Szurszewski, 1981; Simmons, 1985).

REFERENCES

BAHNS E, HALSBAND U, JANIG W (1985). Functional characteristics of sacral afferent fibres from the urinary bladder, urethra, colon and the anus. Pflugers Arch 405: Suppl R51.
BAHR R, BARTEL B, BLUMBERG H, JANIG W (1986a). Functional characterization of preganglionic neurons projecting in the lumbar splanchnic nerves: neurons regulating motility. J Auton Nerv Syst 15: 109-130.
BAHR R, BARTEL B, BLUMBERG H, JANIG W (1986b). Functional characterization of preganglionic neurons projecting in the lumbar splanchnic nerves: vasoconstrictor neurons. J Auton Nerv Syst 15: 131-140.
BAHR, R, BARTEL B, BLUMBERG H, JANIG W (1986c). Secondary functional properties of lumbar visceral preganglionic neurons. J Auton Nerv Syst 15: 141-152.
BARON R, JANIG W, MCLACHLAN EM (1985a). On the anatomical organization of the lumbosacral sympathetic chain and the lumbar splanchnic nerves - Langley revisited. J Auton Nerv Syst 12: 289-300.

BARON R, JANIG W, MCLACHLAN EM (1985b). The afferent and
sympathetic components of the lumbar spinal outflow to
the colon and pelvic organs in the cat. I. The
hypogastric nerve. J. Comp Neurol 238: 135-146.
BARON R, JANIG W, MCLACHLAN EM (1985c). The afferent and
sympathetic components of the lumbar spinal outflow to
the colon and pelvic organs in the cat. II. The lumbar
splanchnic nerves. J Comp Neurol 238: 147-157.
BARON R, JANIG W, MCLACHLAN EM (1985d). The afferent and
sympathetic components of the lumbar spinal outflow to
the colon and pelvic organs in the cat. III. The colonic
nerves, incorporating an analysis of all components of
the lumbar prevertebral outflow. J Comp Neurol 238:
158-168.
BARTEL B, BLUMBERG H, JANIG W (1986). Discharge patterns
of motility-regulating neurons projecting in the lumbar
splanchnic nerves to visceral stimuli in spinal cats. J
Auton Nerv Syst 15: 153-163.
JANIG W (1984). Vasoconstrictor systems supplying skeletal
muscle, skin and viscera. Clin Exp Hyper - Theory and
Practice A6: 329-346.
JANIG W (1985). Organization of the lumbar sympathetic
outflow to skeletal muscle and skin of the cat hindlimb
and tail. Rev Physiol Biochem Pharmacol 102: 119-213.
JANIG W (1986). Spinal cord integration of visceral
sensory systems and sympathetic nervous system reflexes.
In F. Cervero, JFB Morrison (eds), Visceral Sensation,
Progress in Brain Res 67: 255-277.
JANIG W, MCLACHLAN EM (1986a). The sympathetic and sensory
components of the caudal lumbar sympathetic trunk in the
cat. J Comp Neurol 245: 62-73.
JANIG W, MCLACHLAN EM (1986b). Identification of distinct
topographical distributions of lumbar sympathetic and
sensory neurons projecting to end organs with different
functions in the cat. J Comp Neurol 246: 104-112.
KUO DC, HISAMITSU T, DEGROAT WC (1984). A sympathetic
projection from sacral paravertebral ganglia to the
pelvic nerve and to postganglionic nerves on the surface
of the urinary bladder and large intesting of the cat. J
Comp Neurol 226: 76-86.
MORGAN C, DEGROAT WC, NADELHAFT I (1986). The spinal
distribution of sympathetic preganglionic and visceral
primary afferent neurons that send axons into the
hypogastric nerves of the cat. J Comp Neurol 243:
23-40.
SIMMONS M (1985). The complexity and diversity of synaptic
transmission in the prevertebral sympathetic ganglia.

Progr Neurobiol 24: 43-93.
SZURSZEWSKI JH (1981). Physiology of Mammalian
prevertebral ganglia. Ann Rev Physiol 43: 53-68.

Organization of the Autonomic Nervous System:
Central and Peripheral Mechanisms, pages 67–77
© **1987 Alan R. Liss, Inc.**

ANATOMY AND FUNCTION OF THORACIC CARDIAC NEURONS

J. A. Armour

Department of Physiology and Biophysics
Dalhousie University, Halifax, Nova Scotia,
B3H 4H7, Canada

Supported by a Medical Research Council of Canada program
grant (PG-18) and a Nova Scotia Heart Foundation grant.

INTRODUCTION

Recently it has been proposed that intrathoracic
neuronal mechanisms exist which function in concert with
central nervous system ones to regulate cardiovascular
dynamics (1). Anatomical and physiological evidence is
accumulating which demonstrates the complexity of these
local neuronal reflexes.

ANATOMY

Afferent axons arising from canine cardiac receptors
are connected with perikarya located throughout the nodose
ganglia, lesser numbers being located in the C5-T6 dorsal
root ganglia. Canine cardiac efferent postganglionic
sympathetic neurons are located primarily throughout the
middle cervical ganglia and cranial poles of the stellate
ganglia (13). In monkeys these neurons are more evenly
distributed throughout the superior, middle and inferior
cervical ganglia (16). In addition, some of these neurons
are located in the small mediastinal ganglia located along
cardiopulmonary nerves (13). Efferent preganglionic
sympathetic axons are known to synapse on postganglionic
sympathetic neurons via nicotinic cholinergic synaptic
mechanisms. However, other receptor mechanisms may also be
present in thoracic autonomic ganglia. For instance,
neuropeptide Y-, vasoactive intestinal peptide-, and

substance P-like immunoreactivity is present in perikarya
throughout these ganglia (8). Axons containing enkephaline-
like immunoreactivity are also present in these ganglia.
Also SlF cells and interneurons have been located in these
ganglia (18). Thus, anatomical evidence suggests that a
number of synaptic mechanisms may exist in thoracic
autonomic ganglia.

PHYSIOLOGY

A) Function of neurons in thoracic autonomic ganglia.
     Stellate or middle cervical ganglion stimulation
produces generalized augmentation in cardiac chronotropism
and inotropism, whereas stimulation of individual
cardiopulmonary nerves arising from these ganglia can augment
chronotropism and/or inotropism in specific regions of the
heart (16). Following acute decentralization and the
administration of hexamethonium, stimulation of localized
regions within one of these ganglia or a mediastinal
ganglion can also augment cardiac chronotropism and/or
inotropism (11). For instance, stimulation of a locus in
the caudal pole of an acutely decentralized stellate ganglion following the administration of hexamethonium can
augment cardiac chronotropism and/or inotropism to a
considerable degree and occasionally produce ventricular
fibrillation (Fig. 1), even though few if any cardiac
efferent postganglionic neurons are present there (13).
Thus, these data indicate that local circuit neurons in
thoracic autonomic ganglia are involved in cardiac
regulation.
     Some neurons in thoracic autonomic ganglia have
spontaneous activity which is related to cardiac or
respiratory mechanics (5,6,9,10). They can be activated by
mechanical distortion of a limited region of a great
thoracic vessel or the heart, indicating that such neurons
may be influenced by mechanoreceptors in a relatively
limited region (5). They are usually active during one
phase of the cardiac cycle, particularly isovolumetric
contraction (Fig. 2) or relaxation, for up to ~80 cardiac
cycles and only when systolic pressure is ~80-160 mmHg (5).
Such phase-locked pressure-related neural activity persists
following acute (5,6) or chronic (7) decentralization,
suggesting that afferent perikarya exist in thoracic autonomic ganglia. Single supramaximal stimuli (10 V, 1-5 ms)
delivered individually to each major nerve connected with
the middle cervical or stellate ganglia activated only a

small fraction of their neurons, and then rarely after a
fixed latency (5,6,7). In contrast, many of these neurons
were activated during or immediately following trains of
such stimuli. These data imply that the majority of the

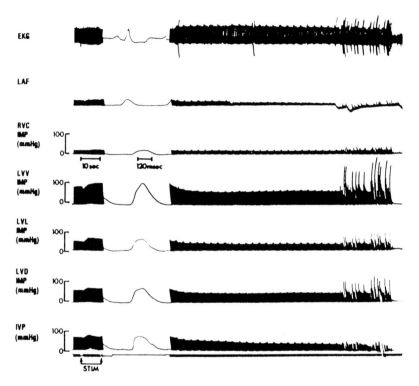

Figure 1. Bipolar stimulation (between arrows) (10 Hz, 4
ms, 4 V) in area A5 of the right middle cervical ganglion
following acute decentralization and the administration of
hexamethonium augmented, from above downward, heart rate,
left (LAF) atrial force, and intramyocardial systolic
pressures in the right ventricular conus (RVC IMP: 20 to 25
mmHg) as well as the ventral (LVV: 80 to 100 mmHg), lateral
(LVL: 50 to 65 mmHg) and dorsal (LVD: 60 to 70 mmHg) walls
of the left ventricle; left ventricular chamber systolic
pressure (IVP: 75 to 85 mmHg) was also augmented. About 10
s after cessation of stimulation an electrical disturbance
occurred in the heart which after ~22 sec was followed by
ventricular fibrillation (far right side).

phase-locked cardiac related neurons do not project axons
out of their respective ganglia and as such are presumably
local circuit neurons. It is concluded that afferent
neurons in thoracic autonomic ganglia which have mechano-
receptor endings in the heart or great thoracic vessels
activate local circuit neurons which, in turn, influence
some of the efferent postganglionic neurons which innervate
the heart or thoracic vasculature.

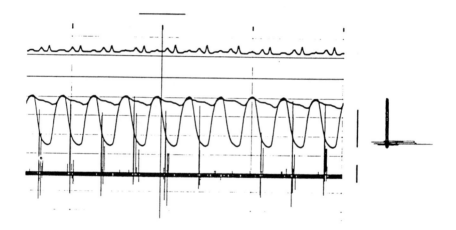

Figure 2. From above down, an EKG, aortic pressure, left
ventricular chamber pressure and neuronal activity recorded
from the in situ middle cervical ganglion illustrating
spontaneous activity from a number of neurons which
occurred during isovolumetric relaxation, as illustrated by
plotting neuronal activity (horizontal axis) versus intraventricular pressure (vertical axis) on the right.
Horizontal bar = 500 ms; vertical bars = 100 mmHg and 0.2
mv.

Electrical stimulation of afferent axons in one
cardiopulmonary nerve (CPN) produces compound action
potentials (CAPs) in efferent postganglionic sympathetic

axons of other CPNs ~20-350 ms later (1,2). Following
acute or chronic decentralization, this activation latency
is reduced to ~20-100 ms (Fig. 3) suggesting that the
production of CAPs with the longest latencies involved

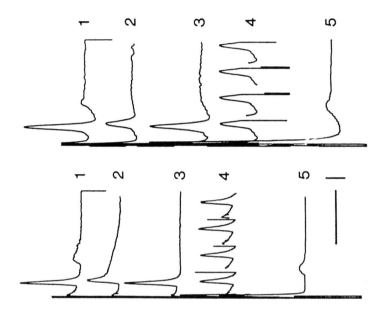

Figure 3. Stimulation (0.5 Hz, 1 ms, 10 V) of afferent
components in the left thoracic vagosympathetic complex
(severed above the middle cervical ganglion and below the
recurrent laryngeal nerve) produced CAPs in the left intermediate medial (left side) and caudal pole (right side)
CPNs (#1). When the left stellate ganglion was stimulated
simultaneously (#2) the first CAPs were reduced in size and
the second suppressed, indicating that efferent preganglionic sympathetic axons can influence local thoracic reflex
mechanisms. Acute decentralization of the stellate and
middle cervical ganglia resulted in abolition of the second
CAPs (#3), presumably because these involved synaptic
mechanisms in the spinal cord. Thereafter, stimulation at
10 Hz reduced the remaining CAPs (#4), indicating that the
synaptic mechanisms involved were modified by the activation frequency. Following the administration of hexamethonium (5 mg/kg i.v.) the CAPs were further suppressed (#5).
Calibrations: vertical bar = 1 mV, horizontal bar = 100 ms.

neurons in the central nervous system (1,4). Despite the fact that axon collaterals arising from a sympathetic neuron can project axons into two different ipsilateral CPNs (17) thus permitting the possibility of axon-axonal reflexes to occur, the production of CAPs was modified by hexamethonium (Fig. 3), atropine (Fig. 4), phentolamine or propranalol (2). Thus, it was concluded that nicotinic and muscarinic cholinergic (2,12,14) as well as alpha and beta

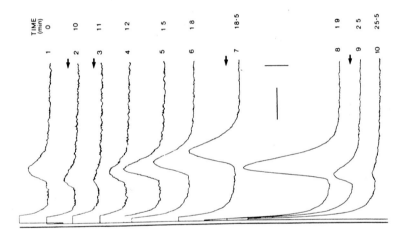

Figure 4. Stimulation of afferent axons in the left inter-mediate CPN produced a CAP in the left caudal pole nerve in an acutely decentralized MCG preparation (line #1). This was suppressed following atropine (0.1 mg/kg i.v., first arrow) (line #2). The CAP was further suppressed (line #3) immediately following another 0.1 mg/kg of atropine (second arrow), the CAP gradually increasing in the following 7 min. It was further enhanced when a total of 0.5 mg/kg of atropine was administered (third arrow before #7). When a total of 1 mg/kg of atropine had been administered (fourth arrow) the CAP was suppressed (lines #9 and 10). Further doses did not alter the CAP. These data indicate that atropine can enhance and/or inhibit thoracic synaptic mechanisms, depending on the dose employed. Calibration bars: 0.1 mV, 20 ms.

adrenergic synaptic mechanisms exist in thoracic ganglia
(2). This picture is further complicated by the fact that
atropine or phentolamine at low doses can enhance such CAPs
(Fig. 4), indicating that these agents may modify inhibitory
mechanisms in these ganglia at lower doses, while blocking
synaptic transmission at higher doses. Due to the fact
that CAPs are generated following the administration of the
four pharmacological agents described above and that these
are transiently abolished by locally injected chymotrypsin
and relatively permanently abolished by local injections of
manganese, it has been proposed that peptide related
synaptic mechanisms also exist in these ganglia (3). This
assumption is supported by the fact that local circuit
neurons in thoracic ganglion can be activated by trains of
stimuli delivered to a CPN or ansa following the administration of hexamethonium, atropine, phentolamine and
propranalol (5,6,7). In fact, these data may, in part,
account for the presence of neuropeptides in thoracic autonomic ganglia (see above). Thus, it appears that five or
more different synaptic mechanisms exist in thoracic autonomic ganglia.

B) Cardiac effects of intrathoracic reflexes
    If local thoracic neural reflexes exist, what is their
potential influence on the heart? In an acutely decentralized preparation, stimulation of afferent components in a
CPN can augment the uptake of 2-[^{14}C] deoxyglucose in the
ventricles, particularly in endocardial regions. This
presumably is due to increased metabolic demand secondary
to increased regional inotropism produced by local thoracic
reflex mechanisms (15). In such experiments metabolism
also increased in the caudal pole of the ipsilateral stellate ganglia where few, if any, efferent postganglionic
neurons are located, thus supporting the contention that
cardiac afferent axons can enhance the activity of thoracic
local circuit neurons independent of neurons in the CNS
(13). Stimulation of the afferent components in a CPN in
an acutely decentralized preparation can also alter cardiac
chronotropism and/or inotropism to a considerable degree
(Fig. 5). Taken together these data imply that intrathoracic cardiocardiac reflexes are capable of functioning
throughout each cardiac cycle to regulate cardiac chronotropism and inotropism.

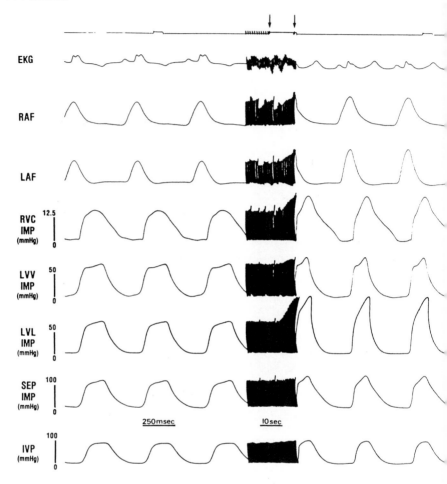

Figure 5. Stimulation (10 Hz, 4 ms, 10 V; between arrows) of the afferent axons in a left vagosympathetic complex of an acutely decentralized left middle cervical and stellate ganglionic preparation produced tachycardia (120 to 134 b/m), and augmentation in right (RAF) and left (LAF) atrial contractile forces as well as intramyocardial pressure in the right ventricular conus (RVC: 15 to 26 mmHg), left ventricular ventral (LVV: 68 to 87 mmHg) and lateral (LVL: 65 to 125 mmHg) walls and intraventricular septum (SEP: 117 to 140 mmHg). Left ventricular chamber pressure was augmented (IVP: 95 to 125 mmHg). This illustrates the magnitude of cardiac changes that can be produced by intrathoracic autonomic reflexes.

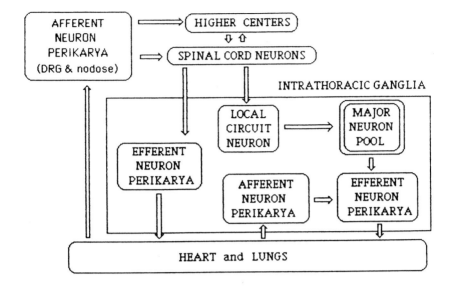

Figure 6. Diagram of the proposed populations of neurons within thoracic autonomic ganglia. The major neuron pool consists of local circuit neurons.

SUMMARY

Afferent (4,7) and efferent perikarya, as well as local circuit neurons (5), may exist in thoracic autonomic ganglia (Fig. 6). These may interact via complex and varied synaptic mechanisms, presumably on a beat-to-beat basis, to regulate the heart and great thoracic vessels primarily when systolic pressure is in the physiological range. This neuronal pool presumably functions to maintain a relatively stable cardiac performance without requiring much input from central nervous system neurons.

ACKNOWLEDGEMENTS

The technical assistance of Richard Livingston and the typing assistance of Joan Livingston are gratefully acknowledged.

REFERENCES

1. Armour, J.A. 1976. Instant-to-instant reflex cardiac regulation. Cardiology 61:309-328.

2. Armour, J.A. 1983. Synaptic transmission to thoracic autonomic ganglia of the dog. Can. J. Physiol. Pharmacol. 61:793-801.

3. Armour, J.A. 1984a. Synaptic transmission in the decentralized middle cervical ganglion of the dog. Brain Res. Bull. 10:103-109.

4. Armour, J.A. 1984b. Synaptic transmission in chronically decentralized middle cervical and stellate ganglia of the dog. Can. J. Physiol. Pharmacol. 6:1149-1155.

5. Armour, J.A. 1985. Activity of in situ middle cervical ganglion neurons in dogs using extracellular recording techniques. Can. J. Physiol. Pharmacol. 63:704-716.

6. Armour, J.A. 1986. Activity of in situ stellate ganglion neurons of dogs recorded extracellularly. Can. J. Physiol. Pharmacol. 64:101-111.

7. Armour, J.A. 1986. Neuronal activity recorded extracellularly in chronically decentralized in situ canine middle cervical ganglia. In Press: Can. J. Physiol. Pharmacol.

8. Armour, J.A., S. Darvesh, D.M. Nance and D.A. Hopkins. 1985. Neuropeptides in canine middle cervical and stellate ganglia. Fed. Proc. 45:781.

9. Bosnjak, Z.J. and J.P. Kampine. 1982. Intracellular recordings from the stellate ganglion of the cat. J. Physiol. (London) 324:273-283.

10. Bosnjak, Z.J., J.L. Seagard and J.P. Kampine. 1982. Peripheral neural input to neurons of the stellate ganglion in dog. Am. J. Physiol. 242:R237-R243.

11. Brandys, J.C., D.A. Hopkins and J.A. Armour. 1984. Cardiac responses to stimulation of discrete loci within canine sympathetic ganglia following hexamethonium. J. Auton. Nerv. Sys. 11:243-255.

12. Brown, A.M. 1967. Cardiac sympathetic adrenergic pathways in which synaptic transmission is blocked by atropine sulphate. J. Physiol. (London) 191:271-288.

13. Hopkins, D.A. and J.A. Armour. 1984. Localization of sympathetic postganglionic and parasympathetic preganglionic neurons which innervate different regions of the dog heart. J. Comp. Neurol. 229:186-198.

14. Jones, A. 1963. Ganglionic actions of muscarinic substances. J. Pharmacol. Exp. Ther. 141:195-205.

15. Kostreva, D.R., J.A. Armour and Z.J. Bosnjak. 1985. Metabolic mapping of a cardiac reflex mediated by sympathetic ganglia in dogs. Amer. J. Physiol. 249: R317-R322.

16. Randall, W.C. ed. 1984. Neural Regulation of the Heart. Oxford Univ. Press, N.Y.
17. Tomney, P.A., D.A. Hopkins and J.A. Armour. 1985. Axonal branching of canine sympathetic postganglionic cardiopulmonary neurons. A retrograde fluorescent labelling study. Brain Res. Bull. 14:443-452.
18. Williams, T.W. 1967. Electron microscope evidence for an autonomic interneuron. Nature (London) 214:309-310.

SECTION II: Spinal Mechanisms

An important source of input to spinal preganglionic neurons are spinal afferents from somatic and visceral nerves, which activate segmental and intersegmental spinal circuits as well as long-loop circuits including supraspinal levels of the central nervous system. An analysis of this circuitry, of obvious importance for understanding the control of the preganglionic neurons, involves defining the chemical mediators of synaptic transmission and the properties of interneurons or projection neurons involved in these pathways. Another important source of input to preganglionic neurons in supraspinal and analysis of the circuits connecting these neurons to supraspinal levels of the CNS with regard to identification of constituent neurons and of transmitters is also of great importance. The five papers of this section offer a very good sample of main experimental approaches to some of these questions.

The paper by deGroat, Kawatani, Houston, Rutigliano and Erdman presents a study of the neuropeptide content of dorsal root ganglion cells sending their axons into pelvic, hypogastric and pudendal nerves. Some of these peptides found in these sensory neurons are known to be excitatory, others inhibitory. On the assumption that the peptides are released by action potentials, that they can act both pre- and post-synaptically, and that their action is likely to be long lasting, their presence adds a potential for "plastic" facilitatory or inhibitory features to the operation of the first order sensory synapse.

The properties of the neurons which connect sensory or centrally-generated input to the output neurons of the autonomic system are an important determinant of the input-output relations of the system. The paper by Foreman, Ammons and Blair focuses on just such neurons and describes spinal neurons in upper thoracic cord segments which receive input from visceral primary afferents travelling in sympathetic nerves. These afferents presumably convey information from the heart or other intrathoracic structures. The paper describes the responses of these neurons, the projection to supraspinal levels and the convergence with afferent input from somatic receptors, as well as from intrathoracic receptors projecting to the brainstem via the vagus nerve. Some of these data seem relevant to the question of how similarities in the organization of sympathetic reflexes evoked by visceral and somatic afferents arises. The basis may be provided by the convergence of these two classes of afferents onto the same spinal interneurons.

The paper by Weaver, Meckler and Stein addresses the question of the heterogeneity of the sympathetic output. Their data show that the background firing of post-ganglionic units in renal, mesenteric and splenic nerves shows differences with respect to dependence on supraspinal input, sensitivity to arterial baroreceptor input and response to input from visceral receptors.

The paper by Schramm and Livingstone explores in the high spinal rat renal nerve activity in spontaneously hypertensive rats (SHR) and age-matched controls. The aim is to search for differences between these two groups which may be attributed to changes in properties of spinal circuits associated with the development of arterial hypertension. They find a relatively lower sensitivity of the SHR to inhibitory inputs, whereas excitatory responses to afferent stimulation and interactions between excitatory and inhibitory responses are similar in SHR and controls.

Finally, the paper by Franz, Steffensen, Miner and Sangdee shows evidence in the high spinal cat that sympathetic preganglionic neuron excitation by descending input, possibly bulbospinal pathways, is controlled through regulation of adenylate-cyclase and cAMP levels by several neurotransmitters.

Organization of the Autonomic Nervous System:
Central and Peripheral Mechanisms, pages 81–90
© 1987 Alan R. Liss, Inc.

IDENTIFICATION OF NEUROPEPTIDES IN AFFERENT PATHWAYS TO THE PELVIC VISCERA OF THE CAT

William C. de Groat, Masahito Kawatani, Mary B. Houston, Michael Rutigliano and Susan Erdman Department of Pharmacology and Center for Neuro- science, University of Pittsburgh, Pittsburgh, Pennsylvania 15261.

INTRODUCTION

Afferent pathways from the pelvic viscera pass to the lumbosacral spinal cord via parasympathetic (pelvic) and sympathetic (hypogastric and lumbar colonic) nerves (de Groat et al., 1981; de Groat and Booth, 1984). Horse- radish peroxidase tracing techniques revealed (Morgan et al., 1981, 1986a, 1986b) that these afferent pathways like visceral afferents at other levels of the spinal cord (de Groat, 1986) have a distinctive pattern of cen- tral termination which is markedly different from the central termination of somatic afferent neurons innervat- ing the skin. One of the most prominent features of the lumbosacral visceral afferent system is the very dense central projection to Lissauer's tract from which axon collaterals pass in a narrow band through lamina I later- ally and medially around the dorsal horn. These projec- tions have been termed, respectively, the lateral and medial collateral pathways (LCP and MCP) of Lissauer's tract (Morgan et al., 1981).

The LCP is very prominent in the sacral spinal cord of the cat and is characterized by a high density of pep- tidergic varicosities (Kawatani et al., 1983, 1985a; Honda et al., 1983; Basbaum and Glazer 1983) many of which (eg., vasoactive intestinal polypeptide, substance P, cholecys- tokinin, dynorphin B, and dynorphin 1-17) arise from pri- mary afferent axons entering the spinal cord via the dor- sal roots. This overlap of peptide immunoreactivity with HRP labeled visceral afferent terminals in the superficial laminae of the dorsal horn has led to speculation that various peptides might be localized in sacral visceral afferent neurons (de Groat et al., 1983, 1986b; Kawatani et al., 1983, 1985a; Honda et al., 1983; Basbaum and Glazer, 1983). This was examined in the present experiments by combining immunocytochemical and axonal tracing techniques to study peptide immunoreactivity in labeled visceral afferent neurons of the cat lumbosacral dorsal root ganglia.

METHODS

As described in detail in recent papers (Kawatani et al., 1985a, 1986) dorsal root ganglion cells (DRG) were retrogradely labelled by fluorescent dyes applied to the pelvic nerves, hypogastric nerves, pudendal nerves, and nerves to the urinary bladder and colon in halothane anesthetized cats. The central ends of the transected nerves were immersed in dye solutions (2-5% fast blue, true blue, diamidino yellow, propidium iodide) and then the animals were maintained for 7-14 days to allow transport of the dyes centrally to the DRG. Colchicine solution (1 mg/ml) was applied topically or injected into the DRG 36-50 hrs before sacrifice to increase peptide immunoreactivity in afferent cells. After perfusion and fixation the DRG were sectioned in a cryostat and sections were processed by indirect immunocytochemical techniques using rabbit or rat antisera for VIP, substance P, CCK, leucine and methionine enkephalin, dynorphin 1-17, and somatostatin at dilutions of 1:500 to 1:3000. Anti-rabbit or anti-rat IgG conjugated with FITC or TRITC was applied to the sections to complete the staining procedure. In some experiments a double staining technique was employed. Two antisera prepared in different species were applied to the same section which was then processed with bridge antibodies linked to different fluorochromes (FITC and TRITC). This allowed two peptides to be identified on the same section. Sections were examined with an epi-illumination fluorescence microscope using a Leitz Ploem-pack A filter for fast blue, true blue, or diamidino yellow, the I_2 filter for FITC and the N_2 filter for TRITC or propidium iodide. Specificity of the antisera was tested with antisera preabsorbed with each peptide (1-50 µg/ml)

RESULTS

Peptides in Sacral Afferent Neurons

Application of fluorescent dyes to the pelvic nerve labeled on the average 2900 DRG cells (range 1968-3720) in segments L_7-Cx_1 (Fig. 1A). As shown in Table 1, a large percentage of these neurons in colchicine treated ganglia exhibited peptide-immunoreactivity. VIP was the most common peptide, occurring in 42% of the neurons followed by leucine enkephalin (LENK), CCK, substance P (SP, Fig. 1B) and methionine enkephalin (MENK). Somatostatin (SS) was detected in a very small percentage of neurons. Dynorphin 1-17 (DYN) was not detected in DRG cells. Peptide immunoreactivity occurred more frequently in pelvic nerve afferents than in pudendal nerve afferents which innervate somatic structures (Kawatani et al., 1986). For example, the sum of the mean percentages of pelvic afferents containing individual peptides was almost double (137%) that of pudendal afferents (70%) (Table 1). The differences were most striking for VIP, CCK and MENK.

The relationship between peptides and specific afferent pathways was also evaluated in the opposite manner by determining the percentage of peptidergic cells which were labeled by tracers applied to the pelvic and pudendal nerves. In the S_2 DRG, which contained the largest number of labeled neurons, pelvic nerve afferent neurons accounted for 70% of the VIP cells and 23% of the substance P cells. Pudendal nerve afferent neurons accounted for approximately 20% of both types of peptidergic cells.

The distribution of peptides in sacral afferent neurons innervating the urinary bladder and colon was determined by applying different dyes to each organ (eg., fast blue to the bladder and diamidino yellow to the colon). The number of labeled neurons innervating each organ (approximately 1000 cells) and the segmental distribution were similar. A small percentage of cells (3-6%) exhibited double dye labeling, suggesting that some afferents send axons to both organs or that dye injected into one organ spread to the other organ. The mean percentage of bladder and colon afferent cells containing peptides was lower than that of the pelvic nerve afferents, however, in both types of afferents VIP (14-25%) and substance P(18-23%) were the most common peptides (Table 1).

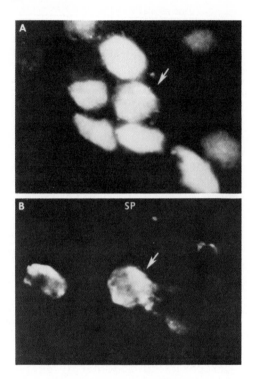

Figure 1. A, photomicrograph of pelvic nerve afferent
neurons in the S_2 DRG labeled with fast blue. B, photomicrograph of the same section showing substance P neurons
(SP) stained with TRITC. Arrow indicates a visceral neuron with substance P immunoreactivity. Reproduced from
the J. Comp. Neurol.

Peptides in Lumbar Visceral Afferent Neurons

Application of fluorescent dyes to the hypogastric
nerve labeled on the average 540 cells in the L_2-L_5 DRG.
As shown in Table 1, VIP, SP, CCK, LENK and MENK were
detected in a large percentage of these neurons, whereas
somatostatin was not detected. The sum of the percentages
of cells containing individual peptides exceeded 100%.

TABLE 1. Percentage of Lumbosacral Afferent Neurons Containing Neuropeptides

	PN	HGN	PUDN	BLD	Colon
VIP	42	45	10	25	14
LENK	30	21	24	5	7
CCK	29	25	12	1	3
SP	24	37	21	23	18
MENK	10	9	3	--	--
SS	2	0	0	2	2
DYN	0	0	0	0	0
Total	137	137	70	56	44

PN - Pelvic Nerve; HGN - Hypogastric Nerve; PUDN - Pudendal Nerve; BLD - Bladder. (--), data not available.

Coexistence of Peptides in Sacral Afferent Neurons

The finding that a large percentage of visceral afferent neurons contain peptides and that the sum of individual percentages for a series of six different peptides exceeded 100% suggested that some peptides must coexist in afferent neurons. This was confirmed using double staining techniques where two peptides could be identified on the same tissue section. Coexistence was examined in the general population of sacral afferent neurons and in bladder, colon and HGN afferent neurons. As shown in Table 2 for colon afferents, coexistence of certain peptides was very common. For example, a large percentage of cells containing LENK exhibited SP, VIP or CCK; and a large percentage (51%) of VIP cells contained SP or LENK. However, LENK was not colocalized with somatostatin. The sum of the mean percentages of LENK cells containing other peptides exceeded 100% indicating that more than two peptides must be contained in one cell. Preliminary studies

of thin serial sections (6 μm) allowing the same DRG cell
to be visualized in three consecutive sections confirmed
that three peptides eg., VIP, SP and CCK could occur in
the same cell. Similar patterns of coexistence were noted
in unlabeled afferents and in dye labeled bladder and HGN
afferents (Kawatani et al., 1985b).

TABLE 2. Summary of Peptide Colocalization in Colon Afferent Neurons

	LENK	SP	VIP	CCK	SS
LENK	--	56	50	6	0
SP	27	--	42	7	--
VIP	51	52	--	--	--
CCK	11	22	--	--	--
SS	0	--	--	--	--

Numbers indicate percentages of neurons in the left
column exhibiting immunoreactivity for other peptides. Each percentage represents the average for
several hundred cells in sacral dorsal root ganglia
of two animals. (--) indicates data not available.

DISCUSSION

The present experiments revealed that lumbosacral
visceral afferent neurons contain a wide spectrum of neuropeptides including those with inhibitory neuronal actions
(the enkephalins) as well as those with excitatory actions
(SP, VIP and CCK). Some peptides, such as VIP and SP
were present in a large percentage of visceral afferent
neurons, whereas other peptides, such as somatostatin,
were rarely present. The prominence of VIP in sacral
afferent neurons is consistent with previous reports of
high densities of VIP terminals in the sacral spinal cord
and provides further support for the view that VIP may be
an important transmitter in afferent pathways from the

pelvic organs. Indeed, it is estimated that approximately 70% of the VIP neurons in the S_2 dorsal root ganglion innervate visceral organs, whereas only 23% of the substance P neurons are visceral.

The large percentage of visceral afferent neurons containing peptides suggested that some peptides must coexist in these cells. This was confirmed with double staining techniques (de Groat et al., 1985). The coexistence of LENK with other peptides (VIP, SP and CCK) was of particular interest since enkephalins and opiate drugs are known to have presynaptic inhibitory actions (Jessel and Iversen, 1977), whereas VIP and substance P are generally considered to have excitatory or facilitatory synaptic actions. LENK was not colocalized with somatostatin, a peptide which also has synaptic inhibitory effects in the spinal cord. However, somatostatin was colocalized with substance P in nonvisceral afferent neurons. Thus both inhibitory peptides coexist with excitatory peptides but not with each other. We have speculated in a recent paper (de Groat et al., 1986a) that opioid inhibitory peptides in afferent pathways might function as mediators of a negative feedback mechanism at primary afferent terminals in the spinal cord and thereby regulate the release of excitatory transmitters (Fig. 2).

Other opioid peptides such as dynorphin B (Basbaum et al., 1986) and dynorphin 1-17 (de Groat et al., 1986a) also appear to be present in afferent terminals in the LCP of the sacral spinal, however their coexistence with other peptides is not known since it has been impossible to demonstrate dynorphin immunoreactivity in dorsal root ganglion cells with immunocytochemical techniques.

In summary, the present histochemical data coupled with recent pharmacological observations (de Groat, 1986, de Groat et al., 1986b) suggest that various neuropeptides may have a role in visceral sensory and reflex mechanisms. The function of opioid peptides may be particularly important since these substances appear to be involved in inhibitory mechanisms in central and peripheral efferent pathways (de Groat et al., 1983, 1986b) in addition to their possible function as inhibitory modulators at primary afferent terminals.

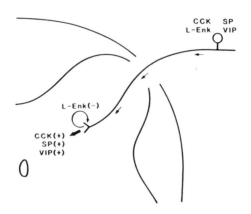

ENKEPHALINERGIC
NEGATIVE FEEDBACK MECHANISM

Figure 2. Diagram illustrating possible function
of leucine-enkephalin (LENK) in primary afferent
neurons. LENK may be released at afferent terminals
in the spinal cord and interact with opioid receptors
on the terminals to mediate feedback inhibition of
the release of excitatory transmitters, such as
substance P (SP), vasoactive intestinal polypeptide
(VIP) and cholecystokinin (CCK). LENK-IR has been
identified in dorsal root ganglion cells containing
either SP, VIP or CCK. However, it is not known
whether all 4 peptides are localized in the same
population of primary afferent neurons. Reproduced
from J. Auton. Nerv. Syst.

ACKNOWLEDGEMENTS

This work was supported in part by NSF Grant BNS
8507113, NIH Grants AM 317888, AM 37241, and Clinical
Research Center Grant MH 30915.

REFERENCES

Basbaum AI, Cruz L, Weber E (1986). Immunoreactive dynorphin B in sacral primary afferent fibers of the cat. J Neurosci 6:127-133.

Basbaum AI, Glazer EJ (1983). Immunoreactive vasoactive intestinal polypeptide is concentrated in the sacral spinal cord: A possible marker for pelvic visceral afferent fibers. Somatosensory Res 1:69-82.

de Groat WC (1986). Spinal cord projections and neuropeptides in visceral afferent neurons. Prog Brain Res 67:165-187.

de Groat WC, Booth, AM (1984). Autonomic systems to the urinary bladder and sexual organs. In Dyck PJ, Thomas PK, Lambert EH, Bunge R (eds): "Peripheral Neuropathy," Vol. I, Philadelphia: W.B. Saunders Co., pp 285-299.

de Groat WC, Nadelhaft I, Milne RJ, Booth AM, Morgan C, Thor K (1981). Organization of the sacral parasympathetic reflex pathways to the urinary bladder and large intestine. J Auton Nerv Sys 3:135-160.

de Groat WC, Kawatani M, Hisamitsu T, Lowe I, Morgan C, Roppolo J, Booth A, Nadelhaft I, Kuo D, Thor K (1983). The role of neuropeptides in the sacral autonomic reflex pathways of the cat. J Auton Nerv Sys 7:339-350.

de Groat WC, Kawatani M, Houston MB, Erdman SL (1985). Colocalization of VIP, substance P, CCK, somatostatin and enkephalin immunoreactivity in lumbosacral dorsal root ganglion cells of the cat. Abstract for Vth International Washington Spring Symposium, May 28-31, Washington, DC.

de Groat WC, Lowe IP, Kawatani M, Morgan CW, Kuo D, Roppolo JR, Thor K, Nagel J (1986a). The identification of enkephalin-like immunoreactivity in sensory ganglion cells. J Auton Nerv Sys (in press).

de Groat WC, Kawatani M, Hisamitsu T, Booth AM, Roppolo JR, Thor K, Tuttle P, Nagel J (1986b). Neural control of micturition: The role of neuropeptides. J Auton Nerv Sys (in press).

Honda CN, Rethelyi M, Petrusz P, (1983). Preferential immunohistochemical localization of vasoactive intestinal polypeptide (VIP) in the sacral spinal cord of the cat: Light and electron, microscope observations. J Neurosci 5:2183-2196.

Jessell TM, Iversen LL (1977). Opiate analgesics inhibit substance P release from rat trigeminal nucleus. Nature (Lond) 268:549-551.

Kawatani M, Lowe I, Nadelhaft I, Morgan C, de Groat WC (1983). Vasoactive intestinal polypeptide in visceral afferent pathways to the sacral spinal cord of the cat. Neurosci Lett 42:311-316.

Kawatani M, Erdman S, de Groat WC (1985a). Vasoactive intestinal polypeptide and substance P in afferent pathways to the sacral spinal cord of the cat. J Comp Neurol 241:327-347.

Kawatani M, Houston MB, Rutigliano M, Erdman SL, de Groat WC (1985b). Colocalization of neuropeptides in afferent pathways to the urinary bladder and colon: Demonstration with double color immunohistochemistry in combination with axonal tracing techniques. Soc Neurosci Abstr 11:145.

Kawatani M, Nagel J, de Groat WC (1986). Identification of neuropeptides in pelvic and pudendal nerve afferent pathways to the sacral spinal cord of the cat. J Comp Neurol (in press).

Morgan C, Nadelhaft I, de Groat WC (1981). The distribution of visceral primary afferents from the pelvic nerve within Lissauer's tract and the spinal gray matter and its relationship to the sacral parasympathetic nucleus. J Comp Neurol 201:415-440.

Morgan C, de Groat WC, Nadelhaft I (1986a). The spinal distribution of sympathetic preganglionic and visceral primary afferent neurons which send axons into the hypogastric nerves of the cat. J Comp Neurol 243:23-40.

Morgan C, Nadelhaft I, de Groat WC (1986b). The distribution within the spinal cord of visceral primary afferent axons carried by the lumbar colonic nerve of the cat. Brain Res (in press).

Organization of the Autonomic Nervous System:
Central and Peripheral Mechanisms, pages 91–100
© 1987 Alan R. Liss, Inc.

CENTRAL ORGANIZATION OF SYMPATHETIC AFFERENT FIBERS

Robert D. Foreman, W. Steve Ammons*, and Robert
W. Blair

Department of Physiology and Biophysics, The
University of Oklahoma Health Sciences Center,
Oklahoma City, Oklahoma 73190

*Department of Physiology, Thomas Jefferson
University, Philadelpha, Pennsylvania

INTRODUCTION

Sympathetic afferent fibers arising from visceral structures transmit impulses to cells located in the gray matter of the spinal cord. Earlier work focused on adequate stimuli for activating afferent fibers and the size of the fibers transmitting the information (Malliani et al. 1982; Nerdrum et al. 1986) and reflexes produced when the receptors of these organs were activated (Longhurst, 1984). This chapter describes the central processing of information arising from sympathetic afferent fibers, particularly, the processing that begins in the upper thoracic (T_1 to T_5) segments of the spinal cord. We will consider viscerosomatic convergence, central pathways, viscero-visceral convergence and vagosympathetic interactions.

VISCERO-SOMATIC CONVERGENCE

Ruch (1961) used viscerosomatic convergence to explain the referred pain of angina pectoris. He hypothesized that both sympathetic and somatic afferent fibers excite the same spinal neuron, resulting in pain that is referred to the somatic regions of the chest, shoulders and arms. In our studies all neurons recorded in the upper thoracic cord received convergent inputs from visceral and somatic afferent fibers, and their axons projected to supraspinal regions. Cervero (1983) observed that some thoracic dorsal horn cells responded only to somatic input, but he did not find any cells responsive only to visceral input. We selected cells differently; ours were found by their response to electrical stimulation of sympathetic afferent fibers, and then testing for somatic input. Furthermore, most of our neurons had identified projections, whereas only a few projecting neurons were examined in Cervero's study.

Projecting neurons were classified according to their ability to respond to somatic manipulation. Manipulations included blowing hair, touching or pinching skin or skin and muscle. Results showed that about 85% of the cells were high threshold or nociceptive specific, 10% were wide dynamic range, that is, they responded slightly to innocuous stimuli and vigorously to noxious stimulation, and about 5% were high threshold but were inhibited by hair movement. About 70% of cells had simple receptive fields limited to the left forelimb and left upper thorax, the area of pain referral often described for angina pectoris. The remainder had complex fields that often extended to the hindlimb and/or were bilateral.

Electrical stimulation of cardiopulmonary sympathetic afferent fibers activated both A-delta and C fibers, which in turn excited spinal neurons (Fig. lA). With weak stimuli an early short latency peak was generated (A-delta peak), and with strong stimuli an additional late (C-fiber) peak was produced (Fig. lA). About 45% of the cells responded only to A-delta input and 55% responded to both A-delta and C fiber input. Why cells respond to inputs from both A-delta and C fibers is unclear.

CENTRAL PATHWAYS

The cells of origin of the spinoreticular (SRT), spinoreticular-thalamic (SRT-STT) and spinothalamic (STT) tracts were distributed from lamina I to lamina VIII. The largest concentration of cells was in lamina V, but many cells were also in lamina IV. The location of cells coincided with the terminal sites for sympathetic afferent fibers and agreed with their location in other thoracic regions (Cervero, 1983).

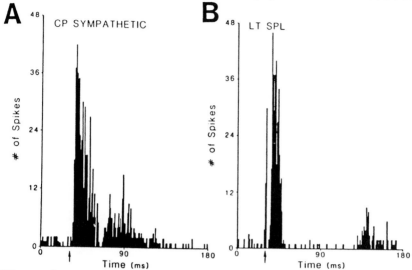

Figure 1

Viscero-visceral convergence onto a dorsal horn cell. A: response to stim. of CardioPulmonary Sympathetic afferent fibers (CP SYMPATHETIC). B: poststimulus histogram of response to stimulation of the left greater splanchnic nerve (LTSPL). Stimulus artifact at the arrow. Histograms are the cumulative responses to 50 stimulus repetitions. (Ammons and Foreman. Exptl. Neurol. 83: 288-301, 1984 by permission of Academic Press, Inc.).

Cells of the upper thoracic spinal cord receive visceral and somatic input and then transmit information in ascending pathways to multiple sites in the brainstem and thalamus. Electrophysiological techniques showed that the same axon could project to both the ipsilateral and contralateral medullary reticular formation and sometimes also projected to the thalamus. Of the cells studied 67% projected only to the reticular formation, 21% projected both to the thalamus and the reticular formation, and 12% projected only to the thalamus. The largest percentage of cells projected to the contralateral reticular formation, where neurons respond to sympathetic input arising from the cardiopulmonary region (Blair, 1985). These SRT and SRT-STT cells are likely associated with cardiovascular adjustments and participate in transmission of information needed for pain perception.

Electrical stimulation of the cardiopulmonary afferent fibers activated spinal neurons projecting to all the sites stimulated in the brainstem and thalamus. A more natural stimulus of coronary afferent endings is brady-kinin because increased amounts are found in the coronary sinus effluent following coronary artery occlusion. Intracardiac injections of bradykinin activated cells in all projection classes, but the percent responses differed (Fig. 2). Cells projecting to the thalamus, ipsilateral

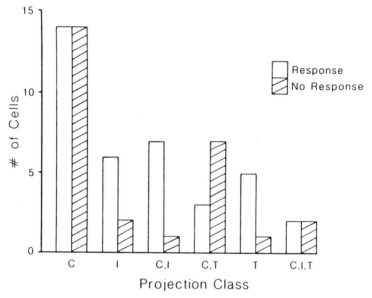

Figure 2
Number of SRT, SRT-STT, and STT cells either re-sponsive or not responsive to intra-atrial injections of bradykinin (2ug/kg). C, Contralateral reticular formation (RF) only; I, ipsilateral RF only; C, I, both contra. and ipsi. RF: C, T, contra. RF and thalamus; T, thalamus only; C, I, T, all three sites. All cells responded to somatic manipulation. (Blair, Weber and Foreman. Am. J. Physiol. 246 (Heart Circ. Physiol. 15): H500-H507, 1984 by permission of the Am. Physiol. Society).

reticular formation or both ipsi- and contralateral formation responded more often to bradykinin. Approxi-mately 60% of the cells projecting to the reticular formation, 83% projecting to the thalamus and 36% projecting both to the thalamus and the reticular formation responded to bradykinin. The varied projections demonstrate that noxious information from the heart reaches widespread regions of the medullary reticular formation and thalamus. These regions are responsible for many functions, such as complex motor interactions to painful stimuli and cardiovascular regulation. The projections of sympathetic afferents from the heart would allow the reticular formation to be involved in reflex cardiovascular or motor adjustments associated with myocardial ischemia or infarction.

VISCEROVISCERAL INTERACTIONS

Anatomical and physiological studies show that sympathetic afferent fibers are segmentally distributed throughout the spinal cord but with some overlap. Since anginal-like symptoms can be associated with gallbladder disease, the following question is raised: Do sympathetic afferent fibers from the splanchnic nerve and gallbladder converge on upper thoracic neurons that also receive input from the cardiopulmonary region?

Recording from upper thoracic dorsal horn neurons showed that electrical stimulation of the splanchnic nerve changed the discharge rate of 84%, excited 60% of the cells, inhibited 14% and both excited and inhibited 10%. Both early and some late responses were observed with electrical stimulation (Fig. 1B). These same cells also were excited by activation of sympathetic afferents in the cardiopulmonary region. Some splanchnic afferent fibers travel rostrally in an extraspinal pathway to upper thoracic neurons. However, fibers enter the spinal cord in the lower thoracic segments and ascend to the T_1 to T_5 segments via intraspinal pathways (Downman, 1955).

Since diseases of the gallbladder can be the source of anginal-like pain, the gallbladder was distended to determine the effects of this stimulus on cell activity in T_2 to T_4 segments of the spinal cord. Responses of a T_3 cell to gallbladder distention is shown in Fig. 3. Cell activity increased during a distention pressure of 20 mm Hg, but this was not associated with increased blood pressure (Fig. 3A). Applying 40 mm Hg distention increased cell activity more and the blood pressure increased slightly (Fig. 3B). Increasing the distention

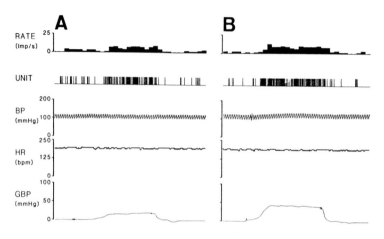

Figure 3

Responses of a dorsal horn cell to gallbladder distension at two pressures, 20 (A) and 40 (B) mm Hg. Top
trace is cell discharge rate with a 1 sec lag; second
trace is cell activity; third trace is blood pressure
(BP); the fourth trace is heart rate (HR); and the bottom
trace is gallbladder pressure (GBP). (Adapted from Ammons
and Foreman. Brain Research 321: 267-277, 1984 by
permission of Elsevier Science Publishers B.V.).

pressure to 80 mm Hg (not shown) further increased both
the cell activity and blood pressure. Approximately 40%
of the cells tested responded to gallbladder distension.
Of this responsive population, 65% were excited and 35%
were inhibited. Thus, gallbladder distention mainly
increases the firing of upper thoracic dorsal horn
neurons.

Cervero (1982) reported that spinal neurons of the
T_9-T_{11} segments of the spinal cord responded only to
noxious levels of gallbladder distention, noxious meaning
an associated increase in blood pressure. In our study,
the gallbladder pressure threshold was less for changing
cell activity than for increasing blood pressure in
approximately 60% of the neurons, was less for increasing
blood pressure in 30%, and was the same for 10% (Ammons

and Foreman, 1984).

Consequently, innocuous levels of gallbladder pressure produce changes in activity of upper thoracic neurons. The different responsiveness between upper and lower thoracic neurons may indicate different organization of sympathetic afferent fibers within a distant segment.

VAGAL-SYMPATHETIC INTERACTIONS

The central organization of the sympathetic afferent fibers involves complex convergent interactions within the spinal cord. Perhaps supraspinal mechanisms modulate the activity of spinal neurons, including vago-sympathetic interactions. Schwartz et al. (1973) showed that vagal stimulation altered the activity of sympathetic pre-ganglionic neurons. Consequently, vagal afferent activity can activate pathways originating in the brainstem which then descend to modify the activity of spinal neurons.

We have studied modulation by vagal afferent fibers of the activity of spinal neurons responding to excitation of sympathetic afferent fibers. A conditioning electrical stimulus was applied to vagal afferents, followed at various intervals by a test electrical stimulus to sympathetic afferent fibers. The conditioning vagal stimulus reduced the response from both A-delta and C fibers to the sympathetic test stimulus with the time course shown in Fig. 4. The response to A-delta sympathetic fiber stimulation (filled circles) was triphasic. The conditioning-test curve for C-fiber input (filled squares) showed maximal inhibition slightly earlier, and more severe inhibition of longer duration than for A-delta input. The long-lasting nature of the inhibition suggests a presynaptic inhibitory mechanism (Schmidt, 1971).

In addition to conditioning-test procedure, the vagus nerve was electrically stimulated during the maximal increase in cell activity following intracardiac injections of bradykinin. Vagal stimulation reduced the enhanced activity of the cell by 60%. The inhibition disappeared after the cervical vagi were transected. Thus, vagal afferent fibers that originate from the cardiopulmonary region can inhibit thoracic spinal neurons.

Excitation of vagal afferent fibers can modulate the input transmitted in sympathetic afferent fibers arising

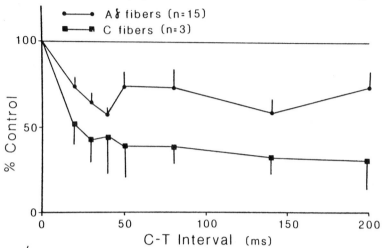

Figure 4

The averaged Conditioning-Test plot for cells responsive to A-delta fibers and to C fibers. Abscissa: interval between the C stimulus applied to thoracic vagus and the T stimulus applied to cardiopulmonary sympathetic afferent fibers (C-T Interval); ordinate: percent of the control test response. (Ammons, Blair and Foreman. Circ. Res. 53: 603-612, 1983 by permission of the American Heart Association, Inc.).

from the heart. Such modulation could reduce the noxious component of pain. Some patients experience a silent infarct, that is, no pain is associated with ischemia and death of the cardiac tissue. In these circumstances overactivity of vagal afferent fibers might prevent noxious information that arises in the heart and travels into the spinal cord in sympathetic afferents from reaching consciousness.

SUMMARY AND CONCLUSIONS

The central projections of sympathetic afferents are complex. The classical view that processing begins only after transmission to areas of the brain is now outdated. Our studies have shown that processing of information occurs in cells of the dorsal horn before any information is transmitted to supraspinal regions by several different pathways. These interactions can arise from other visceral structures, somatic structures and vagal afferents that excite descending pathways. The significance of these interactions will require further intensive study.

ACKNOWLEDGEMENTS

This work was supported by NIH grants HL22730, 27260 and 07430. The authors thank Diana Holston for her technical assistance and Charlene Clark for typing the manuscript.

REFERENCES

Ammons WS, Foreman RD (1984). Cardiovascular and T_2-T_4 Dorsal Horn Cell Responses to Gallbladder Distension in the Cat. Brain Res 321:267-277.

Blair RW (1985). Noxious Cardiac Input onto Neurons in Medullary Reticular Formation. Brain Res 326:335-346.

Downman CBB (1955). Skeletal muscle reflexes of splanchnic and intercostal nerve origin in acute spinal and decerebrate cats. J Neurophysiol 18:217-235.

Cervero F (1982). Noxious intensities of visceral stimulation are required to activate viscero-somatic multireceptive neurons in the thoracic spinal cord of the cat. Brain Res 240:350-352.

Cervero F (1983). Somatic and visceral inputs to the thoracic spinal cord of the cat: effects of noxious stimulation of the biliary system. J Physiol (Lond) 337:51-67.

Longhurst JC (1984). Cardiac receptors: Their function in health and disease. Prog Cardiovas Dis 27(3):201-222.

Malliani A (1982). Cardiovascular sympathetic afferent fibers. Rev Physiol Biochem Pharmacol 94:11-74.

Nerdrum T, Baker DG, Coleridge HM, Coleridge JCG (1986). Interaction of bradykinin and prostaglandin E_1 on cardiac pressor reflex and sympathetic afferents. Am J Physiol 250(5):R815-R822.

Ruch TC (1961). Pathophysiology of pain. In Ruch TC, Patton HD, Woodbury JW, Towe AL (eds): "Neuorphysiology," Philadelphia: W.B. Sanders, pp 350-368.

Schmidt RF (1971). Presynaptic inhibition in the vertebrate central nervous system. Ergeb Physiol 63:20-101.

Schwartz PJ, Pagani M, Lombardi F, Malliani A (1973). A cardiocardiac sympathovagal reflex in the cat. Circ Res 32:215-220.

Organization of the Autonomic Nervous System:
Central and Peripheral Mechanisms, pages 101–109
© **1987 Alan R. Liss, Inc.**

ORGANIZATION OF SYMPATHETIC INFLUENCES ON THE KIDNEY AND
CAPACITIVE CIRCULATION

Lynne C. Weaver, Robert L. Meckler, and Reuben D.
Stein
Department of Physiology, Michigan State University, East Lansing, Michigan 48824-1101 USA

INTRODUCTION

Differences in sympathetic vasoconstrictor outflow to hindlimb cutaneous and muscle vascular beds in response to various somatic and visceral afferent stimuli have been investigated extensively (Jänig, 1985). However, differential reflex responses of abdominal sympathetic nerves have not been well characterized. The kidney contributes to ongoing cardiovascular state directly, as a component of systemic vascular resistance, and indirectly, by its endocrine and excretory functions. In contrast, the spleen and intestine serve as capacitive vascular compartments which can mobilize blood volume, resulting in a rapid increase in cardiac output. Since these viscera perform different functions, sympathetic outflow to the various organs may be expected to react non-uniformly to initiation of reflexes.

Stimulation of mesenteric afferent nerves by serosal application of bradykinin causes greater excitation of mesenteric than renal multifiber nerve activity (Stein et al., 1986). In contrast, this stimulus produces similar magnitudes of excitation of renal and splenic multifiber nerve discharge (Meckler, unpublished observations). Chemical or mechanical stimulation of splenic afferent nerves produces greater excitation of splenic than renal multifiber nerve activity (Calaresu et al., 1984). These viscero-sympathetic reflexes are mediated, at least in part, by spinal neural circuits. Pressor responses usually accompany the neural responses, suggesting that baroreceptor stimulation may contribute to the unequal distribution of reflex responses among the three nerves. However, the character of responses of individual neurons within these nerves remains to be elucidated with respect to these reflex effects. The unequal multifiber response patterns may reflect greater excitation of all neurons in one nerve relative to the excitation of all neurons in another. Alternatively, these differential reflexes may involve heterogeneous responses among subpopulations of neurons comprising one or more of the three nerves.

METHODS

Experiments were done in 32 chloralose-anesthetized, artificially respired cats. The small intestine was externalized via a midline laparotomy and placed in a saline filled plastic dish. The spleen was vascularly isolated as described previously (Calaresu et al., 1984) to allow selective stimulation of splenic receptors. Activity of 23 renal, 16 splenic and 20 mesenteric efferent axons was recorded using standard teased-fiber electro-physiological techniques. The discharge frequency of spontaneously active single fibers was determined by counting output pulses of a window discriminator with a PDP-11/23 microprocessor. Intestinal receptors were stimulated by the serosal application of 10 μg bradykinin in 25 ml saline (Lew and Longhurst, 1986) before and 1 hr after high cervical spinal cord transection. Splenic receptors were stimulated by the injection of 10 μg bradykinin in 0.1 ml saline into the artery of the vascularly isolated spleen. Baroreceptors were stimulated and "unloaded" by intravenous injections of phenylephrine and nitroprusside, respectively. Data are illustrated as the 10-s period of maximum response to these stimuli. In addition, correlation of ongoing neural activity with the arterial pressure pulse was tested.

RESULTS

Fibers of renal, splenic, and mesenteric nerves had similar resting discharge rates that ranged from 0.06 to 6.4 (mean = 1.2 $\pm$ 0.2) spikes/sec. Ongoing activity of 91% (21 of 23) of renal neurons was correlated with the arterial pressure pulse. In contrast, activity of only 56%

(10 of 18) of mesenteric neurons and 50% (8 of 16) of splenic neurons was correlated with blood pressure. These data suggest that activity of mesenteric and splenic neurons is less sensitive than that of renal neurons to tonic influences of baroreceptor stimulation. Representative examples of these correlations are presented in Fig 1. Each panel displays a histogram of unit activity above an average of the arterial pulse wave. Sampling of unit activity was triggered by peak systolic pressure. The top panel shows a histogram of activity of a renal neuron which was correlated with the arterial pressure pulse. The middle and lower panels display relationships between the arterial pulse wave and the discharge of two mesenteric, and two splenic neurons, respectively. The left side of each panel shows histograms of activity of a mesenteric neuron and a splenic neuron which were correlated with the arterial pulse wave. The right side of each panel shows histograms of activity of a mesenteric neuron and a splenic neuron that were not clearly correlated with the arterial pressure pulse.

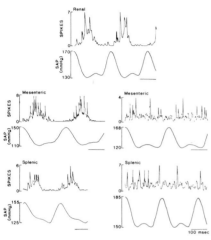

Fig. 1. Relationships between the arterial pulse (SAP) and activity of renal, mesenteric and splenic neurons (spikes).

In addition to testing activity of neurons for correlation with the arterial pressure pulse, responses of 11 mesenteric, 13 renal and 9 splenic neurons to graded decreases and increases in mean arterial pressure were studied (Fig. 2). Nitroprusside caused decreases in mean arterial pressure and significant excitation of activity of fibers from all three groups of nerves. However, activity of mesenteric neurons was affected less than that of renal or splenic neurons to decreases in blood pressure. Whereas activity of mesenteric neurons did not increase until blood pressure was lowered by 30 mmHg, activity of renal and splenic neurons was significantly excited by a 15 mmHg decrease in mean arterial pressure. Similarly, activity of

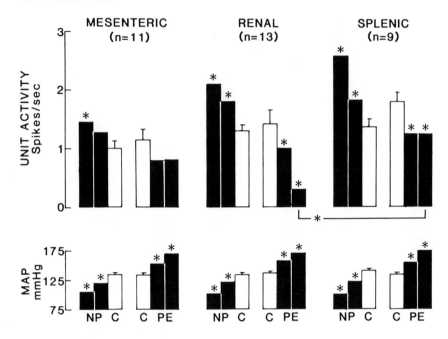

Fig. 2. Changes (black bars) from control (open bars) in activity of mesenteric, renal and splenic neurons (unit activity) and mean arterial pressure (MAP) caused by intravenous injections of nitroprusside (NP) and phenylephrine (PE). Asterisks indicate significant changes from control. Variability indicated by pooled standard error.

mesenteric neurons was less sensitive than that of renal or splenic neurons to increases in mean arterial pressure caused by injection of phenylephrine. A blood pressure increase of 35 mmHg had no significant effect on mesenteric unit activity. In contrast, activity of renal neurons and splenic neurons was significantly decreased by a 20 mmHg increase in mean arterial pressure. Of the three nerves, activity of renal neurons appeared to be most sensitive to increases in blood pressure; when mean arterial pressure was increased by 30-40 mmHg the inhibition of renal unit discharge was significantly greater than that of splenic neurons. In summary, these experiments demonstrate the differential effects of baroreceptor stimulation on the

activity of different visceral sympathetic neurons.
Activity of mesenteric neurons is minimally affected by
baroreceptor input in comparison to the effect on renal or
splenic unit activity. In addition, baroreceptor
stimulation by larger increases in pressure has a greater
inhibitory effect on activity of renal than splenic fibers.

Stimulation of visceral receptors also had unequal
effects on the activity of mesenteric, renal and splenic
neurons. Responses in activity of 17 mesenteric, 23 renal
and 16 splenic neurons, and the pressor responses caused by
stimulation of intestinal receptors are illustrated in
Fig. 3. Serosal application of bradykinin caused increases

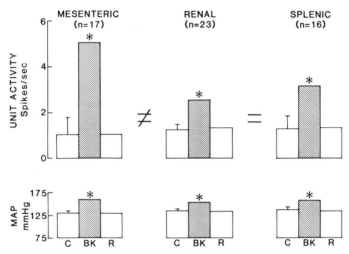

Fig. 3. Responses in activity of mesenteric, renal and
splenic neurons (unit activity) and changes in mean
arterial pressure (MAP) caused by stimulation of intestinal
receptors with bradykinin. C, 2-min control period; BK, 10-
sec period of maximum response; R, 2-min recovery period.
Asterisks indicate significant changes from control.
Variability indicated by pooled standard error.

in the activity of neurons from all 3 groups of nerves and
significant increases in blood pressure. The excitation of
mesenteric neuronal activity was significantly greater than
that of renal and splenic neurons. Since pressor responses
usually accompanied the neural responses, baroreceptor

stimulation may have contributed to the unequal distribution of reflex influences among the three nerves. The role of the baroreceptors may be to attenuate the excitatory reflexes distributed to the kidney and spleen relative to those directed to the intestine. This hypothesis is tenable because similar increases in mean arterial pressure caused by phenylephrine produced significant inhibition of renal and splenic unit activity, while activity of mesenteric neurons was unaffected (Fig. 2).

Alternatively, the unequal neural response pattern could be accounted for by a feature of the functional central organization of autonomic reflexes that potentially provides the largest output to the organ from which the reflex originates. This hypothesis was tested by recording reflex responses of renal and splenic neurons to chemical stimulation of splenic afferent nerves (Fig. 4). This stimulation caused excitation of splenic neuronal activity that was greater than that of renal neurons and caused pressor responses. It is not likely that baroreceptor inhibition of renal unit activity contributed to the unequal nature of this reflex, since the pressor response evoked by spleen stimulation was only 15 mmHg. A similar increase in blood pressure caused by phenylephrine (Fig. 2) produced equivalent inhibition of splenic and renal unit activity. These results imply that viscero-visceral reflexes may be centrally organized to provide the largest output to the organ from which the reflex originates. If the reflex is initiated from an organ with efferent innervation that is not sensitive to baroreceptor influences (e.g., intestine), then concomitant stimulation of baroreceptors may exaggerate the unequal pattern of neural responses.

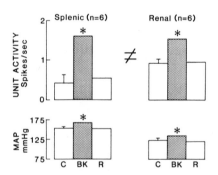

Fig. 4. Responses in activity of splenic and renal neurons and changes in mean arterial pressure caused by stimulation of splenic receptors with bradykinin. Format and abbreviations as in Fig. 3.

Are these viscero-sympathetic reflexes mediated through supra-spinal circuits, or are these unequal response patterns organized within the spinal cord? The central organization of these reflexes was investigated further by studying the reflex responses of mesenteric and renal nerve fibers to stimulation of intestinal afferent nerves before and 1 hr after high cervical spinal cord transection. Whereas spinal transection caused a significant decrease in the spontaneous firing rate of renal neurons, ongoing mesenteric unit activity was not decreased significantly (Fig. 5). Seven of eight (88%) mesenteric neurons, but only 8 of 17 (47%) renal neurons, were spontaneously active after spinal transection. These data suggest that ongoing activity of mesenteric neurons is less dependent upon supraspinal sources of excitation than is ongoing activity of renal neurons. These results are similar to those of a previous study (Meckler and Weaver, 1985) in which spinal transection caused a significant decrease in the spontaneous activity of multifiber renal nerves without affecting the ongoing discharge of multifiber splenic nerves. These two studies demonstrate that the innervation of the splanchnic capacitive circulation is less dependent upon supra-spinal drive than is the innervation of the kidney.

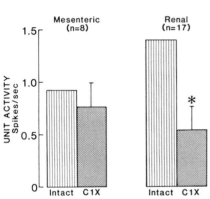

SPONTANEOUS FIRING RATE

Fig. 5. Spontaneous firing rate (unit activity) of mesenteric and renal neurons in cats with intact neuraxes (intact, lined bars) and 1 hr after transection at the first cervical segment (C1X, stippled bars). Asterisk indicates significant differences between firing rate in the intact and spinal states. Variability indicated by pooled standard error.

Stimulation of intestinal receptors with bradykinin in the spinal cats evoked neural and cardiovascular reflexes similar to those produced in cats with intact neuraxes. Responses of mesenteric and renal neurons to this stimulus in cats with an intact neuraxis and in spinal cats are illustrated in Fig. 6.

The bottom panel contains data only from those neurons that were spontaneously active in the spinal state, and, thus, the baseline renal unit activity is not different from baseline activity when the neuraxis was intact. Activity of fibers from both nerves was significantly excited by chemical stimulation of intestinal afferent nerves, both before and 1 hr after transection of the spinal cord. The increase in activity of mesenteric neurons was significantly greater than that of renal neurons following, as well as prior to, spinal cord transection. Therefore, neural circuits within the spinal cord are sufficient for the expression of these differential responses.

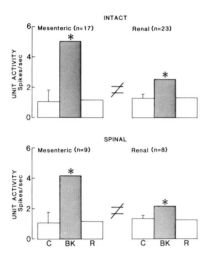

Fig. 6. Responses of mesenteric and renal neurons to stimulation of intestinal receptors with bradykinin in cats with intact neuraxes (top panel) and 1 hr after transection (bottom panel). Format and abbreviations as in Fig. 3.

CONCLUSION

In conclusion, these differential abdominal viscero-sympathetic reflexes are mediated by central neural circuits which are complete within the spinal cord. The stimulation of baroreceptors which results from the concomitant pressor responses may, in some cases, exaggerate the unequal pattern of sympathetic neural responses. Since virtually all neurons responded to the visceral afferent stimulation, the unequal response patterns observed in multifiber nerve recordings do not involve heterogeneous responses among subpopulations of neurons.

REFERENCES

Calaresu FR, Tobey JC, Heidemann SR, Weaver LC (1984).
Splenic and renal sympathetic responses to stimulation of
splenic receptors in cats. Am J Physiol 247 (Regulatory
Integrative Comp Physiol 16):R856.
Jänig W (1985). Organization of the lumbar sympathetic
outflow to skeletal muscle and skin of the cat hindlimb
and tail. Rev Physiol Biochem Pharmacol 102:119.
Lew WYW, Longhurst JC (1986). Substance P,
5-hydroxytryptamine, and bradykinin stimulate abdominal
visceral afferents. Am J Physiol 250 (Regulatory
Integrative Comp Physiol 19):R465.
Meckler RL, Weaver LC (1985). Splenic, renal, and cardiac
nerves have unequal dependence upon tonic supraspinal
inputs. Brain Res 338:123.
Stein RD, Genovesi S, Demarest K, Weaver LC (1986).
Capsaicin treatment attenuates the reflex excitation of
sympathetic activity caused by chemical stimulation of
intestinal afferent nerves. Brain Res:In press.

Organization of the Autonomic Nervous System:
Central and Peripheral Mechanisms, pages 111–120
© 1987 Alan R. Liss, Inc.

PROPRIOSPINAL AND DESCENDING SYSTEMS INHIBITING AND EXCITING
RENAL NERVE ACTIVITY IN HYPERTENSIVE AND NORMOTENSIVE RATS

Lawrence P. Schramm and Renea Livingstone

Department of Biomedical Engineering
The Johns Hopkins University School of
Medicine, Baltimore, MD 21205

INTRODUCTION

The processing of sympathetic activity at spinal
levels is of interest for several of reasons. First, it
seems clear that, although the majority of the regulation
of sympathetic preganglionic neurons comes from supraspinal
systems under normal conditions (Alexander, 1946; Ross, et
al., 1984) the degree to which those supraspinal systems
impinge directly on preganglionic neurons and the degree to
which they act through spinal interneurons is unknown.
Second, spinal systems, left to themselves, are capable of
generating substantial ongoing sympathetic activity. They
also may exhibit hyperactivity and hyperreactivity to
afferent information (see Schramm, 1986 for review). We
have hypothesized that pathological conditions associated
with excessive sympathetic activity, such as some forms of
hypertension, may result from insufficient tonic inhibition
of spinal sympathetic systems or from insufficient
inhibition of afferent activity which excites spinal
sympathetic systems.

Spontaneously hypertensive rats (SHR) of the Okamoto
and Aoki strain (Okamoto, et al., 1967) exhibit abnormally
high splanchnic and renal nerve activity when compared to
normotensive Wistar Kyoto (WKY) rats (Judy, et al., 1976;
Schramm and Barton, 1979; Schramm and Chornoboy, 1982).
Elevated renal nerve activity persists even after spinal
cord transection (Schramm and Chornoboy, 1982). In the
latter study, we showed that spinally-elicited increases in
renal nerve activity were similar in SHR and WKY. However,

renal nerve activity in SHR did not respond as readily to
spinally-elicited sympathoinhibition as that in WKY. This
led us to suggest that a deficit in a spinal or descending
sympathoinhibitory system might, to some extent, be
responsible for sympathetic hyperactivity in SHR.

These studies also raised questions about the nature
of the spinal system which we electrically stimulated to
produce renal nerve sympathoinhibition. We had assumed
that this was a purely descending system, similar to ones
previously described by others (Illert and Gabriel, 1972;
Coote and MacLeod, 1975). However, continued acquaintance
with the system raised a number of questions about its
origin and course which were answered in a subsequent
series of experiments (Schramm and Livingstone, 1986).

We determined that, in the rat, the dorsolateral
spinal sympathoinhibitory system partly descends from
supraspinal levels and is partly propriospinal. It appears
to course in the deep lateral funiculus at cervical levels,
and the propriospinal component consists, in part, of
neurons with somas in the dorsolateral cervical spinal
cord. Its stimulus-response characteristics suggest that
this system is suited to the tonic regulation of ongoing
sympathetic activity. This functional role was supported
by the observation that renal nerve activity could not be
inhibited by dorsolateral spinal stimulation until the
lateral funiculus, rostral to the stimulation sites, had
been bilaterally destroyed.

The present experiments addressed the following
questions. First, is the diminished ability to inhibit
renal nerve activity in SHR, when compared to WKY, due to
an abnormal resistance to inhibition in SHR or to an
abnormal sensitivity to inhibition in WKY? Second, is the
elevated renal nerve activity in SHR a manifestation of
hypersensitivity of spinal sympathetic systems to afferent
input? Finally, how do spinally elicited
sympathoinhibition and sympathoexcitation interact with one
another in normal rats, and is there evidence for an
abnormality of this interaction in SHR?

METHODS

Male, spontaneously hypertensive, Wistar-Kyoto (Taconic

Farms), and Sprague-Dawley (SD) rats (Charles River), weighing between 225 and 350g were anesthetized with 100 mg/kg alpha-chloralose. Arterial and venous cannulae were placed for the measurement of arterial pressure and for infusions, respectively. Rats were paralyzed with gallamine triethiodide (flaxedil), and artificial respiration was administered through a tracheal cannula.

The left renal nerves were dissected through a left laparotomy, cut close to the kidney, and placed on bipolar electrodes. Multiunit renal sympathetic activity was amplified, rectified, and averaged. Averaged activity from SHR and WKY was expressed in identical arbitrary units. Averaged activity from SD was expressed in slightly different arbitrary units.

Rats were placed in a stereotaxic apparatus, and the cervical spinal cord was approached via a laminectomy. Spinal cords were transected at C1. Electrical stimulation was delivered to the surface of the left dorsolateral funiculus (to elicit renal sympathoinhibitions). Deeper portions of the dorsolateral and lateral funiculi were stimulated to elicit renal sympathoexcitations. Stimuli were delivered via either monopolar or concentric electrodes. They consisted of trains of 0.3ms pulses at frequencies between 5 and 100Hz and intensities between 5 and 250 uA. In some rats, the left greater splanchnic nerve was dissected and cut near the left adrenal gland. The proximal portion of the nerve was placed on a bipolar stimulating electrode for eliciting increases in renal sympathetic activity.

RESULTS

Is Spinally-evoked Inhibition Normal in WKY?

To test the hypothesis that ongoing renal nerve activity in WKY is not abnormally sensitive to spinally-evoked inhibition, we compared stimulus-response properties of inhibitions in SD with those previously observed in WKY. Stimuli were delivered at 5,10,20,50, and 100Hz. Stimulation at 5Hz decreased renal nerve activity by even more than the same frequency of stimulation in WKY (Figure 1). Indeed, stimulation was more effective in decreasing renal nerve activity in SD at 5, 10, and 20Hz.

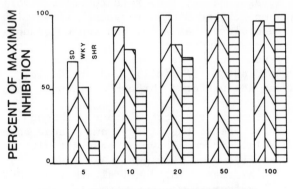

STIMULATION FREQUENCY

Figure 1. The relationship between inhibitory stimulation
frequency and the percent of maximal inhibition in WKY, SD,
and SHR. Data from SHR and WKY are recalculated from the
data of Schramm and Chornoboy (1982).

Are Spinal Sympathetic Systems Supersensitive to Afferents?

We addressed this question by comparing, in SHR and
WKY, the effects on renal nerve activity of low-intensity
(5-40 uA) stimulation of splanchnic afferents at a wide
range of frequencies. As a control, we also replicated the
experiment in which we compared, in SHR and WKY, the
effects on renal nerve activity of sympathoexcitatory
stimulation deep in the dorsolateral funiculus (Schramm and
Chornoboy, 1982). We used much lower stimulus intensities
(10-60uA) than we did in our earlier experiments, and the
evoked responses were correspondingly much smaller, within
the range of normally-observed renal sympathetic activity.
The intensities of the splanchnic and spinal stimuli were
matched to provide an approximately two-fold increase in
renal nerve activity during stimulation of either system at
100Hz.

As previously reported, spinal sympathoexcitatory
stimulation in SHR and WKY elicited similar stimulus-
response relationships (Figure 2) despite our observation
that ongoing renal nerve activity was significantly higher
in SHR than in WKY (107 +/- 13 units vs 62 +/- 10 units).
Of even greater interest was the observation that
stimulation of splanchnic afferents also elicited very

similar increases in renal nerve activity in normotensive
and hypertensive strains (Figure 2).

Note that spinal stimulation was relatively
ineffective at low frequencies. Although each stimulus
elicited a substantial burst of renal nerve activity, these
brief responses were followed by pronounced "silent
periods", during which even ongoing renal nerve activity
was diminished. Responses elicited by higher-frequency
spinal stimulation exhibited smaller "silent periods", and
average activity eventually increased rapidly as a function
of stimulus frequency.

Responses to stimulation of splanchnic afferents were
followed by after-discharges rather than "silent periods".
Thus, renal nerve activity was extremely responsive to this
stimulation.

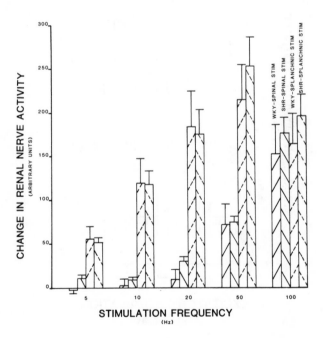

Figure 2. Increases in renal nerve activity elicited by
spinal stimulation and splanchnic afferent stimulation in
SHR and WKY.

Do Inhibition and Excitation Interact Normally in SHR?

How does renal nerve activity change when
sympathoinhibition, elicited by either spinal or splanchnic
afferent stimulation, is paired with spinally-elicited
inhibition? These experiments were initially conducted in
SD. First, we elicited renal nerve sympathoinhibitions and
sympathoexcitations separately. Sympathoinhibitions were
elicited by stimulating the surface of the dorsolateral
funiculus at 20Hz. Sympathoexcitation was elicited by
stimulating spinal and splanchnic systems at three
frequencies (20, 50, and 100Hz) using matched intensities
as described above. Second, we elicited an excitation
during an ongoing inhibition. All stimuli were repeated
five times, and the reported data consist of the averages
of the resulting responses (Figure 3).

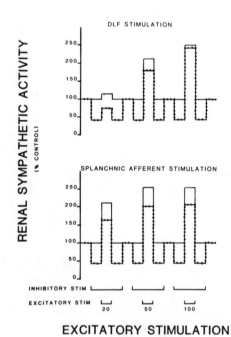

Figure 3. Interaction of Spinally-elicited inhibition with
spinally-and splanchnic-elicited sympathoexcitation.
Solid lines = excitations alone. Dotted lines =
interactions with inhibition.

At 20 Hz, excitatory spinal stimulation did not return renal nerve activity to control levels, although the magnitude of the response to the excitatory stimulation was actually somewhat larger during the inhibitory stimulation than before. The response to spinal excitatory stimulation at 50Hz was almost identical before and during inhibitory stimulation. Therefore, the peak magnitude of the response was diminished by approximately the magnitude of the inhibitory response alone. At 100Hz, spinal excitatory stimulation completely overwhelmed the the inhibitory stimulation, producing an excitation with a peak magnitude as large as that observed without simultaneous inhibitory stimulation. The magnitudes of sympathoexcitations elicited by splanchnic stimulation at all frequencies were unchanged by concomitant inhibition. Therefore, the peak magnitude of each splanchnic response was decreased by an amount equal to the magnitude of the inhibitory response alone.

Identical experiments were conducted in 3 WKY and 5 SHR. Although the numbers of animals were too small to conduct a formal statistical analysis, no differences in the interactions of excitations and inhibitions in SHR and WKY, nor between interactions in these strains and those observed in SD, were seen.

DISCUSSION

Is Spinally-evoked Inhibition Normal in WKY?

Differences between SHR and WKY may represent abnormalities in the WKY strain rather than abnormalities associated with SHR (Judy, et al., 1976). We compared the stimulus-response relationships for inhibition which we had observed in SHR and WKY with relationships from SD. Of the three strains, SD appeared to be the most responsive to inhibitory stimulation. WKY and SHR were both somewhat less responsive, but the stimulus response relationship for the WKY was more similar to that of SD than to that of SHR. It seems clear that the differences in sensitivity to inhibitory stimulation between SHR and WKY do not result from a hypersensitivity in WKY. Indeed, WKY appear to be less sensitive than SD.

Schramm et al., (1986) suggest that the low

recruiting frequency of spinally-elicited inhibition and the prolonged effect of even a single stimulus pulse indicate that this system is well-adapted for the regulation of ongoing sympathetic activity. If this system is, indeed, used for this purpose, then the resistance of spinal sympathetic systems to this inhibition could account for some of the sympathetic hyperactivity exhibited by SHR.

Are Spinal Sympathetic Systems Supersensitive to Afferents?

Our rats were all extensively surgically prepared. Traction was necessary on the abdominal wall and on the kidney in order to record from the renal nerves. Perhaps the elevated renal nerve activity observed in SHR indicated a greater sensitivity of this strain to visceral and somatic afferent stimulation. We tested this hypothesis by comparing the effects of greater splanchnic afferent stimulation on renal nerve activity in SHR and WKY. We used relatively low-intensity stimulation to avoid saturating spinal sympathetic systems. These systems are capable of supporting 7 to 10-fold increases in renal nerve activity (Schramm and Chornoboy, 1982). The largest responses elicited by splanchnic stimulation in this series were approximately twice the level of ongoing renal nerve activity. The similarity of the responses to splanchnic stimulation in SHR and WKY suggested that afferent information was being handled similarly in the two strains.

Do Inhibition and Excitation Interact Normally in SHR?

In intact rats, spinal sympathetic systems are under tonic descending inhibition (see Schramm, 1986, for reviews). In view of the less effective, spinally-elicited inhibition of ongoing renal nerve activity in SHR, discussed above, we hypothesized that this system might also be less effective in inhibiting evoked increases in renal nerve activity in SHR.

We first determined the nature of these interactions in normotensive SD. The results were surprising. Inhibitory stimulation failed to reduce the magnitude of excitatory responses elicited by stimulation of either spinal or splanchnic systems. In most cases, inhibitory stimulation reduced the maximum renal nerve activity

achieved during excitatory stimulation by only the amount
to which it reduced ongoing renal nerve activity. Renal
nerve activity during 100Hz stimulation of the splanchnic
nerve was still reduced by inhibitory stimulation.
However, activity during 100Hz stimulation of spinal
pathways was completely refractory to inhibitory
stimulation.

One explanation for the inability of spinally-elicited
inhibition to reduce spinally-elicited sympathoexcitation
is that spinal sympathoexcitatory stimulation co-activated
the spinal sympathoinhibitory system. Co-activation by the
excitatory stimulus would obviate any additional inhibition
being elicited by the inhibitory stimulus. There are two
reasons to reject this hypothesis. First, spinal
stimulation was conducted deep in the dorsolateral
funiculus and at relatively low intensities. It is
unlikely that this stimulation could have spread to a
superficial, dorsolateral sympathoinhibitory system.
Second, maximal responses of the inhibitory system were
elicited by stimulation at approximately 20HZ. Therefore,
one would not predict a difference in the magnitude of co-
stimulated sympathoinhibition with stimulation of spinal
systems at 50 and 100HZ. Yet, excitation elicited by 50HZ
stimulation <u>was</u> still affected by spinally-elicited
inhibition, and excitation elicited by 100Hz stimulation
<u>was</u> <u>not</u>. The reasons for the differences in the
interactions between spinally-elicited inhibitions and
excitations elicited from splanchnic and spinal systems
remain unknown.

Our small samples of SHR and WKY exhibited very
similar responses to the simultaneous stimulation of
excitatory and inhibitory systems. These responses also
did not differ from those seen in SD. Our interpretation
of these results is that elevated renal nerve activity in
SHR does not result from a failure of this particular
inhibitory system to inhibit either visceral afferent or
descending sympathoexcitation. This inhibitory system
seems to act exclusively on ongoing sympathetic activity of
an unknown source.

ACKNOWLEDGMENT

We would like to thank Evelyn McCann for expert

technical assistance and Kathy Hartzell and Catherine
Palmer for assistance in preparing this manuscript. This
research was supported by grant HL16315 from the National
Institutes of Health.

REFERENCES

Alexander, RS (1946). Tonic and reflex functions of
medullary sympathetic cardiovascular centers. J.
Neurophysiol. 9:205-217.
Coote, JH and MacLeod, VH (1975). The spinal route of
sympatho-inhibitory pathways descending from the medulla
oblongata. Pflugers Arch. 359:335-347.
Illert, M and Gabriel, M (1972). Descending pathways in
the cervical cord of cats affecting blood pressure and
sympathetic activity. Pflugers Arch. 335:109-124.
Judy, WB, Watanabe, AM, Henry, DP, Besch, HR, Jr., Murphy,
WR and Hockel, GM (1976). Sympathetic nerve activity:
role in regulation of blood pressure in the
spontaneously hypertensive rat. Circ. Res. 38(2):21-29.
Okamoto, K, Nosaka, S, Yamori, Y and Matsumoto, M (1967).
Participation of neural factor in the pathogenesis of
hypertension in the spontaneously hypertensive rat. Jpn.
Heart J. 8:168-180.
Ross, CA, Ruggiero, DA, Park, DH, Joh, TH, Sved, AF,
Fernandez-Pardal, J, Saavedra, JM and Reis, DJ (1984).
Tonic vasomotor control by the rostral ventrolateral
medulla: Effect of electrical or chemical stimulation of
the area containing C1 adrenaline neurons on arterial
pressure, heart rate, and plasma catecholamines and
vasopressin. J. Neurosci. 4:474-494.
Schramm, LP (1986). Spinal factors in sympathetic
regulation. In Magro, A (ed): "The Molecular Basis for
the Central and Peripheral Regulation of Vascular
Resistance," New York: Plenum Press.
Schramm, LP and Barton, GN (1979). Diminished sympathetic
silent period in spontaneously hypertensive rats. Am. J.
Physiol. 236(3):R147-R152.
Schramm, LP and Chornoboy, ES (1982). Sympathetic
activity in spontaneously hypertensive rats after spinal
transection. Am. J. Physiol. 243:R506-R511.
Schramm, LP, Livingstone, SR, Taylor, RF and Palmer, CE
(1986). Sympathoinhibition mediated by dorsolateral
spinal cord in the rat. Society for Neuroscience
Abstracts.

Organization of the Autonomic Nervous System:
Central and Peripheral Mechanisms, pages 121–130
© 1987 Alan R. Liss, Inc.

NEUROTRANSMITTER REGULATION OF EXCITABILITY IN SYMPATHETIC
PREGANGLIONIC NEURONS THROUGH INTERACTIONS WITH ADENYLATE
CYCLASE

Donald N. Franz, Scott C. Steffensen, Lewis C.
Miner, and Chaichan Sangdee

Department of Pharmacology, University of
Utah, Salt Lake City, Utah 84132, U.S.A.

INTRODUCTION

Sympathetic preganglionic neurons (SPGNs) appear to
be innervated by an assortment of bulbospinal and local
pathways containing monoamines and neuropeptides (Holets
and Elde, 1982; Bjorklund and Hokfelt, 1984; Krukoff,
Ciriello, and Calaresu, 1985) and probably by excitatory
and inhibitory amino acids. Terminations of bulbospinal
norepinephrine (NE), epinephrine (EPI), and serotonin (5-
HT) pathways and of enkephalin neurons are especially
prominent. This paper summarizes the results of studies
which suggest that the excitability of SPGNs is regulated
in part by intraneuronal cyclic AMP, the levels of which
are controlled by positive and negative coupling of
neurotransmitter receptors to adenylate cyclase.

METHODS

Adult cats were made spinal at C1 under brief ether
or methohexital anesthesia, carotid and vertebral arteries
were occluded to render the brain ischemic, tracheal and
carotid cannulae were placed for respiratory support and
blood pressure monitoring, and muscular paralysis was
induced by gallamine triethiodide. Sympathetic discharges,
recorded from upper thoracic preganglionic white rami, were
evoked by biphasic, tungsten microelectrode stimulation
(0.1 Hz) of intraspinal excitatory pathways in the
dorsolateral funiculus of the cervical spinal cord at C2-3
(Fig. 2D). Drugs were administered either intravenously or
by air-pressure microinjection into the SPGN neuropil of
the T3 segment while recording transmission simultaneously
from T2 and T3 preganglionic rami (Fig. 3D). Drugs,
dissolved in artificial CSF, were microinjected by
controlled air pressure from glass micropipettes in volumes
of 1-5 μL. Transmission was not affected by vehicle

injections below 15 μl. Sizes of evoked discharges were
analyzed every 5 or 10 min by signal averaging of 16
consecutive responses for at least 1 hr before and for
several hours after drug administration. Blood pressure,
respiration, and body temperature were monitored and
maintained optimal throughout surgical and experimental
procedures.

RESULTS

Intravenous injection of 0.5-2 mg/kg of desipramine
(Fig. 1A) or d-amphetamine (Fig. 1B) rapidly and markedly
enhanced transmission, and this enhancement was promptly
blocked by 1-3 mg/kg of chlorpromazine (CPZ). CPZ alone
(Fig. 1C) or reserpine after 36-hr pretreatment with
divided doses of alphamethyl-paratyrosine (Fig. 1D; AMPT)
depressed intraspinal transmission to 40-50% of control but
even higher doses did not block transmission completely.
Transmission was not significantly affected by haloperidol
(0.25-2 mg/kg) or bromocriptine (0.5-1 mg/kg); apomorphine
(0.25-1 mg/kg) only gradually and modestly decreased
transmission. These results suggested that bulbospinal NE
pathways are excitatory to SPGNs.

The possibility that NE might act by increasing
cyclic AMP was assessed by testing the effects of
phosphodiesterase (PDE) inhibitors on intraspinal
transmission. Intravenous injection of aminophylline (50
mg/kg) isobutylmethylxanthine (1 mg/kg; IBMX), or the
selective inhibitor of cyclic AMP PDE, RO 20-1724 (1
mg/kg), rapidly enhanced transmission by about 80% before
declining to control levels within 3 hr (Fig. 2). One-half
of these doses enhanced transmission by only about 50%.
Pretreatment with CPZ or AMPT and reserpine delayed and
restricted enhancement by 1 mg/kg of IBMX to only 15-20%.
Neither prazosin (0.1-1 mg/kg) nor propranolol (2-5 mg/kg)
depressed transmission or restricted enhancement by IBMX.
These results suggest that NE pathways activate receptors
that are positively coupled to adenylate cyclase thereby
increasing intraneuronal cyclic AMP levels and enhancing
SPGN excitability, probably through phosphorylation of
membrane proteins.

Further support for an excitatory role of cyclic AMP
was obtained from the results of microinjection studies
(Fig. 3). Microinjection of the stable cyclic AMP analogs,
dibutyryl cyclic AMP (Fig. 3A) or 8-bromo-cyclic AMP (Fig.
3B), or the direct activator of adenylate cyclase,
forskolin (Fig. 3C), into the SPGN neuropil at T3 increased
transmission through the T3 segment by 100% or more for

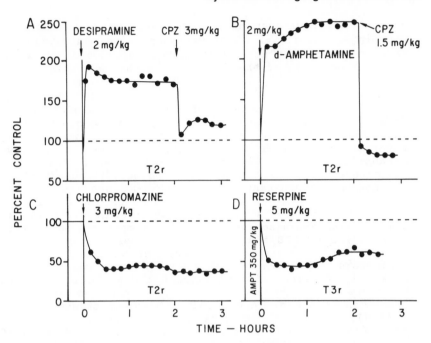

Figure 1. Enhancement of intraspinal transmission by desipramine (A) or d-amphetamine (B) and antagonism of enhancements by chlorpromazine (CPZ). CPZ (C) and reserpine after 36-hr pretreatment with AMPT (D) reduced transmission. Responses were recorded from T2 or T3 preganglionic rami in separate experiments.

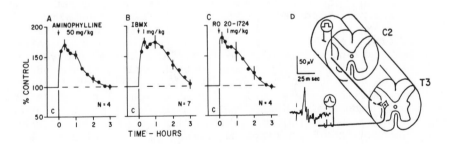

Figure 2. Enhancement of intraspinal transmission by three PDE inhibitors (A-C). D illustrates electrode placement and a typical control response. N = number of experiments; vertical bars represent S.E.M.

several hours without affecting transmission through T2. Microinjection of 1-2 µL of methylene blue indicated that injected solutions were distributed rostrocaudally along the SPGN neuropil of the T3 segment within a volume of 15-20 µL.

Clonidine, opiates, and 5-HTP have been shown to reduce intraspinal transmission in a dose-dependent manner and these effects of clonidine and opiates are readily reversed to original control levels by their respective antagonists (Madsen et al., 1981; Franz, Hare, and McCloskey, 1982); no antagonists have been found effective against the depressant effects of 5-HT precursors. As shown in Fig. 4, intravenous injection of clonidine, methadone, or 5-HTP markedly depressed intraspinal transmission and also prevented all or most of the typical enhancement by PDE inhibitors; lower doses produced less depression and permitted some enhancement by PDE inhibitors. L-tryptophan (150 mg/kg) after pargyline (30 mg/kg) also depressed transmission and markedly retarded enhancement by IBMX. In contrast, diazepam depressed transmission but did not affect subsequent enhancement by IBMX (Fig. 4E). Respective alpha-2 receptor or opiate antagonists not only antagonized the depressant effects of clonidine (Fig. 4A and B) or methadone (Fig. 4C) but also restored the ability of the PDE inhibitors (which were still present) to enhance transmission to levels well above control. Microinjection of 1-3 µg of clonidine, methadone, or 5-HT into the T3 segment produced prolonged depression of intraspinal transmission through that segment. Microinjection of leu- or met-enkephalin (2-5 µg) also produced transient depression.

In contrast to the usual brief 3-hr duration of enhancement produced by IBMX or RO 20-1724 alone (Fig. 2), the maximal enhancements were increased to 200% - 300% of control levels with no decline for up to 5 hr after pretreatment with yohimbine (Fig. 5A). These observations suggested that the increases in SPGN excitability produced by the PDE inhibitors are normally limited by activation of an inhibitory system which involves alpha-2 receptors and their endogenous ligand. The results of a previous study in which two selective PNMT inhibitors produced a linear enhancement of intraspinal transmission to 200% - 250% during 4 hr (Sangdee and Franz, 1982) and other studies showing a close association between brain EPI and alpha-2 receptors (U'Prichard, 1984) suggested that alpha-2 receptors on SPGNs may be normal substrates for bulbospinal EPI pathways. Like pretreatment with yohimbine,

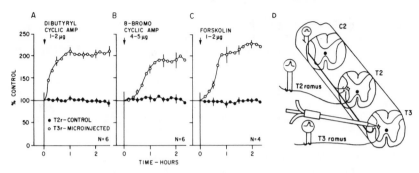

Figure 3. Enhancement of intraspinal transmission through T3 by cyclic AMP analogs (A, B) or forskolin (C), microinjected into the T3 SPGN neuropil as illustrated in D. Transmission through T2 was not affected.

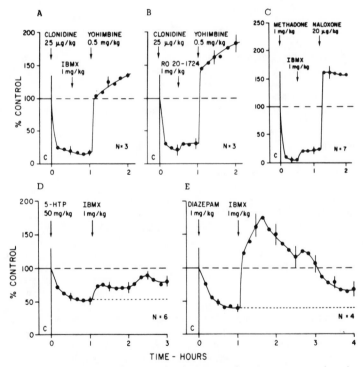

Figure 4. Depression of intraspinal transmission and prevention of enhancement by PDE inhibitors after clonidine (A,B), methadone (C), or 5-HTP (D). Antagonists in A-C reversed depression and restored enhancement by PDE inhibitors. Diazepam produced depression but did not affect enhancement by IBMX.

pretreatment with the PNMT inhibitor, LY134046, for 4 hr to deplete central EPI levels also intensified and greatly prolonged enhancement of transmission by RO 20-1724 (Fig. 5B) or by IBMX.

The possibility that acetylcholine, released locally from SPGNs or their axon collaterals, might trigger the apparent inhibitory system was tested with cholinergic antagonists. Although atropine (2 mg/kg) did not alter the normal transient time course of enhancement by the PDE inibitors, dihydro-beta-erythroidine, a centrally acting nicotinic antagonist, did prevent the early termination of enhancement by both RO 20-1724 (Fig. 5C) and IBMX. Predictably, pretreatment with the cholinesterase inhibitor, physostigmine, markedly restricted both the duration and the maximal enhancement produced by RO 20-1724 (Fig. 5D) or IBMX.

The possible presence of an inhibitory interneuron in the inhibitory circuit was tested by pretreating with subconvulsive doses of strychnine or picrotoxin. Picrotoxin (0.5 mg/kg) but not strychnine (0.05 mg/kg) markedly prolonged enhancement by IBMX. Although the early enhancement was less than half of normal, enhancement continued to increase for more than 4 hr (average, 185% of control, N=6).

DISCUSSION

The present results provide evidence for modulation of SPGN excitability over a wide range by neurotransmitter regulation of adenylate cyclase and intraneuronal cyclic AMP levels as depicted in Fig. 6A. The enhancement of intraspinal transmission by the PDE inhibitors can best be attributed to preservation of cyclic AMP because RO 20-1724 is highly selective for cyclic AMP PDE and does not block adenosine receptors, and the potency ratio of aminophylline and IBMX is not consistent with antagonism of adenosine receptors (Daly, 1977; van Caulker, Muller, and Hamprecht, 1979). The marked and prolonged enhancement of intraspinal transmission by microinjection of forskolin or cyclic AMP analogs provides additional strong support for the proposal that activation of adenylate cyclase increases cyclic AMP levels which lead to increased SPGN excitability.

Adenylate cyclase appears to be activated by NE pathways that innervate receptors which are positively coupled to the enzyme and are blocked by CPZ. Although some dopamine pathways also appear to innervate SPGNs, the marked enhancement of transmission by desipramine (Sangdee

and Franz, 1979), which selectively blocks NE but not
dopamine reuptake, and the absent or inconclusive effects
of haloperidol, apomorphine, or bromocriptine do not
support such a role for dopamine. The inability of
prazosin or propranolol to depress transmission indicates
that the NE receptors are neither alpha-1 or beta
receptors. Perhaps they represent a third type of
adrenergic receptor which is positively coupled to
adenylate cyclase as described in the rat limbic forebrain
(Mobley and Sulser, 1979). The inability of CPZ or
AMPT/reserpine pretreatment to block intraspinal
transmission completely infers activation by other
descending excitatory pathways, possibly mediated by
neuropeptides or excitatory amino acids. Nevertheless,
both pretreatments markedly impaired enhancement by the PDE
inhibitors; the modest enhancements observed may reflect
preservation of basal levels of cyclic AMP.

The marked depression of both intraspinal
transmission and its enhancement by PDE inhibitors produced
by clonidine, methadone, and 5-HTP or L-tryptophan suggest
that alpha-2, opiate, and 5-HT receptors are negatively
coupled to adenylate cyclase, thereby preventing synthesis
of cyclic AMP and reducing SPGN excitability. The
tentative axosomatic locations of alpha-2, opiate, and 5-HT
receptors as shown in Fig. 6A are based largely upon the
apparent close apposition of EPI, enkephalin, and 5-HT
terminals to SPGNs (Holets and Elde, 1982; Bjorklund and
Hokfelt, 1984; Krukoff, Ciriello, and Calaresu, 1985) and
the results of iontophoretic studies (Guyenet and
Stornetta, 1982). NE terminals have been described as

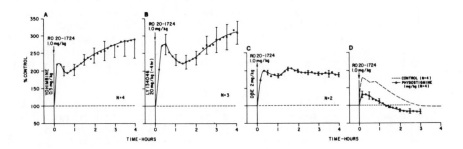

Figure 5. Pretreatment with yohimbine (A), LY 134046 (B),
or dihydro-beta-erythroidine (C) prolonged and increased
enhancement of intraspinal transmission by RO 20-1724.
Pretreatment with physostigmine (D) markedly reduced
enhancement by RO 20-1724.

primarily axodendritic (Glazer and Ross, 1980). As shown in other biological systems that are regulated by receptor coupling to adenylate cyclase (Rodbell, 1980), the respective receptors on SPGNs are most likely coupled by stimulatory (Ns) and inhibitory (Ni), GTP-dependent regulatory proteins. This arrangement would permit independent regulation of SPGN excitability by each of the neurotransmitters acting upon their respective receptors.

The early termination of enhancement by the PDE inhibitors was prevented in nearly identical fashion by alpha-2 receptor blockade with yohimbine, by depletion of central EPI with LY-134046, or by nicotinic receptor blockade with dihydro-beta-erythroidine. On the other hand, the intensity and duration of enhancement were markedly reduced by the acetylcholinesterase inhibitor, physostigmine. These results suggest that rapid increases in the excitability of SPGNs produced by cyclic AMP are limited by an unusual type of local inhibition which is mediated sequentially by release of acetylcholine, activation of nicotinic receptors, release of EPI, and activation of alpha-2-receptors which are negatively coupled to adenylate cyclase (Fig. 6B). Acetylcholine, released from SPGNs, may activate nicotinic receptors on EPI terminals to release EPI by mechanisms similar to those operating at the adrenal medulla.

The possibility for the presence of a GABA inhibitory interneurone in the inhibitory pathway gains some support from the prolongation of IBMX enhancement by subconvulsive doses of picrotoxin which alone did not enhance transmission. However, the enhancement by IBMX after picrotoxin followed a rather different course than produced by the other pretreatments shown in Fig. 5A-C. The prolongation of enhancement by picrotoxin may reflect additive excitation with IBMX rather than blockade of GABA receptor complexes. More definitive evidence for a GABA link is clearly warranted.

Although axon collaterals from SPGNs injected with HRP have been detected in pigeons (Cabot and Bogan, this volume), similar studies of cat SPGNs have revealed only spinelike protuberances along the course of axons in the ventral horn which may represent presynaptic boutons (Dembowsky, Czachurski, and Seller, 1985). These findings therefore provide potential anatomical support for some kind of inhibitory circuitry, but definitive evidence for recurrent inhibition from classical conditioning studies

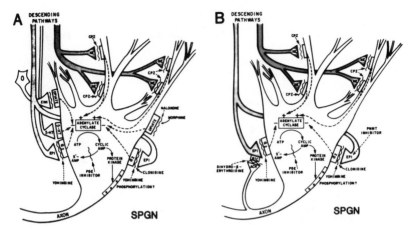

Figure 6. A, diagramatic representation of modulation of SPGN excitability by monoaminergic and enkephalin pathways through positive or negative receptor coupling to adenylate cyclase. B, representation of proposed recurrent inhibitory pathway that limits SPGN excitability.

remains elusive (Polosa, Schondorf, and Laskey, 1982). Such standard approaches would not be expected to activate a local inhibitory mechanism that is triggered primarily by large, rapid increases in intraneuronal cyclic AMP. This inhibitory mechanism may be intrinsically important for limiting excessive and sustained hyperexcitability of central sympathetic activity.

This work was supported by HL-24085 and GM-07579 and by the Utah and Montana Heart Associations. We thank Eli Lilly, Roche, and Merck for supplies of LY-134046, RO 20-1724, and dihydro-beta-erythroidine, respectively.

REFERENCES

Bjorklund A, Hokfelt T (1984). "Handbook of Chemical Neuroanatomy, Volume 2, Classical Transmitters in the CNS, Part I." New York:Elsevier.
Daly J (1977). "Cyclic Nucleotides in the Nervous System." New York:Plenum Press.
Dembowsky K, Czachurski J, Seller H (1985). Morphology of sympathetic preganglionic neurons in the thoracic spinal cord of the cat: An intracellular horseradish peroxidase study. J Compar Neurol 238:453.
Franz DN, Hare BD, McCloskey KL (1982). Spinal sympathetic neurons: Possible sites of opiate-withdrawal suppression by clonidine. Science 215:1643.

Glazer EJ, Ross LL (1980). Localization of noradrenergic terminals in sympathetic preganglionic nuclei of the rat: Demonstration by immunocytochemical localization of dopamine-β-hydroxylase. Brain Res 185:39.

Guyenet PG, Stornetta RL (1982). Inhibition of sympathetic preganglionic discharges by epinephrine and α-methylepinephrine. Brain Res 235:271.

Holets V, Elde R (1982). The differential distribution and relationship of serotonergic and peptidergic fibers to sympathoadrenal neurons in the intermediolateral cell column of the rat: A combined retrograde axonal transport and immunofluorescence study. Neurosci 7:1155.

Krukoff TL, Ciriello J, Calaresu FR (1985). Segmental distribution of peptide and 5HT-like immunoreactivity in nerve terminals and fibers in the thoracolumbar sympathetic nuclei of the cat. J Compar Neurol 240:103.

Madsen PW, Hare BD, Sangdee C, Franz DN (1981). Contrasting effects of clonidine and 5-hydroxytryptophan on spinal sympathetic pathways. Clin Exp Hypertension 3:1151.

Mobley PL, Sulser F (1979). Norepinephrine stimulated cyclic AMP accumulation in rat limbic forebrain slices: Partial mediation by a subpopularion of receptors with neither α nor β characteristics. Eur J Pharmacol 60:221.

Polosa C, Schondorf R, Laskey W (1982). Stabilization of the discharge rate of sympathetic preganglionic neurons. J Auton Nerv Syst 5:45.

Rodbell M (1980). The role of hormone receptors and GTP regulatory proteins in membrane transduction. Nature 284:17.

Sangdee C, Franz DN (1979). Enhancement of central norepinephrine and 5-hydroxytryptamine transmission by tricyclic antidepressants: A comparison. Psychopharmacology 62:9.

Sangdee C, Franz DN (1983). Evidence for inhibition of sympathetic preganglionic neurons by bulbospinal epinephrine pathways. Neurosci Lett 37:167

U'Prichard DC (1984). Biochemical characteristics and regulation of brain alpha-2 receptors. Ann NY Acad Sci 430:55.

van Calker D, Muller M, Hamprecht B (1979). Receptors regulating the level of cyclic AMP in primary cultures of perinatal mouse brain. In Meisami E, Brazier MAB (eds): "Neural Growth and Differentiation", New York: Raven Press, p. 11.

SECTION III: Sympathetic Tone and Periodicities

The background discharge of sympathetic and parasympathetic nerves shows rhythmic components of various frequencies.

The first three papers of this section are concerned with description of these rhythmic signals. The paper by Gootman, Cohen, DiRusso, Sica, Cohen, Eberle, Rudell and Gootman presents a survey of the various periodicities which characterize sympathetic activity in most laboratory animals, while Czyzyk, Fedorko and Trzebski describe in the rat the pattern of sympathetic neuron activity in relation to the central respiratory cycle. Koizumi and Kollai record simultaneously the activity of sympathetic and parasympathetic nerves. The relation to the central respiratory cycle of their activities is compared and contrasted.

The question of how these rhythmicities appear in the discharge of autonomic neurons is the topic of the next three papers, which are all concerned with the respiratory modulation of autonomic neuron activity. Wurster and Connelly emphasize the importance of the baroreceptor reflex in producing changes in sympathetic activity, locked to the respiratory cycle, which are secondary to the changes in systemic arterial pressure produced by the centrally-generated respiratory modulation of sympathetic activity. Koepchen, Abel and Klüssendorf, in contrast, focus on the central mechanisms of generation. They present views on the generation of the respiratory rhythm and of the respiratory modulation of sympathetic activity which attempt to reconcile the hypothesis that each is generated by an independent neural oscillator with the hypothesis of "irradiation" of activity from the respiratory oscillator to the sympathetic system. Bachoo and Polosa are also concerned with the central mechanism of generation of respiratory modulation and discuss the properties of the inspiration related and cardiac related sympathetic rhythms in relation to the properties to be expected if these rhythms were generated as the result of the coupling of two oscillators.

Finally, some of the rhythms which are relatively specific to sympathetic neurons may be used as markers for tracing connections within the CNS of the preganglionic neurons with the antecedent neurons which carry the rhythmic input to them. The paper by Varner, Gebber, Barman and Huang is an example of this application. They demonstrate a correlation betwen unit activity in the medial thalamus and sympathetic slow wave activity, suggesting a role for this structure in the generation of this type of quasi-rhythmic sympathetic activity.

Organization of the Autonomic Nervous System:
Central and Peripheral Mechanisms, pages 133-142
© 1987 Alan R. Liss, Inc.

PERIODICITIES IN SPONTANEOUS PREGANGLIONIC SYMPATHETIC DISCHARGE

Phyllis M. Gootman, Morton I. Cohen, Steven M. DiRusso, Anthony L. Sica, Howard L. Cohen, Larry P. Eberle, Alan P. Rudell, Norman Gootman

Dept. of Physiology, State University of New York, Health Sciences Center at Brooklyn, New York 11203, Dept. of Physiology and Biophysics, Albert Einstein College of Medicine, Bronx, New York 10461, and Schneider Children's Hospital, Long Island Jewish Medical Center, New Hyde Park, New York 11042

INTRODUCTION

While carrying out an extensive study of brain stem influences on the efferent discharge of the greater splanchnic nerve (Gootman, 1967), the presence of a number of different periodicities was noted and detailed quantitative analyses were performed (Cohen & Gootman, 1970; Cohen et al., 1980; Gootman & Cohen, 1970, 1971, 1973, 1974, 1980, 1981, 1983; Gootman et al., 1975a,b, 1980). To further investigate the nature of such periodicities in spontaneous efferent sympathetic (SYMP) discharge, we also examined activity from other SYMP nerves, e.g., cervical sympathetic (Cohen et al., 1980; Gootman & Cohen, 1973, 1980, 1981, 1983; Gootman et al., 1975a,b, 1980). More recently, our studies include examination of activity in neonatal mammals, e.g., Sus scrofa (Cohen et al., 1986; Gootman, 1986; Gootman et al., 1981, 1983, 1984). We have found common periodicities in spontaneous efferent SYMP discharge; however, differences between different nerve outputs and ages have also been noted.

METHODS

Experiments were performed on decerebrate-unanesthetized or urethane-anesthetized adult cats and on halothane or Saffon (Glaxo)-anesthetized neonatal swine (birth to 1 month of age), with neuromuscular blockade, bilateral pneumothorax, and artificial ventilation. Further details of methods have been given in earlier papers.

Recordings were made on magnetic tape of: a) efferent left greater splanchnic activity (SPL), b) efferent cervical sympathetic activity (CS), c) efferent phrenic activity (PHR), d) EKG, e) aortic blood pressure (AoP), f) intratracheal pressure (ITP), g) end-tidal CO_2, h) derived pulses marking times in the cardiac or central respiratory cycles. SPL and CS discharges were monophasically recorded with bipolar electrodes; a relatively wide amplifier bandpass (0.2-1000 Hz) was used in order to allow faithful reproduction of slow potential changes. PHR discharge was recorded mono- or biphasically with a bandpass of 10 Hz-10 KHz.

Relative changes of SYMP and PHR activity were examined by integration procedures. The periodicities in spontaneous SPL and CS activity were studied by auto- and cross- correlation methods, power spectral analysis and averaging techniques using a PDP 11/45 computer. Further details of data analysis are given in earlier papers.

RESULTS

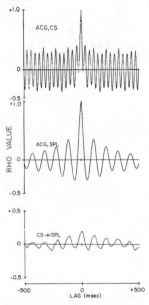

Fig. 1. Autocorrelograms (**ACG**) of simultaneously recorded **CS** (<u>top</u>) and **SPL** (<u>middle</u>) activity from an unanesthetized decerebrate cat. <u>Bottom Trace:</u> crosscorrelation histogram between CS and SPL activities. Bandpass 1-100 Hz, 500 2-msec bins, 10,000 data points.

Adult Studies. Spontaneous SPL and CS activity consisted predominantly of slow waves having amplitudes in the range of 10-30 uV, with faster activity superimposed. The predominant frequency in the SPL nerves was about 10/sec (Fig. 1); less commonly, waves with the frequency of the cardiac cycle (3-5/sec) were observed (cf. Fig. 6, Cat B). A prominant frequency in the CS nerve was about 30 Hz (Fig. 1); in addition 10/sec activity was observed.

Neonatal Studies. Examination of power spectra and autocorrelation histograms (ACH) of spontaneous efferent SPL and CS activity revealed peak frequencies at ca. 20 and 30 Hz (Fig. 2). In addition, 5/sec waves were occasionally observed in SPL discharge and ca. 10/sec in CS.

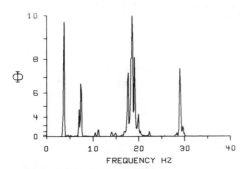

Fig. 2. Power spectrum (Φ) of efferent SPL activity from a 2 day old piglet. Sampling rate 128 Hz with 20 epochs of 1024 data points. Signal filtered with a 1-40 Hz bandpass. (From Gootman, 1986.)

Vasomotor Nature of Discharge. When a noticeable spontaneous change in SPL discharge occurred, there followed an alteration of AoP. Spontaneous changes in PHR and SYMP discharge in adult cats and neonatal swine are shown in Figs. 3 and 4, respectively. Note that in both examples the increase in spontaneous SYMP discharge is followed by an increase in AoP. The relationship between changes in SYMP discharge, AoP and PHR activity was also apparent following induced cardiovascular alterations, e.g., bolus epinephrine (EPI) injection. As shown in Fig. 5, the rise in AoP consequent to the injection produced depression of CS activity and of the central respiratory rhythm generator (RRG) for > 1 min in neonatal swine. Thus changes in baroceptor activity have profound effects on both the central SYMP generator and the RRG even in newborns.

Cardiac and Respiratory Modulation of Sympathetic Activity. Spontaneous activity in efferent SYMP discharge usually oscillated in phase with both the cardiac and central respiratory cycles; signal averaging and crosscorrelation techniques were used to show such modulation.

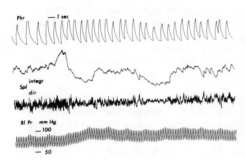

Fig. 3. Events associated with a spontaneous **AoP** rise in an adult cat. Polygraph traces of integrated **PHR** discharge (100 msec time constant); **SPL** discharge integrated (**integr**) (440 msec time constant); **SPL** potentials directly recorded (**dir**), negativity upward (vertical bar, voltage calibration); blood pressure (**Bl Pr**). (From Gootman & Cohen, 1970.)

Fig. 4. Events associated with a spontaneous **AoP** rise in a 23 day old swine. Polygraph traces of **ITP**, integrated **PHR** and **CS** discharges (100 msec time constants) and **AoP**.

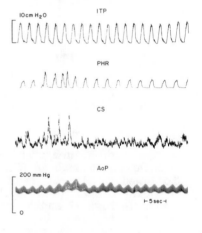

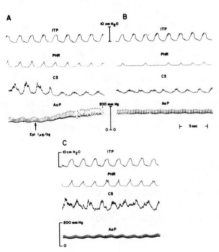

Fig. 5. Effect of epinephrine (1 ug/kg, iv) on integrated **PHR** and **CS** discharges (100 msec time constants), EKG and **AoP**. Panel A: at time of injection, Panel B: 32 sec after injection, Panel C: 6 1/2 min after injection.

The degree of locking of two periodic signals, evaluated by auto- and cross- correlation functions, could differ, as shown in Fig. 6. In Cat A the 10/sec periodicity was locked in a 3:1 relation to the cardiac cycle, as shown by the EKG-triggered histograms in Fig. 6, Cat A. In Cat B, the slow waves were locked in a 1:1 relation to the cardiac cycle. In contrast to Cat A, Cat C showed no locking of the 10/sec waves to the EKG. Similar findings were observed in CS discharge from neonatal swine. Thus, prominent periodicity can exist with different degrees of synchronization to the cardiac cycle.

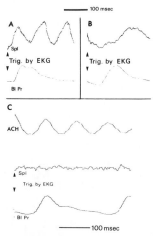

Fig. 6. Two common patterns of cardiac modulation of SPL discharge (Cats A and B). Traces are computer readouts of summed SPL activity and aortic blood pressure (**Bl Pr**), triggered from EKG-derived pulses. 1-msec bins; 500 epochs. Bottom Panel: Comparison (in Cat C) between ACH of SPL activity (top trace) and CCH of SPL and EKG-derived pulses (middle trace). Bottom trace: CCH of AoP and EKG-derived pulses. (Adapted from Cohen & Gootman, 1970).

One possible mechanism of such differences in locking to the cardiac cycle may be the relation between cardiac cycle duration and period of SYMP oscillation. In Cat A the heart period was almost exactly 3 times the SPL oscillation period, while in Cat C the two periods had a nonintegral ratio (265 vs. 100 msec) (Cohen & Gootman, 1970).

An example of cardiac modulation of SPL activity in newborn swine is shown in Fig. 7; the crosscorrelation histograms (**CCH**) show that minimum SPL activity occurred during systole. The similarity of the two CCHs in this figure, each based on a different sample, verifies that the cardiac modulation is real and not a spurious periodicity due to insufficient averaging of a sample of finite length containing frequencies which are near to the scanning frequency (Gootman et al., 1984).

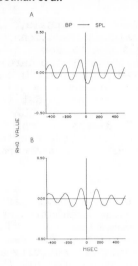

Fig. 7. Normalized CCHs between AoP (**BP**) and **SPL** activity from 13 day old piglet, each based on a different sample. 500 2-msec bins; 20,000 data points. SPL signal filtered with a 2.5-40 Hz bandpass. Zero time represents peak systole during cardiac cycle. (From Gootman et al., 1984.)

Respiratory modulation of SYMP activity was present in both cat and swine and in both adults and neonates. Quantitative examination of the repiratory modulation was obtained from normalized CCHs (Fig. 8); note the increase in SYMP activity during inspiration and the decrease during the expiratory phase.

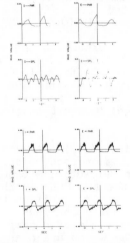

Fig. 8. Normalized CCH of **PHR** and **SPL** activities (after processing through an 80 Hz high pass filter and half-wave rectifier) vs. I- (left) or E- (right) derived pulses. Data from a 13 day old piglet (top traces) and an adult cat (bottom traces). 500 10-msec bins; 20,000 data points. (Adapted in part from Gootman et al., 1984.)

Examination of pulmonary afferent influences on respiratory modulation of SYMP discharge was carried out systematically in adult cats (Gootman & Cohen, 1983; Gootman, et al., 1980). We have also begun to examine the

effects of alterations in pulmonary afferent activity in
neonates   (Fig. 9). This activity produces inhibition of
SYMP discharge as shown by the observation   in Fig. 9

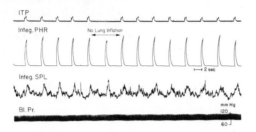

Fig. 9. Effects of **No Lung Inflation Test** monitored
by ITP) on integrated **PHR** and **SPL** activities (time
constants 0.1 sec) and on **AoP** from a 6 day old
piglet.

that the No Inflation Test produced an   increase in SPL
activity in piglets; similar observations were made in
adult cats.

The effects of stresses, e.g., hypercapnia, on
periodicities in SYMP discharge were also investigated. As
can be seen in the ACHs of Fig. 10, increasing the CO_2
level resulted in an increase of the 10/sec component of
the activity. In contrast, asphyxia in newborn piglet
(Fig. 11) did not cause any significant change in the
power distribution of SPL activity.

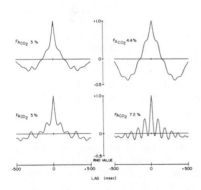

Fig. 10. Effect of CO_2 level
on 10/sec periodicity of **SPL**
discharge (bandpass 1-100 Hz)
in adult cat. Each trace is
the normalized **ACH** of **SPL**
activity at a different end-
tidal CO_2. 500 2-msec bins;
10,000 data points.

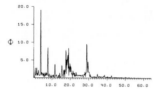

Fig. 11. Effect of asphyxia on the power spectra (Φ) of SPL discharge from a 2 day old piglet. Sampling rate 128 Hz with 15 epochs of 1024 data points; signal filtered with a 1-64 Hz bandpass.

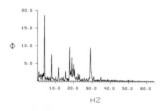

DISCUSSION

Periodicities Common to Different Ages. Analysis of the periodicities found in the discharge of preganglionic SYMP nerves is an essential prelude to understanding the central organization of the autonomic nervous system, since these periodicities can furnish information about the neuronal relations within the SYMP generating system as well as its relations with other systems, e.g., the RRG. In addition, examination of the changes in periodicities ocurring postnatally is essential to our understanding of the postnatal development of the neuronal networks making up the SYMP generating system.

Three major types of periodicity were observed in SYMP discharge: a) slow rhythms (periods of several seconds) synchronized to a greater or lesser extent with the central respiratory oscillator (Fig. 8); b) fast rhythms (2-6/sec), which were usually synchronized in a 1:1 relation with the cardiac cycle (Fig. 6, Cat B) by baroreceptor input, and c) still faster rhythms (> 10/sec, Fig. 1), which may lock to the cardiac cycle in an N:1 relation (Fig. 6, Cat A).

In monophasic recordings of whole nerve activity, the fluctuations of potential are due to the summated activity of individual fibers. However, the faster (2-10/sec) rhythms are not necessarily produced by random summation of activities of different fibers having similar discharge frequencies, since they are common (as indicated by crosscorrelation) to several SYMP outflows; these are driven by correlated inputs from supraspinal systems (Gootman & Cohen, 1980, 1981; Jänig, 1984).

The SYMP recordings from neonatal swine indicate that spontaneous efferent activity was similar in many respects to SYMP discharge in adult cats. Such recordings have also been done in 2 day old rat pups (Smith, 1986; Smith et al., 1982). One marked age difference observed was the occurrence of higher frequencies in neonatal SPL discharge (19 and 29 Hz) as compared with those in adults (10/sec) (Figs. 2 and 11 vs. Figs. 1 and 10), although higher frequencies (27-32 Hz, Fig. 1) are observed in adult cat CS discharge. The fact that the fast SYMP rhythms can vary systematically with physiological conditions and developmental level suggests that they are intimately related to the functional state of the SYMP generating systems.

Acknowledgment. This research was supported by N.I.H. grants HL-20864 (P.M.G.), and HL-27300 (M.I.C.).

REFERENCES

Cohen, HL, Sica, AL, Gootman, PM, Griswold, PG, Rao, PP, Gandhi, M (1986). Spontaneous efferent cervical sympathetic activity in neonatal swine. Neurosci Abst 12: in press.

Cohen, MI, Gootman PM (1970). Periodicities in efferent discharge of splanchnic nerve of the cat. Am J Physiol 218:1092.

Cohen, MI, Gootman, PM, Feldman, JL (1980). Inhibition of sympathetic discharge by lung inflation. In: Sleight, P (ed): "Arterial Baroreceptors and Hypertension," New York: Oxford Univ Press, p.161.

Gootman, PM (1967). Brain stem influences on efferent splanchnic discharge. Ph D thesis, Albert Einstein College of Medicine, New York.

Gootman, PM (1983). Neural regulation of cardiovascular function in the perinatal period. In: Gootman, N, Gootman, PM (eds): "Perinatal Cardiovascular Function," New York: Marcel Dekker, p.265.

Gootman, PM (1986). Development of central autonomic regulation of cardiovascular function. In Gootman, PM (ed): "Developmental Neurobioilogy of the Autonomic Nervous System," New Jersey: Humana Press, p. 279.

Gootman, PM, Cohen, HL, DiRusso, SM, Rudell, AP, Eberle, LP (1984). Characteristics of spontaneous efferent splanchnic discharge in neonatal swine. In Usdin, E, Dahlstrom, A, Engel, J, Carlsson, A (eds): "Catecholamines: Basic and Peripheral Mechanisms," New York: Alan R. Liss,p 369.

Gootman, PM, Cohen, MI (1970). Efferent splanchnic activity and systemic arterial pressure. Am J Physiol 219:897.

Gootman, PM, Cohen, MI (1971). Evoked potentials produced by electrical stimulation of medullary vasomotor regions. Exp Brain Res 13:1.

Gootman, PM, Cohen, MI (1973). Periodic modulation (cardiac and respiratory) of spontaneous and evoked sympathetic discharge. Acta Physiol Pol 24:99.

Gootman PM, Cohen, MI (1974). The interrelationships between sympathetic discharge and central respiratory drive. In: Umbach, W, Koepchen, HR (eds): "Central Rhythmic and Regulation," Stuttgart, Hippokrates,p.195.

Gootman, PM, Cohen, MI (1980). Origin of rhythms common to sympathetic outflows at different spinal levels. In: Sleight, P (ed): "Arterial Baroreceptors and Hypertension," New York, Oxford Univ Press, p. 154.

Gootman, PM, Cohen, MI (1981). Sympathetic rhythms in spinal cats. J Auton Nerv Syst 3:379.

Gootman, PM, Cohen, MI (1983). Inhibitory effects on fast sympathetic rhythms. Brain Res 270:134.

Gootman, PM, Cohen, MI, Piercey, MP, Wolotsky, P (1975a). A search for medullary neurons with activity patterns similar to those in sympathetic nerves. Brain Res 87:395.

Gootman, PM, Cohen, MI, Rudell, AP (1975b). Criteria for identification of brain stem sympathetic related neurons. Neurosci Abst 1:418.

Gootman, PM, Feldman, JL, Cohen, MI (1980). Pulmonary afferent influences on respiratory modulation of sympathetic discharge. In: Koepchen, HP, Hilton, SM, Trzebski, A (eds): "Central Interaction Between Respiratory and Cardiovascular Control Systems," New York: Springer-Verlag, p.172.

Gootman, PM, Gootman, N, Buckley, BJ (1983). Maturation of central autonomic control of the circulation. Federation Proc 42: 1648.

Gootman, PM, Gootman, N, Turlapaty, P, Yao, AC, Buckley, BJ, Altura, BM (1981). Autonomic regulation of cardiovascular function in neonates. In: Burnstock, G (ed): "Ciba Foundation Symposium 83. Development of the Autonomic Nervous System," London: Pitman Medical, p. 70.

Jänig, W (1984). Vasoconstrictor systems supplying skeletal muscle, skin, and viscera. Clin Exp Hyper-Theory Prac A6:329.

Smith, PG (1986). Relationship between the sympathetic nervous system and functional development of smooth muscle end organs. In: Gootman, PM (ed): "Developmental Neurobiology of the Autonomic Nervous System," New Jersey: Humana Press, p. 251.

Smith, PG, Slotkin, TA, Mills, E (1982). Development of sympathetic ganglionic neurotransmission in the neoatal rat. Pre- and postganglionic nerve response to asphyxia and 2-deoxyglucose. Neuroscience 7:501.

Organization of the Autonomic Nervous System:
Central and Peripheral Mechanisms, pages 143–152
© 1987 Alan R. Liss, Inc.

PATTERN OF THE RESPIRATORY MODULATION OF THE SYMPATHETIC
ACTIVITY IS SPECIES DEPENDENT: SYNCHRONIZATION OF THE
SYMPATHETIC OUTFLOW OVER THE RESPIRATORY CYCLE IN THE RAT

Maria F. Czyzyk, Ludwik Fedorko and Andrzej
Trzebski
Department of Physiology, Medical Academy,
Warsaw 00-927

INTRODUCTION

Very little is known on the oscillations of the
sympathetic activity related to the respiratory cycle in
species other than cats. The purpose of this study was to
analyze the central respiratory modulation of sympathetic
discharge in the rat. Spontaneously hypertensive rats
(SHRs) provide a unique experimental model for the study of
genetically controlled hypertension, the basis of which is
known to be sympathetic overactivity. Our previous study
indicated an augmented respiratory drive in SHRs
(Przybylski et al., 1982). Respiratory related rhythmical
sympathetic discharges account for a significant fraction
of the total vasoconstrictor sympathetic output (Lioy et
al., 1978, Polosa et al., 1980, Lioy and Trzebski, 1984,
Millhorn, 1986). Therefore an analysis of the respiratory
modulated sympathetic discharges in the rat seems
particularly interesting. In cats numerous studies
demonstrated that respiratory periodicities of the
sympathetic activity are characterized by inspiratory
related discharge. This has been found by recording the
efferent activity of whole sympathetic nerves (Adrian et
al., 1932, Cohen and Gootman, 1970, Koepchen et al., 1981,
Trzebski and Kubin, 1981), by recording the activity of
single sympathetic fibers (Koizumi et al., 1971, Preiss et
al., 1975, Janig et al., 1980, Kollai and Koizumi, 1980),
by measuring rhythmical shifts in antidromic latency
indicating membrane depolarization of the spinal
preganglionic neurons during inspiration (Lipski et al.,
1977). Recently Bainton et al. (1985) found some

depression of sympathetic activity at the onset of the
phrenic burst with a rapid increase to the peak in late
inspiration and a strong depression in stage I expiration.
In dogs respiratory modulation of sympathetic discharge is
variable and an increase may occur also in expiration
(Okada and Fox, 1967, Trzebski, 1980) especially during the
late expiratory phase (Kollai and Koizumi, 1981). In
neonatal swine the pattern is similar to that of the cat
(Gootman et al., 1984). In rabbits with increasing
respiratory frequency sympathetic discharge shifts to the
expiratory period (Hukuhara, 1984). Also in cats the
frequency of the respiratory oscillator was reported to
influence the timing of the sympathetic discharge within
the respiratory cycle (Barman and Gebber, 1976). In
conscious humans increased sympathetic discharge in muscle
nerves appears to be synchronous with expiration (Eckberg
et al., 1985) although a secondary respiratory related
reflex feedback from the pulmonary stretch receptors and/or
arterial baroreceptors has not been excluded.

METHODS

Experiments were performed on 17 rats weighing 250-350
g anaesthetized with intravenous urethane (1.0 g/kg),
paralyzed with pancuronium bromide and artificially
ventilated. In 11 animals the carotid sinus nerves and
vagi were cut. The activity of the cut right phrenic and
cervical sympathetic nerves was recorded. Phrenic nerve
activity was rectified and then averaged (Rc. phren.).
Sympathetic efferent activity (SA) was processed by moving
averager and averaged again over 16 respiratory cycles
(M.A. symp) using as a trigger the onset or the termination
point of the rectified phrenic burst. Central respiratory
frequency was changed over the range 20-80 min^{-1} by hypo-
and hypertermia and/or hyper- and hypocapnia. Short
respiratory arrest was produced by nasopharyngeal
stimulation with tap water (experimental diving reflex).
To stop the respiratory oscillator hyperventilation in air
causing hypocapnia was used. Periodicities of the
sympathetic activity collected over 10 s periods at 2.5 kHz
sampling were studied off-line by power density spectral
analysis using a MERA computer. Arterial blood pressure in
the femoral artery and heart rate by ECG limb electrodes
were continuously recorded. Student's test for statistical
evaluation of the significance of differences between
groups was used.

RESULTS

In all experiments both in intact and sino-aortic
denervated animals a similar pattern was observed over a
range of central respiratory frequencies between 20 and 80
min^{-1}: a peak of sympathetic activity occurred in stage I
expiration and a second peak in the late expiratory phase.
The latter effect was more pronounced during hypercapnia.
At the onset of inspiration sympathetic activity was
rapidly depressed reaching its minimum in the middle or in
the first half of the inspiratory phase. The activity
gradually rose in late inspiration (Fig. 1).

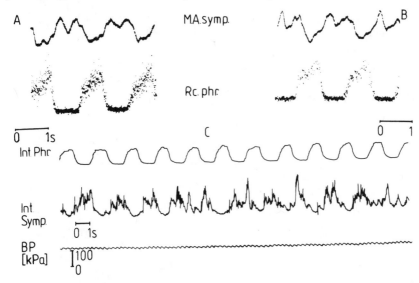

Figure 1. Pattern of averaged sympathetic activity (SA) in
the rat. Averaging was triggered by onset of inspiration
(A) and expiration (B). C - original record of integrated
activities. BP - arterial blood pressure in mmHg.
Mid-inspiratory depression and biphasic expiratory
facilitation of SA.

In hypercapnia a distinct burst occurred in early
expiration close to the inspiratory-expiratory transition.
Hypocapnia reduced both phrenic activity and the magnitude
of respiratory related sympathetic oscillations (Fig. 2).
Changing T_I and/or T_E had little effect on the timing of

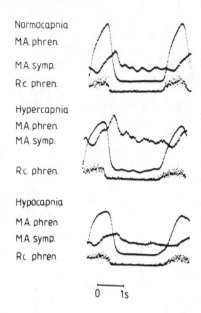

Normocapnia
M.A. phren.
M.A. symp.
Rc. phren.

Hypercapnia
M.A. phren.
M.A. symp.

Rc. phren.

Hypocapnia
M.A. phren.
M.A. symp.
Rc. phren.

0   1s

Figure 2. Effect of hypercapnia and hypocapnia upon SA
synchronization over the
respiratory cycle. Hypercapnia produces an addi-
tional early expiratory peak
of SA and augments the magnitude of expiratory SA whereas
hypocapnia reduces it. SA
timing related to expiratory-
inspiratory and inspiratory-
expiratory transition points
remains unchanged.

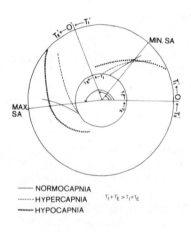

NORMOCAPNIA
HYPERCAPNIA
HYPOCAPNIA

$T_I + T_E > T_I + T_E$

Figure 3. Circles $T_I' + T_E'$ and
$T_I + T_E$ represent the time
duration of the longest and
the shortest respiratory
cycles (T_{TOT}). Each respiratory cycle starts at 0 and
runs anticlockwise. Curves on
the right represent relative
delays of minimal SA from T_E -
T_I transition or 0 as
percentage as of respective
T_I. Curves on the left
represent relative delays of
maximal SA from T_I - T_E
transition or 0'. The radial
lines show the hypothetical
phase-relation that would exist if phase-locked delays were
proportional to the absolute value of T_I and T_E. The
observed delays of the minima and maxima of SA deviate
significantly from this hypothetical phase-relation. The
delays tend to maintain a constant value and therefore to
represent a smaller and smaller fraction of T_I and T_E as
the respiratory cycle lengthens.

the early inspiratory depression and early expiratory discharge following the expiratory-inspiratory and inspiratory-expiratory transition. The delays of the minimum and maximum sympathetic activity respectively from the onset and from the termination of phrenic burst did not change with changes in duration of T_I and T_E thus the sympathetic oscillations exhibited a phase-spanning rather than phase-locked pattern (Fig. 3). In the rats with intact carotid sinus, aortic and vagus nerves slight respiratory sinus arrhythmia was observed with inspiratory cardioacceleration and expiratory cardiac slowing (Fig. 4). Bilateral vagotomy abolished respiratory modulation of the heart rate.

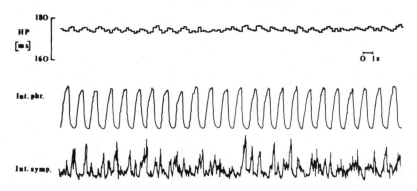

Figure 4. Respiratory sinus arrhythmia in the rat. From the top: HP - heart period recorded continuously as R-R interval of ECG. Int. Phr. - integrated phrenic nerve activity, Int. symp. - integrated activity of the sympathetic cervical trunk. Shortening of HP is synchronous with phrenic burst whereas HP prolongation occurs in expiration.

Nasopharyngeal superfusion with water produced a short reflex apnoea and increased sympathetic activity. The first phrenic burst after the apnoea was associated with marked sympathetic depression (Fig. 5). In the power density spectra of sympathetic activity distinct peaks of frequencies in the range of cardiac (5-7 Hz) and respiratory (0.3 - 0.7 Hz) frequencies were usually observed. 3 multiples (harmonics) of the respiratory frequency occurred in the spectrum suggesting that

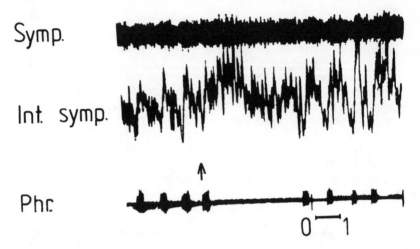

Figure 5. Diving reflex. ↑-superfusion of the nasopharyngeal cavities. Inhibition of augmented SA synchronous with
first post-apnoea phrenic burst.

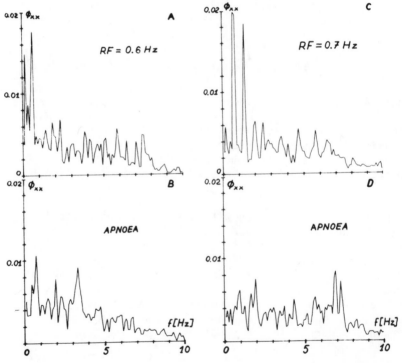

Figure 6. Averaged power density spectra of sympathetic

oscillations. RF - respiratory frequency. A - vagotomized rat with carotid sinus nerves cut. A peak corresponding to the respiratory frequency (0.6 Hz) is followed by 2 harmonics (1.2 and 1.8 Hz). Cardiac frequency in the range of 5 Hz insignificant. B - hypocapnic apnoea in the same animal. Respiratory related frequencies still present. A new peak in the range of 3-4 Hz. C - rat vagotomized with both carotid sinus nerves intact. Respiratory related frequencies and its harmonics present. Cardiac frequencies in the range 5 Hz. D - the same animal with hypocapnic apnoea. Respiratory related frequency and its harmonics reduced yet not abolished. Cardiac frequency in the spectrum shifted to the higher range of 7 Hz corresponding to hypocapnic increase in the heart rate.

sympathetic oscillations were entrained to the respiratory cycle in a 3:1 ratio. In sinoaortic denervated animals cardiac frequencies were significantly reduced. In hypocapnic apnoeic animals respiratory frequencies were depressed yet not entirely abolished. Other frequencies were also present (Fig. 6).

DISCUSSION AND CONCLUSIONS

Our data indicate that the pattern of rhythmical sympathetic activity over the respiratory cycle in rats is different and opposite to that known in cats. As this pattern of an augmented sympathetic discharge in expiration and of inspiratory depression is constant over a wide range of respiratory frequencies and occurs in a phase-spanning rather than phase-locked manner it is suggested that some subpopulations of phase-spanning respiratory related neurons are the source of this modulation, a suggestion made earlier in relation to the respiratory sympathetic oscillations of the cat (Cohen and Gootman, 1970, Bainton et al., 1985). In cats a strong depression of sympathetic activity in phase I expiration was explained as a possible influence of inhibitory neurons related to post-inspiratory activity (Bainton et al., 1985). In rats there is no sympathetic depression at this stage, on the contrary, a sympathetic discharge occurs. We were unable to record any postinspiratory activity of the phrenic nerve in the rat which makes sense in this species in which the respiratory frequency is very high, expiratory period short and any slowing of expiratory flow could impede ventilation.

Our results are consistent with the concept of Bainton et al. (1985) that both respiratory related central inhibition (in rats in early inspiration) and central facilitation (in rats during expiration) contribute to shaping the pattern of rhythmical sympathetic discharge.

As the sympathetic oscillations near respiratory frequency and its harmonics still occur during hypocapnic apnoea it seems that intrinsic sympathetic oscillations are entrained to some neuronal subpopulations of respiratory oscillator, a suggestion similar to that of Barman and Gebber (1976). Gilbey et al. (1985) observed 2 kinds of sympathetic preganglionic neurons in rats firing either in inspiration or in expiration. They did not report, however, if inspiratory related activity occurred in the early or in the late inspiration, where we observed also a gradual increase in the sympathetic activity.

Expiratory related sympathetic discharge may be of functional significance in the rat which seems to be a diving animal exhibiting a strong diving reflex (Lin 1974). Characteristic feature of the diving reflex is an expiratory apnoea (Angell-James et al., 1981). Reflex sympathetic response would be reinforced by expiratory related sympathetic discharge augmenting the peripheral vasoconstriction, an oxygen saving mechanism of functional adaptation to diving. Vagally mediated respiratory sinus arrhythmia exhibits a pattern similar to that in other species, a finding which indicates some co-activation of rhythmical vagal and sympathetic discharge in the rat, the former being dominant in controlling heart rate.

REFERENCES

Adrian ED, Bronk DW, Phillips G (1932). Discharges in mammalian sympathetic nerves. J Physiol (Lond) 74: 115-153.
Angell-James JE, Elsner R, de Burgh Daly M (1981). Lung inflation: effects of heart rate, respiration, and vagal afferent activity in seals. Am J Physiol 240: H190-H198.
Bainton CR, Richter DW, Seller H, Ballantyne D, Klein JP (1985). Respiratory modulation of sympathetic activity. J Aut Nerv System 12:77-90.
Barman SM, Gebber GL (1976). Basis for synchronization of sympathetic and phrenic nerve discharges. Am J Physiol 231:1601-1607.

Cohen MI, Gootman PM (1970). Periodicities in efferent discharge of splanchnic nerve of the cat. Am J Physiol 218:1092-1101.

Eckberg DL, Nerhed C, Wallin BG (1985). Respiratory modulation of muscle sympathetic and vagal cardiac outflow in man. J Physiol (Lond) 365:181-196.

Gilbey MP, Jordan D, Numao Y, Spyer KM, Wood LM (1985). Respiratory modulation of cervical sympathetic preganglionic neurones in the anaesthetized rat. J Physiol (Lond) 369:145P.

Gootman PM, Cohen MI, Di Russo SM, Rudel AP, Eberle LP (1984). Characteristics of spontaneous efferent splanchnic discharge in neonatal swine. In Usdin E, Dahlstrom A, Engel B, Carlsson A (eds) "Catecholamines: Basic and Peripheral Mechanisms" New York: Alan R Liss p 369.

Hukuhara T (1984). Cross-correlation analysis of phase relation between respiratory volleys in the phrenic sympathetic and vagus nerve activities under varied rhythm conditions. In Miyakawa K, Koepchen HP, Polosa C (eds) "Mechanisms of Blood Pressure Waves" Tokyo Berlin Heidelberg New York: Japan Scientific Societies Press, Springer Verlag, p. 65.

Janig W, Kummel H, Wiprich L (1980). Respiratory rhythmicities in vasoconstrictor and sudomotor neurones supplying the cats' hindlimb. In Koepchen HP, Hilton SM, Trzebski A (eds) "Central Interaction Between Respiratory and Cardiovascular Control System", Berlin Heidelberg New York: Springer Verlag, p. 128.

Koepchen HP, Klussendorf D, Sommer D (1981). Neurophysiological background of central neural cardiovascular-respiratory coordinations: basic remarks and experimental approach. J Aut Nerv System 3:335-368.

Koizumi K, Seller H, Kaufman A, McC Brooks C (1971). Patterns of sympathetic discharges and their relation to baroreceptor and respiratory activities. Brain Res 27:281-294.

Kollai M, Koizumi K (1980). Patterns of single unit activity in sympathetic postganglionic nerves. J Aut Nerv System 1:305-312.

Lin YC (1974). Autonomic nervous control of cardiovascular response during diving in the rat. Am J Physiol 227:601-605.

Lioy F, Hanna BD, Polosa C (1978). CO_2 dependent component of the neurogenic vascular tone in the cat. Pflugers Arch 374:187-191.

Lioy F, Trzebski A (1984). Pressor effect of CO_2 in the rat: different thresholds of the central cardiovascular and respiratory responses to CO_2. J Aut Nerv System 10:43-54.

Lipski J, Coote JH, Trzebski (1977). Temporal patterns of antidromic invasion latencies of sympathetic preganglionic neurons related to central inspiratory activity and pulmonary stretch receptor reflex. Brain Res 135: 162-166.

Millhorn DE (1986). Neural respiratory and circulatory interaction during chemoreceptor stimulation and cooling of ventral medulla in cats. J Physiol (Lond) 370: 217-231.

Okada H, Fox JJ (1967). Respiratory grouping of abdominal sympathetic activity in the dog. Am J Physiol 213:48-56.

Polosa C, Gerber U, Schondorf R (1980). Central mechanisms of interaction between sympathetic preganglionic neurons and the respiratory oscillator. In Koepchen HP, Hilton SM, Trzebski A (eds): "Central Interaction Between Respiratory and Cardiovascular Control Systems" Berlin Heidelberg New York: Springer Verlag, p 137.

Preiss G, Kirchner F, Polosa C (1975). Patterning of sympathetic preganglionic neuron firing by the central respiratory drive. Brain Res 87: 363-374.

Przybylski J, Trzebski A, Czyzewski T, Jodkowski J (1982). Altered ventilatory and circulatory responses to hyperoxia, hypoxia, hypercapnia and almitrine in spontaneously hypertensive rats. Bull Europ Physiopath Respirat 11:145-154.

Trzebski A (1980). Introduction. In Koepchen HP, Hilton SM, Trzebski A (eds) "Central Interaction Between Respiratory and Cardiovascular Control Systems" Berlin Heidelberg New York: Springer Verlag, p. 127.

Trzebski A, Kubin L (1981). Is the central inspiratory activity responsible for pCO_2-dependent chemical drive of the sympathetic activity? J Aut Nerv System 3:401-412.

**Organization of the Autonomic Nervous System:
Central and Peripheral Mechanisms, pages 153–167**
© **1987 Alan R. Liss, Inc.**

CARDIORESPIRATORY RELATIONSHIPS: CORRELATION BETWEEN THE
ACTIVITY OF CARDIAC VAGUS, SYMPATHETIC AND PHRENIC NERVES

Kiyomi Koizumi and Mark Kollai
Department of Physiology,
State University of New York
Health Science Center at Brooklyn
450 Clarkson Avenue, Brooklyn, NY 11203, USA

INTRODUCTION

In the past, little attention has been paid to the various manifestation, in which the modulation of autonomic nerve activity by the respiratory function can become apparent. Previous work suggested that during inspiration central inspiratory activity facilitates discharges in the majority of sympathetic preganglionic neurons and, at the same time, exerts an inhibitory influence on the firing of cardiac parasympathetic preganglionic neurons: during expiration, the sympathetic neurons are disfacilitated and the parasympathetic neurons are disinhibited (Preiss, Kirchner and Polosa, 1975; Polosa, Gerber and Schondorf, 1980; Spyer, 1981, 1982).
In reality, however, respiratory function is not a simple succession of uniform inspiratory and expiratory phases. Recently a third phase of the normal respiratory cycle was recognized, the "post-inspiratory" period or stage I expiration, which is characterized by a gradually declining pattern in phrenic activity (Richter, 1982). Also, it is common knowledge that the length and intensity of inspiration can vary from cycle to cycle, and that voluntary changes in respiration can produce changes in cardiac function, e.g., breath holding results in bradycardia. Recent research findings suggest that variations in breathing pattern may often modulate cardiovascular functioning in every day life (Hirsch and Bishop, 1981). In certain pathological conditions, such as cerebral hypoxia or ischemia, cardiovascular parameters fluctuate with a slow rhythm (e.g., Mayer waves) and a fluctuation with the same

period is also present in the phrenic activity (Koizumi, Terui and Kollai, 1984).

The aim of this study was a more detailed description of the central respiratory-cardiac relationship in the anesthetized dog. We simultaneously monitored the activity of peripheral respiratory and autonomic nerves and compared the activity patterns in a variety of situations occurring spontaneously.

METHODS

Preparation

Twenty eight dogs (12-16 kg in body weight) were anesthetized initially with ketamine hydrochloride (20 mg/kg) given intraperitoneally. The trachea was cannulated, catheters were inserted into the left femoral artery for blood pressure recording, in the femoral vein for drug and fluid administration, and through a branch of the femoral artery to obtain blood samples for pH and blood gas analyses. When the effect of the short-acting anesthetic, ketamine, began to wear off, alpha-chloralose (5% solution in 3% sodium-borate) was administrated intravenously until a dosage of 80-100 mg/kg was reached. Supplemental injections of chloralose (10-20 mg/kg i.v.) were given whenever necessary. Succinylcholine chloride (1 mg/kg) was injected intravenously when recording of nerve activity started.

The chest was opened under artificial ventilation using a mixture of room air and O_2. A pressure of 3cm H_2O was applied on the expiration side of the respiratory pump. The amounts of O_2 mixed in the inspired air as well as the ventilatory volume were adjusted according to results of the blood gas analyses. The arterial pO_2 and pCO_2 were maintained at normal levels. When needed, bicarbonate solution (4.2%) was given intravenously to adjust the acid base balance. Body temperature, measured intraesophageally, was maintained at 38-38.5°C by heating the table top and by use of an overhead lamp.

Nerve Recordings

The cardiac vagal and sympathetic nerves as well as the phrenic nerve and the internal branch of the 6th intercostal nerve were dissected on the right side of the chest. All efferent branches of the right stellate ganglion were severed in order to eliminate the activity of sympathetic fibers present in the vagal nerves. The ventral branch of the ansa subclavia was prepared for recording. The cranio-vagal or caudo-vagal nerves (Mizeres, 1955) were dissected as close as possible to the heart and left intact except for one or two small branches which were cut and used for recording. In this way vagal influence on the heart was not much disturbed. Nerve activities were recorded by standard electrophysiological techniques.

Record Analysis

For quantitative measurement of the nerve activities the following methods were used. Since in vagal, phrenic and expiratory nerve recordings separate action potential could be recognized, the number of spikes were counted. Sympathetic discharges were also counted as above if the nerve activity had spiky appearance; when the activity consisted of compound action potentials, it was integrated by an area integrator. In a few instances, the sympathetic nerve recordings were made first from a whole nerve and the activity was quantified by use of the area integrator. Then the nerve was split into multifiber preparations so that individual action potentials could be counted. The results indicated that, as far as the type of experiments carried out in this study was concerned, changes measured by both methods were similar. Therefore, we used either method of assessing changes in sympathetic activity and in comparing sympathetic with vagal activity. Occasionally the nerve activities were integrated by a leaky integrator (time constant, 0.1-0.005 sec). The integrated or counted records obtained every 1 or 2 sec were displayed on a Grass polygraph on which blood pressure, heart rate (by a tachograph, triggered by the pressure pulse), the level of CO_2 in the end-expired air and trachea pressure were also recorded. All data were recorded on magnetic tape and histograms were produced offline (Nicolet 170).

RESULTS

1. Two Types of Respiratory-modulated Discharge Patterns in Cardiac Nerves. Their Relation to Post-inspiratory Phrenic Nerve Activity

During our earlier work we observed that the distri-

bution of cardiac vagal and sympathetic discharges during
the respiratory cycle could vary greatly from experiment to
experiment. The present study revealed a distinct relationship between cardiac autonomic discharge pattern and the
presence or absence of post-inspiratory phrenic activity.
Out of 28 experiments, in 12 no phrenic activity was observed in expiration (type 1), while in 10 experiments
phrenic activity was present in early expiration (type 2).
In the remaining 6 the post-inspiratory phrenic activity

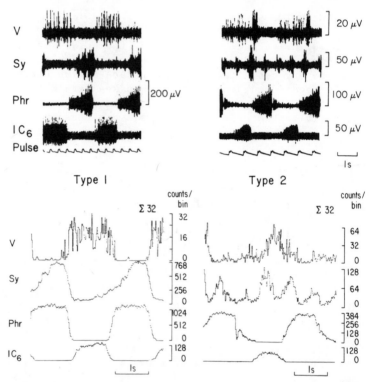

Figure 1. Type 1 and type 2 patterns in ongoing autonomic
and respiratory nerve activities. Upper part: Electrical activity in cardiac vagal, cardiac sympathetic, phrenic and
expiratory intercostal (IC6) nerves (from top downwards).
These abbreviations apply to all subsequent figures. Bottom
trace is arterial pulse. Lower part: Time histograms of ongoing discharges in nerve listed above, triggered from the
rising phase of RC integrated phrenic discharges (time constant 0.1 s); 32 sweeps, 20 ms bins. Note difference in
magnitude of count/bin for type 1 and 2.

was present during some cycles only. Cardiac autonomic
activity was found to exhibit characteristic differences in
type 1 and type 2 cases (Fig. 1).

In the type 1 case, vagal discharges started to appear
immediately after the cessation of phrenic discharges, and
exhibited a steady firing rate throughout expiration. Expiratory nerve activity appeared in a fashion similar to
that of vagal discharges (Koizumi, Terui and Kollai, 1983),
while sympathetic activity was mostly in phase with phrenic
activity. This is more or less the "classic" picture,
which has been reported by several laboratories in the past
(Koizumi, Seller, Kaufman and Brooks, 1971; Preiss,
Kirchner and Polosa, 1975; Preiss and Polosa, 1977; Polosa,
Gerber and Schondorf, 1980; Spyer, 1981, 1982).

In the type 2 case phrenic activity, after it subsided,
increased again in early expiration and this "afterdischarge" was often separated from the main phrenic activity
which occurred during inspiration by a short silent period.
The afterdischarge usually lasted for nearly one third of
the expiratory period. Respiratory physiologists refer to
this period as post-inspiration or stage-1 expiration
(Richter, 1982). Vagal nerve activity invariably showed
the following characteristic pattern in the type 2 case:
Relatively little activity was present during the post-inspiratory period, then, as phrenic-afterdischarge gradually
subsided, the magnitude of pulse synchronous vagal bursts
started to increase, reaching the maximum level toward the
later phase of expiration. As for sympathetic activity, the
picture was less uniform. The pattern shown in Fig. 1 was
observed in about half of type 2 cases; sympathetic activity
was less during post-inspiration, then reached its maximum
during the later phase of expiration from where it fell
gradually till the next expiration. In the rest of type 2
cases there was a second peak in sympathetic activity during
late inspiration which equalled or exceeded the one during
expiration.

Additional observations were made relative to the type
1 and the type 2 case. First, using standard preparative
and recording procedures phrenic activity, measured as the
average number of spikes counted per unit time, was always
stronger (or higher) in the cases with the type 1 than in
those with the type 2 pattern. Second, mean vagal firing
rate was usually higher in the type 2 compared to the type
1 and neurons were regularly active not only during the expiratory phase but also during the first quarter of inspiration. Comparison of activity levels recorded from nerve

bundles in different experiments would not be ordinarily
permissible, but the fact that heart rate was always significantly lower in the type 2 than the type 1 (82 ± 19 vs.
152 ± 36 beats/min, mean ± SE), made the higher vagal
activity level likely. Third, respiratory cycle length in
the type 2 case was often an integer multiple of cardiac
cycle length. This ratio made possible the formation of
pulse synchronous groups in the histograms of Fig. 1, when
the histograms were triggered from the rising phase of RC-
integrated phrenic activity. The apparent synchronization
of cardiac and respiratory cycle length could be explained
as a result of baroreceptor interference with the relatively weak inspiratory activity, i.e., central inspiratory
drive was able to commence its rise only in the absence of
baroreceptor firing. Baroreceptor activity has been reported to inhibit respiratory activity (Brunner, et al.
1982).

2. Alternating Phrenic Discharges

    In most of the experiments phrenic activity was regu-
lar, and with the vagi intact, the rate was set by the
respiratory pump. Occasionally, however, after cardiovascular tests were applied or anesthetics were administered, or laryngeal afferents were stimulated, at other

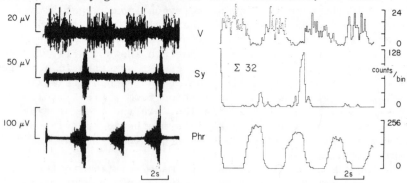

Figure 2. Discharge patterns of cardiac vagal and sympathetic nerves associated with alternating phrenic activity.
Left panel: nerve activity recordings. Right panel: time
histograms (32 sweeps, 80 ms bins), triggered from the peak
of the RC integrated large phrenic bursts (time constant
0.1 s).

times without any obvious reason, periods of transient irregularity occurred. The pattern shown in Fig. 2 was triggered by the injection of 10 mg/kg chloralose, given in order to maintain the proper level of anesthesia, and persisted for several minutes. The intensity of phrenic discharges alternated, weaker and stronger bursts followed each other in regular succession. Vagal firing was inhibited in each period of phrenic activity regardless of its intensity. Since the inhibition was near complete during both weak and strong phrenic activity, no alternating pattern appeared in vagal firing. Sympathetic activity, on the other hand, followed the phrenic pattern in such a way that only strong phrenic activity was associated with a substantial level of sympathetic activity, during weak phrenic activity sympathetic fibers remained almost silent. It is of interest that "weak" and "strong" phrenic discharge did not differ much in terms of quantity in nerve activity; the histograms of Fig. 2, which were triggered by the peak of the RC-integrated "strong" phrenic burst, demonstrate that the total number of active fibers was not much different during weak and strong phrenic firing. This is probably due to recruitment of a few large diameter phrenic axons producing large spikes at the later part of the strong phrenic discharge, when most of the sympathetic facilitation occurred. It should be noted, that with the appearance of phrenic activity vagal discharges were inhibited first and sympathetic discharges appeared later.

3. Effect of Lung Inflation

Pulmonary stretch receptors are activated at each stroke of the respiratory pump, therefore it was of interest to determine to what extent did pulmonary stretch receptors contribute to the modulation of cardiac autonomic activity. We studied those situations when the pump cycle period became dissociated from the phrenic cycle. In these cases it was frequently observed that phrenic cycle period was a multiple integer of the former and the rhythm became entrained by the pump, as it did in Fig. 3, which was reported to occur at higher levels of pCO_2 (Bainton, Kirkwood and Sears, 1978). This configuration had the advantage of showing the effect of lung inflation alone and also the simultaneous effect of lung inflation and central inspiratory activity, representing a condition closer to normal. Inflation of the lung alone produced inhibition in both vagal and sympathetic activities. When inflation of the

lung alone produced inhibition in both vagal and sympathetic activities. When inflation of the lung coincided with
the phrenic discharge the inhibition of the vagal activity
became more accentuated and lasted longer. For the sympathetic activity the inhibition became shorter and was confined to the early phase of inspriation. As the rate of
phrenic discharges increased in the later part of inspiration, sympathetic activity also increased.

    We must emphasize that the recordings in Fig. 3 show a
clear example, but the effect of lung inflation generally
was weak and variable, in some cases it had no inhibitory
effect at all, unless the gas volume inflating the lung was
increased several times.

4. Quasi-continuous Phrenic Activity

    The behavior of cardiac autonomic activity during slow
wave fluctuations of blood pressure and heart rate (e.g.,
Mayer waves) was described in our recent work (Koizumi,
Terui and Kollai, 1984). The present re-examination revealed that changes in respiratory activity were also involved
in the phenomenon. A single cycle from a long-lasting
fluctuation is illustrated in Fig. 4. The cycle started
with a depression of vagal activity and an augmentation of

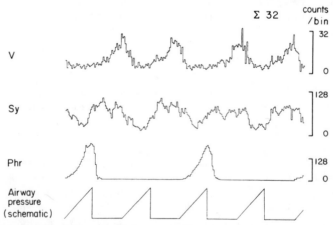

Figure 3. Effect of lung inflation of cardiac vagal, cardiac sympathetic and phrenic nerve activities (32 sweeps, 50
ms bins). The sweep was triggered from the rising phase in
airway pressure (bottom trace) produced by the respiratory
pump. Schematic diagram of airway pressure was drawn from
polygraph tracings.

sympathetic activity resulting in a wave of tachycardia and
blood pressure elevation. Simultaneously phrenic activity
exhibited characteristic changes; during inspiration phrenic activity increased considerably compared to previous
levels and in addition a moderate level of phrenic activity
was present during the expiratory period, where there was
complete silence before. This meant that phrenic activity
was present continuously for three respiratory cycles, and

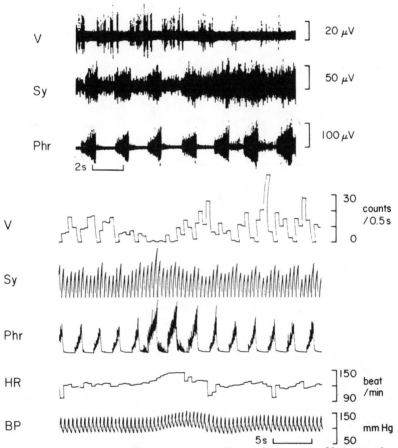

Figure 4. One cycle of cardiovascular slow wave fluctuation.
Upper panel: recordings from cardiac vagal, cardiac sympathetic and phrenic nerves. Lower panel, from top to bottom:
counted action potentials of vagal nerve, area integram of
sympathetic nerve activity, RC integram of phrenic nerve
activity (time constant 5 ms), heart rate and arterial blood
pressure.

only its intensity changed during inspiratory and expiratory phases. Therefore we called this phrenic pattern "quasi-continuous". As for the secondary changes, vagal activity increased afterwards, presumably as a result of the pressor response. It appears likely that the continuously active inspiratory neurons contributed to the creation of suppressed vagal and increased sympathetic activity during this slow wave pressure.

DISCUSSION

Critique of Methods

The experiments were done in animals with the vagi and carotid sinus nerves intact. Such preparation has the advantage of preserving tonic cardiac vagal discharges, which was essential in the present study, since the existence of the vagal activity was found to depend on the integrity of peripheral baroreceptor function (Kunze, 1972; Kollai and Koizumi, 1979). At the same time, the preparation presents the problem, as to what extent the observed respiratory autonomic patterns are the products of central interactions or the products of reflex effects from pulmonary stretch receptors and arterial baroreceptors.

We observed that inflation of the lung had inhibitory influence on both the cardiac sympathetic and parasympathetic activity. This, usually weak and variable effect, was reported earlier, separately for the sympathetic and parasympathetic system (Daly and Robinson, 1968; Gandevia, McCloskey and Potter, 1978; Potter, 1981). The inhibitory influence might have been a factor that contributed to the shaping of the autonomic discharge profile along the respiratory cycle, though probably not a relevant one. In the present experiments the airway pressure wave either coincided with or lagged behind, the phrenic discharge contour (Breuer-Hering reflex). When the airway pressure wave coincided with the peak of phrenic discharge contour the inhibitory effect of lung inflation on vagal activity probably added little to the inhibition that was deriving from central inspiratory activity (Potter, 1981). It might have, however, contributed to the development of inhibtion of sympathetic activity in the early inspiratory period, that was detected in some of the type 2 pattern. When the peak airway pressure lagged behind the peak of phrenic activity, the effect of lung inflation might have contributed to the depression of the autonomic activity during the post-inspiratory period in the type 2 case, but it did not seem to affect the commencement of vagal firing. We concluded that the influence of lung inflation was probably minor, since when the respirator was turned off, little change was observed in the autonomic nerve activity pattern during the next few respiratory cycles. As for the modulatory influence of arterial baroreceptor activity due to respiratory related fluctuations in systemic arterial pressure, our present data do not allow us to discuss their possible contribution in the formation of respiratory related cardiac autonomic patterns. Nevertheless, the basic forms of the type 1 and 2 patterns were clearly observed in nerve recordings when arterial pressure remained fairly constant. Also, our preliminary findings with controlled baroreceptor activity indicate that the arterial baroreceptor reflex is relatively unimportant in this respect (Kollai and Koizumi, in preparation).

Different Types of Respiratory-Autonomic Activity Patterns

Variability in respiration-related autonomic activity patterns is evident in the documentation of many earlier works, even though these differences have rarely been discussed. In vagal activity, both the type 1 and the type 2 patterns could be identified in earlier records (Jewett, 1964; Davidson, Goldner and McCloskey, 1976); in studies done in cats the type 1 pattern dominated, which might be partly the consequence of experimental procedures, i.e., vagal activity was induced by local application of exciting amino acids (McAllen and Spyer, 1978). Variability in sympathetic activity was reported in the form of changes in the phase-relationship between slow waves in sympathetic and respiratory nerve activities (Barman and Gebber, 1976). In respiratory activity, the post-inspiratory phase was emphasized only later (Richter, 1982); in earlier reports it was often difficult to judge the presence of post-inspiratory activity since most integrams were presented with slow time constants (usually 0.1 sec), which probably masked the declining pattern of post-inspiratory activity, if it was present at all.

Based on our results and data of the literature it seems likely that the changing qualities of central respiratory activity contributed in creating different autonomic patterns; the time course of central inspiratory activity defined the period when vagal activity was inhibited, and its intensity determined whether and when sympathetic activity was facilitated. In the type 1 pattern, inspiratory activity (assessed by monitoring phrenic discharges) was strong and ended abruptly, resulting in facilitation of sympathetic activity during inspiration and prompt resumption of vagal firing at the end of inspiration. In the type 2 pattern inspiratory activity was relatively weaker, therefore it did not facilitate or entrain sympathetic activity and post-inspiratory activity allowed vagal firing to occur only during later expiration. Activity patterns associated with alternating phrenic discharges or slow wave fluctuations could be interpreted on a similar basis.

Discussion of the type 1 and 2 patterns inevitably leads to the question, under what conditions would they occur, or which one is normal. It may be that the type 1 pattern reflects the slight hypoxic condition of certain brainstem areas due to impaired local circulation, even in the face of normal blood gas values. Such situations could develop in long experiments which are necessary to perform these studies. This assumption is supported by the observations that in these type 1 cases discharge rates of both inspiratory and expiratory nerves were higher than those observed in the type 2, and also the post-inhibitory period, which is regarded to be part of a normal respiratory cycle (Richter, 1982), was missing. In a few experiments we indeed observed that lowering the arterial pO_2 tended to turn the type 2 pattern into the type 1, but raising the arterial pO_2 rarely changed the type 1 into the type 2 pattern. Supporting this argument is the report that hyperventilation, which diminished phrenic activity, produced phase shift between phrenic activity and the slow wave component of the sympathetic activity (Barman and Gebber, 1976). In many of the earlier studies where mostly the type 1 pattern was reported, artificial respiration was adjusted to maintain normal end tidal CO_2 levels. At present it is well established that with normal end tidal CO_2 values arterial pO_2 can reach critically low levels, especially when extensive thoracic surgery was performed. In brief, we regard the type 2 pattern to be a closer representation of normal conditions.

SUMMARY

1. The respiratory-cardiac relationship was investigated by studying cardiac autonomic nerve discharges.

Activity in cardiac sympathetic and parasympathetic nerves as well as in phrenic and expiratory spinal nerves was recorded simultaneously in chloralose anesthetized and paralyzed dogs, ventilated with a mixture of room air and O_2.

2. Patterns of activity in cardiac sympathetic and vagal nerves in relation to the respiratory cycle was found to depend on the presence or absence of phrenic after-discharge during early expiration.

3. When the intensity of phrenic firing varied to a great extent the intensity of sympathetic activity was modulated accordingly. The period of vagal inhibition during the inspiratory phase was determined only by the duration of phrenic firing.

4. Inflation of the lung produced inhibition in both cardiac sympathetic and vagal activity, though the effect was usually weak and variable.

5. During the slow wave of blood pressure and heart rate fluctuations (e.g., Mayer wave) phrenic activity tended to become continuous, sympathetic activity increased and vagal activity diminished.

6. It was concluded that the primary factor in creating different patterns in cardiac autonomic activity was the varying parameters of central inspiratory activity: its time course defined the period when vagal activity was inhibited and its intensity modulated the level of sympathetic facilitation.

ACKNOWLEDGEMENT

This work was supported by a grant from the U.S. Public Health Service, National Institute of Health, NS-00847.

REFERENCES

Bainton CR, Kirkwood A, Sears TA (1978). On the transmission of the stimulating effects of carbon dioxide to the muscles of respiration. J Physiol (Lond) 280:249-272.

Barman, SM, Gebber GL (1976). Basis for synchronization of sympathetic and phrenic nerve discharges. Am J Physiol 231:1601-1607.

Brunner MJ, Susman MS, Green AS, Kallman CH, Shoukas AA (1982). Carotid sinus baroreceptor control respriation. Circ Res 51:624-636.

Daly M De B, Robinson BH (1968). An analysis of the reflex systemic vasodilator response elicited by lung inflation in the dog. J Physiol (Lond) 195:387–406.

Davidson NS, Goldner S, McCloskey DI (1976). Respiratory modulation of baroreceptor and chemoreceptor reflexes affecting heart rate and cardiac vagal efferent nerve activity. J Physiol (Lond) 259:523–530.

Gandevia SS, McCloskey DI, Potter EK (1978). Inhibition of baroreceptor and chemoreceptor reflexes on heart rate by afferents from the lungs. J Physiol (Lond) 276:369–381.

Gilbey MP, Jordan D, Richter DW, Spyer KM (1984). Synaptic mechanisms involved in the inspiratory modulation of vagal cardioinhibitory neurones in the cat. J Physiol (Lond) 356:65–78.

Hirsch J, Bishop B (1981). Respiratory sinus arrhythmia in humans: How breathing pattern modulates heart rate. Am J Physiol 241:H620–H629.

Jewett DL (1964). Activity of single efferent fibers in the cervical vagus nerve of the dog, with special reference to possible cardioinhibitory fibers. J Physiol (Lond) 175:321–357.

Koizumi K, Terui N, Kollai M (1983). Neural control of the heart; significance of double innervation re-examined. J Auton Nerv Syst 7:279–294.

Koizumi K, Terui N, Kollai M (1984). Relationships between vagal and sympathetic activities in rhythmic fluctuations. In Miyakawa K, Koepchen HP, Polosa C (eds): "Mechanisms of Blood Pressure Waves." Tokyo: Japan Sci Soc Press and Berlin: Springer-Verlag, pp 43–56.

Kollai M, Koizumi K (1979). Reciprocal and non-reciprocal action of the vagal and sympathetic nerves innervating the heart. J Auton Nerv Syst 1:33–52.

Kunze DL (1972). Reflex discharge patterns of cardiac vagal efferent fibres. J Physiol (Lond) 222:1–15.

McAllen RM, Spyer KM (1978). The baroreceptor input to cardiac vagal motoneurones. J Physiol (Lond) 282:365–374.

Mizeres NJ (1955). The anatomy of the autonomic nervous system in the dog. Am J Anat 96:285–318.

Polosa C, Gerber Y, Schondorf HR (1980). Central mechanisms of interaction between sympathetic preganglionic neurones and respiratory oscillator. In Koepchen HP, Hilton SM, Trzebski A (eds): "Central Interaction Between Respiratory and Circulatory Control Systems," Berlin: Springer-Verlag, pp. 137–143.

Potter EK (1981). Inspiratory inhibition of vagal responses to baroreceptor and chemoreceptor stimuli in the dog.

J Physiol (Lond) 316:177-190.
Preiss G, Kirchner F, Polosa C (1975). Patterning of sympathetic preganglionic neuron firing by the central respiratory drive. Brain Res 87:363-374.
Preiss G, Polosa C (1977). The relation between end-tidal CO_2 and discharge patterns of sympathetic preganglionic neurons. Brain Res 122:255-267.
Richter DW (1982). Generation and maintenance of the respiratory rhythm. J Exp Biol 100:93-107.
Spyer KM (1981). Neural organization and control of the baroreceptor reflex. Review in Physiology, Biochemistry and Pharmacology 88:23-124.
Spyer KM (1982). Central nervous integration of cardiovascular control. J Exp Biol 100:109-128.

Organization of the Autonomic Nervous System:
Central and Peripheral Mechanisms, pages 169–178
© 1987 Alan R. Liss, Inc.

PHASE CHANGES OF SYMPATHETIC ACTIVITY WITH RESPIRATION
BEFORE AND AFTER PONTINE LESIONS

R.D. Wurster and C.A. Connelly.

Department of Physiology, Loyola University
Medical Center, Maywood, IL 60153 and
Rehabilitation Research and Development Center,
Hines VA Center, Hines, IL 60141

INTRODUCTION

Sympathetic nerve activity demonstrates different
types of rhythmic activity. One of the major, characteristic
rhythms is often synchronized with respiration and is called
the sympathetic respiratory-like slow wave activity(Fig. 1).

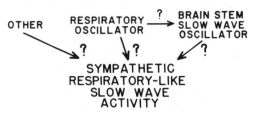

Figure 1. Possible sources of sympathetic respiratory-like
slow wave activity.

Brain stem respiratory oscillatory circuits, as well as
other inputs, may impart this slow rhythm to sympathetic
central nervous system networks(Koepchen,1983). Alternately,
Barman and Gebber(1976) have proposed that this rhythm is
due to a hypothetical slow sympathetic oscillator of brain
stem origin. This oscillator has a period similar to that of
respiration and is referred to here as the sympathetic brain
stem slow wave oscillator. Although this oscillator may be
usually synchronized to the respiratory oscillator, it was
proposed that it could be separated or revealed following
hyperventilation to apnea. However, Connelly and Wurster

(1985) were unable convincingly to separate the slow wave activity from the respiratory cycle during hyperventilation. Futhermore, midline medullary lesions, which interrupt respiratory activity but not sympathetic reflexes, did not reveal a separate brain stem slow wave oscillator (Kubin et al, 1985 and Connelly and Wurster, 1984). Another way to separate these oscillators may be to produce apneustic breathing patterns by placing lesions in the parabrachial regions, resulting in slow breathing patterns with long inspiratory periods.

METHODS:

In eleven, alpha chloralose (40-60 mg/Kg) anesthetized cats, phrenic and inferior cardiac sympathetic neurograms were recorded by means of bipolar electrodes, AC amplifiers and "leaky" integrators(time constant 0.5 to 0.005 sec). Each cat was vagotomized, paralyzed (iv succinyl choline, 6 mg/kg.hr) and artificially ventilated. End-tidal pCO2 was monitored, as well as arterial pO2 and pH. To maintain blood gases and pH in a normal range (pO2>100 mmHg, pH = 7.34-7.40 and end-expiratory %CO2 = 4.5%), respirator frequency and depth were varied and 8.4% sodium bicarbonate was administered intravenously. Rectal temperature was maintained at 38 $\pm$ 1 C with a servo-regulated heating pad. Arterial blood pressure was monitored via a femoral arterial cannula, pressure transducer and oscillograph. After securing the head in a stereotaxic frame, a craniotomy was performed and bipolar coaxial lesioning electrodes were placed in the pontine parabrachial region of both sides. Following control measurements, bilateral pontine parabrachial area lesions were made using direct current (2 milliamps for 15 seconds). The lesions sites were histologically verified following the experiment. Spectral analysis was performed on the sympathetic activity (0 to 20 Hz, bin width = 0.05 Hz, 16 averages/spectrum). Baroreflex sensitivity was assessed by noting the pressor reflex responses to baroreceptor hypotension produced by bilateral carotid artery occlusion.

RESULTS:

From the phrenic neurogram, three phases of the respiratory cycle were noted: inspiration, post-inspiration and expiration (Fig. 2)(Richter and Ballantyne, 1983).

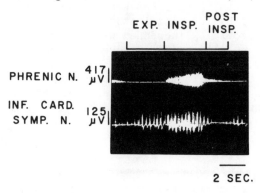

Figure 2. Oscilloscope tracings of phrenic and inferior cardiac sympathetic (INF. CARD. SYMP. N.) neurograms. The three phases of respiratory cycle are indicated: expiration (EXP.), inspiration (INSP.) and post-inspiration (POST INSP.)

Following a very brief inhibition at the beginning of inspiration as noted by Bainton et al(1985), sympathetic activity increased with the initiation of inspiration, markedly decreased during post-inspiration, and returned to preinspiratory levels during expiration. In most cats, the inspiratory-related increase in sympathetic activity was followed 2-5 seconds later by an increased arterial blood pressure. This reflexly induced inhibition of sympathetic activity coincided with the post-inspiratory phase (Fig. 3).

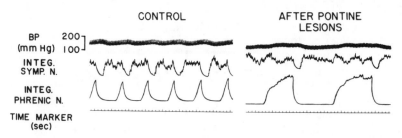

Figure 3. Integrated sympathetic and phrenic neurograms and blood pressure changes before (CONTROL) and after pontine lesions.

Following lesions of the parabrachial area, classic apneustic breathing patterns were produced, which were characterized by long inspiratory periods (Fig. 3). Sympathetic activity increased with the beginning of inspiration resulting in an increased blood pressure after a few seconds. The blood pressure changes induced a reflex inhibition of sympathetic activity which after another delay resulted in a decreased blood pressure. This decreased blood pressure could induce another increase of sympathetic activity in some cats (Fig. 4).

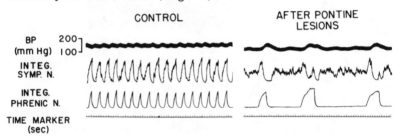

Figure 4. Integrated phrenic and sympathetic neurograms and blood pressure before (CONTROL) and after bilateral pontine lesions- reflex secondary oscillations of blood pressure and sympathetic activity.

Hence, oscillations of sympathetic activity and blood pressure were induced with a period approximately equal to twice the delay time between sympathetic activity and blood pressure changes. These oscillations often had frequencies quite similar to the respiratory frequencies before pontine lesions were made (Fig. 5).

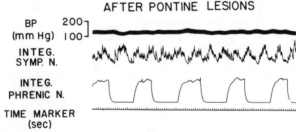

Figure 5. Integrated phrenic and sympathetic neurograms and blood pressure after bilateral pontine lesions - sustained sympathetic and blood pressure oscillations similar to pattern before lesions.

To analyze the low frequency characteristics of the sympathetic neurograms, spectral analysis was performed before and after the bilateral pontine lesions (Fig. 6). Due to the band pass filters of the AC amplifier and integrator circuit, marked attenuation of frequencies greater than about one Hz occurred. In all cats a very large slow spectral peak occurred at a frequency identical to the respiratory cycle. Another characteristic peak had a frequency similar to the cardiac cycle but was greatly attentuated due to the low pass filter.

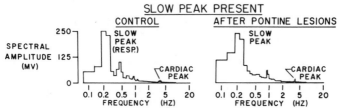

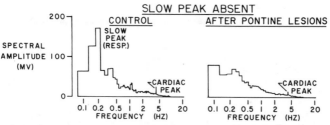

Figure 6. Spectral analysis of sympathetic nerve activity representing two groups of cats before (CONTROL) and after bilateral pontine lesions. The amplitudes of the higher frequencies are attenuated by the low pass filter of the recording system.

Six out of eleven cats had marked attenuation of the slow respiratory-like peak (Fig. 6, bottom). In the five other cats, the slow wave component showed little or no change from eupnic breathing patterns before the lesion to apneustic breathing patterns following the bilateral parabrachial area lesions (Fig. 6, top).

In some animals, the sympathetic-baroreflex oscillations were slower than the respiratory frequency and so large that they dominated over the respiratory pattern of the sympathetic nerve activity (Fig. 7). Thus, the respiratory effects on sympathetic activity were modulated by the phase relationship of the sympathetic-baroreflex oscillations.

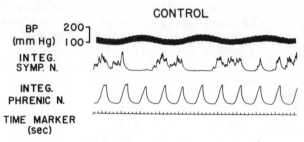

Figure 7. Baroreflex-modulation of the respiratory effects on sympathetic activity in a control.

In other cats, the sympathetic-baroreflex oscillation was so dominant that no apparent association was readily discernible between phrenic and sympathetic neurograms (Fig. 8).

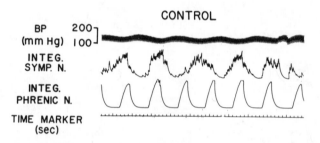

Figure 8. Disassociation of slow-wave activity and respiration in a control cat.

The induced blood pressure oscillations were typically 5 to 20 mm Hg. These sympathetic oscillations were characteristic particularly of cats with marked baroreceptor responses. When baroreflexes diminished, the slow wave oscillation diminished. These oscillations also disappeared during bilateral carotid occlusion although the respiratory-related activity was still able to induce some increases and decreases of sympathetic activity. Furthermore, testing of the reflex responses to bilateral carotid occlusion (baroreceptor hypotension) indicated that the pressor reflex was statistically greater in those cats which had an independent slow wave activity following parabrachial area lesions than those which lost their slow wave component (75 versus 60 mm Hg arterial pressure

increment, p<0.05). These observations support the notion
that the slow wave activity of sympathetic nerves often may
not represent an independent brain stem oscillator but
rather represent an oscillation due to the delayed
inhibitory feedback from the baroreceptors. Depending on the
delay loop time, these oscillations may mimick frequencies
of the respiratory oscillator and may often be synchronized
with the respiratory oscillator.

DISCUSSION:

Since the early recordings of sympathetic activity,
investigators recognized the importance of the respiratory
cycle on sympathetic activity. In 1932 Adrian et al recorded
sympathetic nerve activity in anesthetized cats. They noted
that the sympathetic activity increased corresponding with
the inspiration. Several other groups have studied the
relationship between respiratory activity and sympathetic
nerve activity (Okada and Fox, 1967; Seller et al, 1968;
Koizumi et al, 1971; Gootman and Cohen,1974; Preiss et al,
1975; Lipski et al, 1977; Kubin et al, 1979; Polosa et al,
1980). Koepchen(1983) has skillfully reviewed and
synthesized much of this literature.
Recordings of sympathetic activity of unanesthetized
human demonstrate similar responses. Hagbarth and Vallbo
(1967) found that sympathetic activity increased during
expiration. Delius et al(1972) also recorded from human
sympathetic fibers and noted "no rhythmic fluctuations in
the vasoconstrictor outflow that occurred independently of
preceding blood pressures waves". Janig et al (1983)
compared the sympathetic activity of anesthetized cats with
unanesthetized humans. They stated that the respiratory
modulations of sympathetic discharge has two components: one
related to respiratory-induced blood pressure changes and
the second due to central neuronal coupling of respiratory
and "vascular" neurons.
Much of the slow wave sympathetic rhythms and the
phase relationship between the phrenic and sympathetic
activity will vary depending upon the respiratory frequency,
pattern (eg. apneustic patterns) and depth and baroreflex
sensitivity. It is impressive that these oscillations or
phase changes may be mediated by rather small phasic blood
pressure changes. Hence, demonstration of a slow wave
independent sympathetic oscillator of brain stem origin
requires the elimination of the possible

sympathetic-baroreflex oscillations. Even baroreceptor activity from non-carotid or aortic receptors may be capable of establishing these oscillations. Thus, it may be difficult to remove all of the cardiovascular afferent feedback producing by slow wave activity.

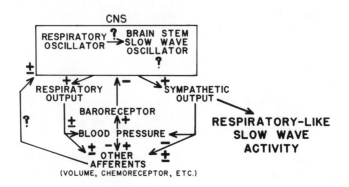

Figure 9. Schematic summary of generation of respiratory-like slow wave activity of sympathetic nerves.

In conclusion, the phase relationship of sympathetic and respiratory activities, as well as much of the slow wave sympathetic activity, may depend upon the nature of the respiration and the baroreflex rather than on an independent brain stem oscillator(Fig. 9). The mechanics of respiration may also produce changes of blood pressure providing feedback inhibition of sympathetic activity via various afferents. This does not entirely eliminate the possibility that other slow wave sympathetic oscillations may be due to other reflexes or a separate brain stem oscillator in the experimental preparations. However, it is clear that the two major causes for respiratory-like slow activity of sympathetic nerves is due to activity from the respiratory oscillator and baroreflexes.

REFERENCES

Adrian ED, Bronk DW, Phillips (1932). Discharges in mammalian sympathetic nerves. J Physiol (Lond.) 74: 115-153.

Bainton CR, Richter DW, Seller H, Ballantyne D, Klein JP (1985). Respiratory modulation of sympathetic activity. J Auton Nerv Syst 12: 77-90.

Barman SM, Gebber GL (1976). Basis for synchronization of sympathetic and phrenic nerve discharges. Am J Physiol 231: 1601-1607.

Connelly CA, Wurster RD (1984). Effects of midline medullary lesions on the respiratory modulation of sympathetic nerve activity. Fed Proc 43: 402.

Connelly CA, Wurster RD (1985). Sympathetic rhythms during hyperventilation-induced apnea. Am J Physiol 249: R424-R431.

Delius W, Hagbarth KE, Hongell A, Wallin BG (1972). General characteristics of sympathetic activity in human muscle nerves. Acta Physiol Scand 84: 65-81.

Gootman PM, Cohen MI (1974). The interrelationships between sympathetic discharge and central respiratory drive. In Umbach W, Koepchen HP(eds): "Central-Rhythmic and Regulation," Stuttgart: Hippokrates-Verlag, pp 195-209.

Hagbarth KE, Vallbo AB (1968). Pulse and respiratory grouping of sympathetic impulses in human muscle nerves. Acta Physiol Scand 74: 96-108.

Jänig W, Sundlöf G and Wallin BG (1983). Discharge patterns of sympathetic neurons supplying skeletal muscle and skin in man and cat. J Auton Nerv Syst 7: 239-256.

Koepchen HP (1983). Respiratory and cardiovascular "centres": Functional entirety or separate structures?. In Schläfke ME, Koepchen HP and See WR (eds): "Central Neurone Environment," Berlin: Springer Verlag, pp 221-237.

Koizumi K, Seller H, Kaufman A, McC Brooks C (1971). Pattern of sympathetic discharges and their relation to baroreceptor and respiratory activities. Brain Res 27: 281-294.

Kubin L, Trzebski A, Lipski J (1985). Split medulla preparation in the cat: arterial chemoreceptor and respiratory modulation of the renal sympathetic nerve activity. J Auton Nerv Syst 12: 211-225.

Lipski J, Coote JH, Trzebski A (1977). Temporal patterns of antidromic invasion latencies of sympathetic preganglionic neurons related to central inspiratory activity and pulmonary stretch receptor reflex. Brain Res 135: 162-166.

Okada H, Fox IJ (1967). Respiratory grouping of abdominal sympathetic activity in the dog. Amer J Physiol 213: 48-56.

Polosa C, Gerber U, Schondorf R (1980). Central mechnisms of interaction between sympathetic preganglionic neurons and the respiratory oscillator. In Koepchen HP, Hilton SM and Trzebski A(eds): "Central Interaction Between Respiratory and Cardiovascular Control Systems," Berlin: Springer Verlag, pp 137-143.
Preiss G, Kirchner F, Polosa C (1975). Patterning of sympathetic preganglionic neuron firing by the central respiratory drive. Brain Res 87: 363-374.
Richter DW, Ballantyne D (1983). A three phase theory about the basic respiratory pattern generator. In Schläfke ME, Koepchen HP, See WR (eds): "Central Neurone Environment," Berlin: Springer Verlag, pp 163-174.
Seller H, Langhorst P, Richter D, Koepchen HP. Über die Abhängigkeit der pressoreceptorischen Hemmung der Sympathicus von der Atemphase und ihre Auswirkung in der Vasomotorik. Pflügers Arch ges Physiol 302: 300-314.

Organization of the Autonomic Nervous System:
Central and Peripheral Mechanisms, pages 179–188
© **1987 Alan R. Liss, Inc.**

BRAIN STEM GENERATION OF SPECIFIC AND NON-SPECIFIC RHYTHMS

H.P. Koepchen, H.-H. Abel, D. Klüßendorf

Institute of Physiology, Free University Berlin

Arnimallee 22, D-looo Berlin 33, FRG

There is general agreement that several rhythms with different frequencies are generated within the brain stem. Speaking of specific and non-specific rhythms we have to clear in advance the nomenclature. Since many rhythms appear in several outputs, a meaningful denomination can be given only according to the appearance in the efferent innervation projecting on a special target organ. Thus e.g. central rhythm becomes sympathetic, vasomotor or respiratory only when it appears in sympathetic or vasomotor fibres or respiratory motor nerves respectively, but not before in brain stem neurons only on the basis of its frequency. It is important to keep this in mind, when we confine our considerations in the following to the rhythmic oscillations of cardiovascular innervation with respiration or phrenic discharge related frequencies, especially when we ask for the cause-effect relationships. Usually it is tacitly presumed that cardiovascular rhythmicity with respiratory-related rhythm is generated by that oscillator the functional destination of which is the production of respiratory movements. This is implied in the classical term "irradiation" as well as in the modern question from which respiratory neurons the cardiovascular rhythm takes its origin. Here we are confronted with an unfortunate change of the meaning of "respiratory", when within the central nervous system we call "respiratory" every neuron with any relation to phrenic rhythm. Therewith we have passed over from a functional definition to a classification derived from the discharge pattern. When we accept this, the statement that respiration-related rhythm in cardiovascular innervation stems from respiratory neurons becomes tautological. In the very common case of synchrony between e.g. vasomotor and respiratory oscillations, why are we used to call the vasomotor fluctuations "respiratory" but not conversely the respiration "vasomotor"? This anparently strange question points to a dogmatic presumption, namely that of the obligatory primacy of respiratory rhythm which is due to the teleological consideration that respiration needs rhythm for its peripheral function, but vasomotion does not; the latter again a non proven presumption. The reasons why we take up again this theme which has a more than loo years old history are the following:

1) It provides important information on the functional relation of autonomic to other control systems;
2) It is a paradigm for the general question of specificity;
3) Analysis of cardiovascular rhythmicity gains growing application in clinical medicine;
4) The controversy on the dependency of respiration-related fluctuations in autonomic innervation on the respiratory brain stem oscillator continues since more than loo years up to the present meeting.

Thus we have to look not only for the cause-effect relations between the respective rhythms, but have to ask why two opposite interpretations could persist simultaneously with changing preponderance for such a long time. The two controversial standpoints may be characterized as follows:

A) Respiration-related rhythm in autonomic outputs is a secondary phenomenon caused by the respiratory oscillator in the sense of "irradiation".
B) Cardiovascular rhythms, even those in the frequency range of respiration, are centrogenic rhythms in their own right which have been synchronized by entrainment with the respiratory rhythm. This implies the existence of sliding coordinations and integer multiple frequency relations.

Interestingly the majority even of those authors advocating the second concept still ascribe the leading role to the respiratory rhythm. We have to consider the arguments and evidences of both parties. Starting with the more complex concept B, there have been reported many observations indicating the existence of sliding coordinations, entrainment and multiple integer relations (Barman and Gebber, 1976; Koepchen, 1962; 1984), so that there is no doubt that such mechanisms do exist. One characteristic example (Fig. 1) is taken from an extensive study in anaesthetized and curarized dogs, where respiratory feedback afferences were excluded by diffusion respiration, i.e. abolition of respiratory mechanics. In this case respiratory rhythm recorded in the phrenic discharge temporarily stopped after injection of succinylcholine, but

the previously respiration synchronous blood pressure oscillations continued with the previous frequency. Lateron phrenic rhythm reappears and interferes in various ways with the
blood pressure rhythm. The transitory state of 2:1 relation
in the second half of the registration period and the jump
in both frequencies with deceleration of phrenic and accel-
eration of blood pressure rhythm resulting in a state of final synchrony with an intermediate frequency are especially
informative. Such examples clearly demonstrate that synchrony is the result of mutual interaction between two faculta-
tively independent rhythms.

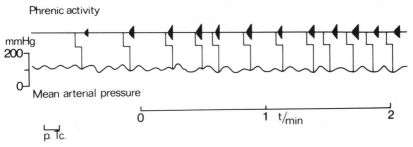

Fig. 1. Time course of mean arterial blood pressure and
phrenic nerve activity in an anaesthetized dog after injection of succinylcholine under diffusion respiration. p.Tc.:
Previous respiratory cycle duration (modified redrawing from
Koepchen, 1961).

Fig. 2 gives a schematic compilation of the findings
from the mentioned study in anaesthetized dogs under diffusion respiration. It symbolizes in each of the sections one
of the experimentally observed states of rhythm coordination.
Most remarkable was the observation that one state of rhythm
coordination could switch over to another one spontaneously
within the same experiment. This whole complex was called
"common central rhythmicity" (Koepchen, 1962). The entirety
of these findings lead to the recognition that a certain
rhythm can variably encompass the output network of different
peripheral systems. In other words, a central rhythm does not
obligatorily belong to a special output and consequently a
central neuron cannot be attributed to the central control
system for a special peripheral function on the basis of a
rhythm found in its discharge pattern. This of course applies
to the brain stem neurons with respiratory discharge pattern
as well as to those with e.g. "sympathetic" or "EEG" rhythm.

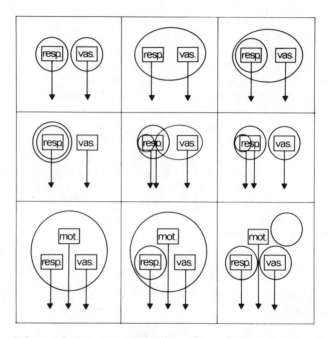

Fig. 2. Schematic representation of various states of rhythm
coordination during diffusion respiration in anaesthetized
dogs. The squares symbolize the output to respiratory (resp),
vasomotor (vas) and somatomotor (mot) innervation. Each circle or ellipse indicate a rhythm encompassing the respective
output neurons. Two circles enclosing or overlapping each
other indicate the occurrence of two superimposed rhythms in
the respective target system. A circle which does not touch
one of the squares means a rhythm which does not appear in
one of the three recorded systems.

Let us consider now the arguments of those authors who
stress the irradiation concept A with the primacy of respiratory rhythm and unidirectional cause-effect relation and an
always leading role of the respiratory oscillator. The most
striking evidence seems to come from the classic experiment
of Hering (1869), i.e. the curarized anaesthetized animal
after cessation of artificial ventilation, where periodic
blood pressure increases follow the manifestation of rudimentary respiratory movements or - in more advanced experiments -

the discharge bursts of the phrenic nerve. Since the time order is the main argument for the cause-effect relation in these experiments, we have to take into account that the latencies between central activation and phrenic activity or respiratory movement respectively on the one hand and blood pressure increase on the other hand are quite different. We have recalculated these latencies using own previous measurements in dogs and values from the literature and have drawn in this into a copy of the original registration of Hering (Fig. 3). The surprising result is, that the central excitations causing the blood pressure increases do precede and not follow the central inspiratory bursts. The same time order results when we reexamine more recent registrations with phrenic nerve recordings. Thus the time order does not support the dogma of the obligatory primacy of respiratory rhythm.

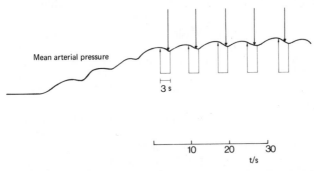

Fig. 3. Modified redrawing of the registration of the classic experiment of Hering (1869). The original marks of Hering above the registration indicate the occurrence of rudimentary respiratory movements in an incompletely curarized dog. The calculated latencies between central excitation and its manifestation by blood pressure increase are marked below the record.

There are further arguments in favour of central excitation preceding the start of inspiration:
1) The observation that with general central excitation (occurring spontaneously or evoked by stimulation) autonomic effects precede the respiratory and behavioural ones (Heinemann et al., 1973; Schulz et al., 1986 in press).
2) The phenomenon that after hyperventilation with reincreasing chemical drive sympathetic activation precedes the start of the first phrenic burst (Koepchen et al., 1981; Trzebski and Kubin, 1981).

3) The time course of the known respiration synchronous fluctuations of baroreceptor reflex sensitivity, where the decrease of baroreceptor efficiency starts clearly before the beginning of the next phrenic burst (Koepchen et al., 1961). This applies to the heart rate effect as well as to sympathetic inhibition (Seller et al., 1968). From all these observations the picture emerges that there is a central oscillatory process leading the final respiratory rhythmic innervation, whereby the efferent sympathetic outflow has a lower threshold to follow the central oscillator than the respiratory innervation. When this is true, conditions are conceivable, where the threshold for the autonomic output is reached, but not that for the respiratory output. We have described this long ago in experiments on dogs, where the baroreceptor-heart rate reflex shows oscillations without a corresponding phrenic discharge (Koepchen et al., 1961), but exactly at that time when the latter was expected to occur according to the previous respiratory rhythm. Under these conditions the expected bimodal frequency distribution of cycle durations could be found in respiration. Such excitation of one output remaining occasionally subthreshold for another one is general basis for the frequent phenomenon of multiple integer relations between various rhythms in the target organs. Following further this idea, there have to be postulated states where the threshold is never reached in the higher threshold output. This corresponds exactly to those periods of an experiment where the "respiratory" rhythm goes on in other outputs, as manifested e.g. in the blood pressure oscillations at the beginning of the registration in Fig. 1, or the continuation of "respiratory" sinus arrhythmia during voluntary apnea in man. One very instructive example in this context is shown in Fig. 4.

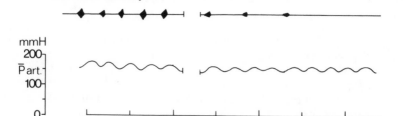

Fig. 4. Variable forms of coordination between phrenic and mean arterial blood pressure rhythms in an anaesthetized dog under diffusion respiration (modified redrawing from Koepchen, 1962).

In the first part of this registration blood pressure oscillates with the rhythm of phrenic activity, i.e. "respiratory" blood pressure waves according to the classical nomenclature, occur. Thereafter during hyperventilation phrenic activity after a period of 2:1 coordination disappears entirely. Nevertheless, blood pressure oscillations continue, demonstrating that they are not "respiratory". With our above interpretation we can state that, in this case, hypocapnia has lowered so much the threshold of the final respiratory premotor network that it is never reached during the positive phase of the oscillation.

This throws new light on the function of this premotor respiratory network. Comparing the discharge pattern of those sympathetic outputs which show respiratory related rhythmicity with the phrenic pattern, the main difference - apart from various deviations in phase - is the sharp onset and cutoff of the phrenic pattern with a distinct zero phase. Thus the special function of the respiratory premotor network is the sharpening of the more smooth preoscillation. Consequently this can be called a rhythm transformer. There is experimental evidence in favour of such a discrimination between rhythm generation and rhythm transformation. Interference with the common drive as e.g. lesions or cooling at certain sites of the ventral medulla or change of P_{CO_2} act on the activity and rhythm of sympathetic as well as respiratory outputs. On the other hand the region ventrolateral to the solitary tract (vlNTS) is crucial in the determination of inspiratory duration. Its lesion can lead to states of "medullary apneusis" with huge increase of net phrenic output, but without corresponding sympathetic activation (Koepchen et al., 1981). In special cases of apnea local intramedullary cooling at special sites could restore respiratory rhythm, i.e. bring the respiratory output from zero to normal values. This again was not accompanied by any change in systemic arterial pressure. Such manipulations can be interpreted as interferences with the rhythm transformer in the final respiratory part of the network. This part - in our interpretation the rhythm transformer - providing the typical on-off pattern of respiratory outputs can be really called specific.

As to the characterization of a "respiratory" and a "cardiovascular" or "sympathetic" frequency range of rhythmicity, there is no doubt that favourite frequencies can be demonstrated statistically, e.g. very clearly in the power spectra of heart beat interval variations (Koepchen et al., 1985). As a rule respiratory frequency and one part of heart rate rhythmicity lie in a higher frequency range (mean period duration T   lo-15 s). It has to be stressed, however, that these are only preferential and not rigid obligatory frequency ranges and that vasomotor or sympathetic rhythms also in the higher frequency range can be found as well as respiratory rhythm in the lower one. Thus in humans during spontaneous slowing of respiration down to the lower frequency range the higher previously "respiratory" frequency range of heart rate variations does not disappear nor even diminish. In the Hering type of experiment and in the similar conditions in the first period of Fig. 4 respiration has slowed down to the lower frequency range. Therefore misunderstandings can be avoided when the corresponding frequency ranges are not called "cardiovascular", "sympathetic" or "respiratory" but simply are classified according to their frequency band. The vasomotor or respiratory events in one of the frequency ranges depends not at least on the time properties of the effector system with the slow follower range of vascular smooth muscle (Koepchen, 1984), whereas respiratory frequency is essentially determined by the time properties of the central rhythm transformer which can hardly follow beyond a certain frequency range.

Finally we have to ask whether there does exist any kind of "irradiation" from the specific respiratory part of the network, i.e. the rhythm transformer, to other systems apart from the variable synchrony given by the dependency on common preoscillators. There are indeed many phenomena which indicate direct influences from the final respiratory rhythm transformer on sympathetic outputs, as e.g. phrenic-like discharge patterns of single cervical sympathetic fibres (Preiss et al., 1975) or the postinhibitory inhibition in sympathetic outputs or reticular activity (Bainton et al., 1985) which is strongly correlated to the phrenic discharge. Thus the final respiratory rhythm transformer acts back on the general brain stem activity from which reversely it receives its activating general drive. We call this the "irradiation paradoxon". These bidirectional actions of course complicate the functional structure, and we suggest that this is the reason why the controversy between the advocates of the sliding entrainment concept and those of the irradiation concept could continue over the decades and is acute again at this symposium. One part of the authors look to the one complex of phenomena, the other to the other complex, where some selection according to the theoretical concept may come

into play in addition. Moreover, two factors tend to strengthen the irradiation phenomena:
1) In anaesthetized animals under strongly reduced and normalized experimental conditions a scarcely variable synchrony as the final result of mutual entrainment is the most frequently found state.
2) Automatic averaging methods with phrenic activity as a trigger signal introduce the presumption of primacy of respiratory rhythm in advance into the evaluation enhancing selectively those phenomena which are tightly bound to the final respiratory pattern transformer, i.e. the "irradiation".

Thus it is our final conclusion that one or several variably coupled brain stem oscillators act on the final respiratory as well as on the various sympathetic and other output networks being unspecific unless they appear in a distinct peripheral innervation. One of the output networks which is specific respiratory transforms the rhythm into the functionally necessary sharp respiratory discharge pattern and in addition "irradiates" backwards into reticular networks reaching among others also sympathetic outputs. Thus both controversial concepts - mutual entrainment and irradiation - do not exclude each other and can be joint to a general picture which is in agreement with all observed phenomena.

References

Bainton CR, Richter DW, Seller H, Ballantyne D, Klein JP (1985). Respiratory modulation of sympathetic activity. J Aut Nerv Syst 12:77-9o.
Barman SM, Gebber GL (1976). Basis for synchronization of sympathetic and phrenic nerve discharges. Am J Physiol 231:16o1-16o7.
Heinemann H, Stock G, Schaefer H (1973). Temperal correlation of responses in blood pressure and motor reaction under electrical stimulation of limbic structures in unanaesthetized, unrestrained cats. Pflügers Arch 343:27-4o.
Hering E (1869). Über Atembewegungen des Gefäßsystems. Sber Akad Wiss Wien, Math-naturwiss Kl 2, 6o:829-856.
Koepchen HP (1962). "Die Blutdruckrhythmik". Darmstadt: Dr. Dietrich Steinkopff Verlag.

Koepchen HP (1984). History of studies and concepts of blood pressure waves. In Miyakawa K, Koepchen HP, Polosa C (eds): "Mechanisms of Blood Pressure Waves", Berlin Heidelberg New York Tokyo: Springer-Verlag, p.3.

Koepchen HP, Abel HH, Klüßendorf D (1985). Heart-rate dynamics in healthy humans before, during and after a mental test. Pflügers Arch 4o5 (suppl 2):R 5o.

Koepchen HP, Klüßendorf D, Sommer D (1981). Neurophysiological background of central neural cardiovascular-respiratory coordination: Basic remarks and experimental approach. J Aut Nerv Syst 3:335-368.

Koepchen HP, Wagner PH, Lux HD (1961). Über die Zusammenhänge zwischen zentraler Erregbarkeit, reflektorischem Tonus und Atemrhythmus bei der nervösen Steuerung der Herzfrequenz. Pflügers Arch 273:443-465.

Preiss G, Kirchner F, Polosa C (1975). Pattering of sympathetic preganglionic neuron firing by the central respiratory drive. Brain Res 87:363-374.

Schulz G, Lambertz M, Stock G, Langhorst P (1986 in press). Neuronal activity in the amygdala related to somatomotor and vegetative components of behaviour in cats. J Aut Nerv Syst.

Seller H, Langhorst P, Richter D, Koepchen HP (1968). Über die Abhängigkeit der pressorezeptorischen Hemmung des Sympathikus von der Atemphase und ihre Auswirkung in der Vasomotorik. Pflügers Arch 3o2:3oo-314.

Trzebski A, Kubin L (1981). Is the central inspiratory activity responsible for pCO_2-dependent drive of the sympathetic discharge. J Aut Nerv Syst 3:4o1-42o.

Organization of the Autonomic Nervous System:
Central and Peripheral Mechanisms, pages 189–202
© 1987 Alan R. Liss, Inc.

LACK OF EVIDENCE OF COUPLED OSCILLATOR MECHANISMS IN
THE GENERATION OF SYMPATHETIC RHYTHMS

Manjit Bachoo and Canio Polosa

Department of Physiology, McGill
University,
Montreal, Quebec H3G 1Y6

INTRODUCTION

Under usual experimental conditions, the background
discharge of sympathetic preganglionic or postganglionic
neurons, in preparations with intact CNS, shows
periodicities time-locked to the central respiratory cycle
or to the cardiac cycle. One possible explanation of these
periodicities is that sympathetic preganglionic neurons
(SPN) activity is modulated by the rhythmic output of
brainstem respiratory neurons (respiratory periodicity) or
by rhythmic inhibition from arterial baroreceptor afferents
(cardiac periodicity). This explanation implicitly
excludes the possibility that the SPN themselves, or the
associated antecedent circuitry, have intrinsic
rhythmicity, i.e. rhythmicity independent of that
resulting from these two periodic inputs. It has been
reported, however, that in particular experimental
conditions sympathetic discharge can show periodicities
similar to, but independent of, the central respiratory
(Koepchen, 1962; Barman & Gebber, 1976) and cardiac
(Gebber, 1980) rhythms. These observations have raised the
possibility that these sympathetic periodicities result
from an intrinsic rhythmicity of neuron networks antecedent
to the SPN (i.e. of "sympathetic" oscillators, Gebber,
1980). It has been proposed that under most experimental
conditions such intrinsic rhythms may become entrained to
the rhythm of activity of arterial baroreceptor afferents
or of brainstem respiratory neurons. Thus, the SPN and
antecedent circuitry may be viewed as a system made of an

oscillator which receives rhythmic input from external sources. Such a system is referred to as a coupled oscillator system.

There is ample theoretical (Pavlidis, 1973; Stein, 1977; Segundo & Kohn, 1981) and experimental (Pinsker & Ayers, 1983) literature describing the behaviour of systems of coupled oscillators in biology. A comparative survey of a variety of such systems involving nerve or cardiac cells will be presented to illustrate their main features. Experimental tests will be described of whether or not the respiratory rhythm of sympathetic discharge conforms with these features. In addition, published experimental evidence, which has been used as basis for the hypothesis that an independent sympathetic oscillator generates the cardiac modulation of sympathetic discharge, will be examined in search of the essential features of oscillator behaviour.

GLOSSARY

An attempt has been made to use in this paper terminology consistent with that used in oscillator literature (Pavlidis, 1973; Pinsker, 1977b). Some terms and concepts are defined here. A neural oscillator is a single neuron, or a network of neurons, which generates a rhythmic output in the absence of rhythmic input. An oscillation is a cyclical change in a variable (e.g. neural activity) with relatively constant waveform and period. The free-run or intrinsic frequency of an oscillator is the frequency in the absence of periodic input. When considering two oscillators, coupling between the two exists if perturbing the rhythm of one resets the rhythm of the other. For neural oscillators coupling is provided by synaptic connections. Coupling can be weak or strong, depending on the strength of the synaptic connection. The relationship between two oscillators can be described by the temporal relationship of their respective waveforms, expressed in real time as delay or normalized to cycle duration as phase angle. Entrainment refers to a condition in which an oscillator (the follower) is driven at a frequency different from its free-run frequency by a rhythmic input originating from another oscillator (the driver) to which it is coupled or from an external periodic input, e.g. from a sensory source: a constant phase angle between oscillator input and output is evidence of entrainment.

COUPLED OSCILLATOR PROPERTIES

Any input which produces a transient perturbation of an oscillator free-run period (i.e. a phase-shift) can entrain that oscillator (which becomes a follower) at frequencies higher or lower than its free-run frequency. The input produces the entrainment by either phase-advancing or phase-delaying, on a cycle by cycle basis, the follower oscillator (a phase-advance occurs when the onset of the cycle occurs earlier than predicted from the free-running frequency, a phase-delay when the onset of the cycle occurs later than predicted). A phase response curve (PRC) describes the just mentioned phenomenon, i.e. the change in oscillator cycle duration produced by a single discrete input, as a function of the time of the cycle at which the input occurs. The maximum phase advance or phase delay caused by the input defines the limits within which the frequency of an oscillator can be modified by that input. For known neural oscillators these limits define a narrow range of frequencies around the free-run frequency (see below).

In the steady-state, as a consequence of the properties disclosed by the PRC (1) an oscillator coupled to a rhythmic synaptic input can be stably entrained to the frequency of the perturbing external source in a one to one ratio only over a narrow range of frequencies (2) at each frequency in the one to one range the equality of the period of the driven oscillator with the input period is achieved by the input occurring at a unique phase of the cycle, such that the input-output phase difference may span the entire free run cycle duration of the driven oscillator (3) when the frequency of the driving input exceeds the limits of the one-to-one range, different entrainment patterns involving small integer ratios are established between the frequency of the input and the frequency of the driven oscillator. For instance, beyond the boundaries of the 1:1 entrainment ratio, the entrainment pattern assumes a 2:3, 1:2 etc., ratio, as the input frequency is increased and 3:2, 2:1 etc, ratio as the input frequency is reduced. Under these conditions the phase relation varies on a cycle to cycle basis in an orderly, repeating manner. The range of ratios outside the 1:1 range is also described as relative coordination (von Holst, 1939). At frequencies of the input which are at the boundary between ranges giving stable entrainment, the driven oscillator may exhibit transient irregular dynamics with no fixed phase relation to the input.

BEHAVIOUR OF COUPLED BIOLOGICAL OSCILLATORS

The above mentioned features of coupled oscillators, namely limited range of frequencies over which a stable one-to-one relation is maintained and different phase-relation between respective waveforms at different frequencies within the one-to-one range, are derived from both theoretical considerations (Pavlidis, 1973; Stein, 1977; Glass & Mackey, 1979; Winfree, 1980; Segundo & Kohn, 1981) and experimental observations (see below). They apply to oscillators with free run periods from milliseconds (Perkel et al., 1964; Guevara et al., 1981) to circadian (Enright, 1965; Moore-Ede et al., 1982; Turek, 1985). The generality of these features is illustrated by examples of coupled oscillators drawn from single pacemakers neurons (Perkel et al., 1964; Pinsker, 1977a), simple neural network oscillators in invertebrates (Stein, 1976; Ayers & Selverston, 1979; Peterson & Calabrese, 1982), complex neural network oscillators in vertebrates (von Holst, 1939; Petrillo et al., 1983) and cardiac pacemaker cells (Levy et al., 1972; Guevara et al., 1981; Jalife, 1984). Although this list of examples is by no means exhaustive (for comprehensive reviews see Pinsker and Ayers 1983; Selverston and Moulins, 1985; Winfree, 1980) it illustrates the principle that, at least qualitatively, the dynamics of coupled oscillator behaviour is predictable and applies to a wide variety of biological oscillators.

Entrainment of single pacemaker neurons by rhythmic electrical stimulation of an excitatory or inhibitory synaptic input has been well characterized in a number of preparations. Pinsker (1977a) demonstrated the range of stable 1:1 entrainment of an endogenously bursting neuron of Aplysia by an inhibitory input to be limited to 6% above and 30% below its free-run frequency. At each frequency the burst of the pacemaker neuron assumed a unique phase-relation to the rhythmic driving stimulus. Similar findings have been described by Ayers and Selverston (1979) in the stomatogastric neural network of the lobster in response to stimulation of inhibitory or excitatory interneurons. Peterson and Calabrese (1982) reported that the neural network generating the rhythm of the heart beat in the leech could be synaptically driven by rhythmic electrical stimulation of an antecedent neuron, at rates different from its free-run frequency.

They noted stable locking of the cardiac neural oscillator rhythm to the driving frequency within well defined limits (10% above and 40% below the free-run frequency). Stein (1976) has shown a similar phenomenon for neural oscillators which govern limb movement in crayfish, while v. Holst (1939) reported similar findings for central locomotor pattern generators in the spinal cord of the dogfish. An example of this phenomenon in vertebrates is provided by the effects of vagus nerve stimulation on the period of the cardiac sinus rhythm. Over a restricted range of frequencies, both above and below the intrinsic sinus node frequency, the sinus rhythm can be entrained to the period of the vagal stimulus, with a unique phase relation of the stimulus to the cardiac cycle at each frequency (Levy et al., 1972; Slenter et al., 1984). A more detailed analysis of the behaviour of cardiac pacemaker cells entrained by rhythmic intracellular current pulses (Guevara et al., 1981) or iontophoretic pulses of acetylcholine (Michaels et al., 1984) has been reported, again with very similar results to those described above. Jalife (1984) developed an in vitro cardiac preparation which is instructive in defining the essential elements involved in the behaviour of coupled oscillators. His data shows that the range of frequencies over which two independent pacemaker centers in the rabbit sino-atrial node can be stably entrained is a function of the strength of the coupling between the two centers. The coupling strength was manipulated by a variable shunt resistance connecting the two autonomous pacemaker populations. With infinitely high shunt resistance (zero coupling) each pacemaker had its intrinsic frequency and was not affected by changes in the frequency of the other. With intermediate values of shunt resistance, mutual 1:1 entrainment occurred which was limited to a range of frequencies bordering the intrinsic frequency of the pacemakers and was characterized by a unique phase-relation at each frequency. At frequencies beyond those characterizing the 1:1 range, mutual entrainment involved integer ratios. With zero shunt resistance, i.e. with infinitely tight coupling, the two pacemaker centers assumed an identical frequency and behaved as a single pacemaker. In vertebrates, the brainstem neural network generating the rhythmic central respiratory drive for motoneurons of the respiratory muscles (which will be referred to as the respiratory oscillator) can be entrained by rhythmic sensory input, presumably from pulmonary

stretch receptors, associated with lung inflation produced
by a mechanical ventilator. Thus, the situation is
analogous to that of two coupled oscillators, i.e. there
is a rhythmic synaptic input acting on an intrinsically
rhythmic neural network. A number of investigators
(Vibert et al., 1981; Pham Dihn et al., 1983; Petrillo &
Glass, 1984) have described the entrainment behaviour of
the respiratory oscillator to the mechanical ventilator.
One of the most detailed accounts of this behaviour is by
Petrillo et al (1983). Their data show that it is
possible to entrain the frequency of the respiratory
oscillator to that of the mechanical ventilator such that
it may be speeded up or slowed down with respect to its
free-run frequency. The 1:1 entrainment is limited to a
narrow range of frequencies and within this range each
frequency is obtained by the lung inflation occurring at a
specific phase of the respiratory cycle. The described
dynamic characteristics of coupled biological oscillators
are observed in experimental situations, with the
exception of the data by Jalife (1984), in which
entrainment is unidirectional. However, two or more
oscillators may be mutually entrained such that their
phase-relation is the result of the interplay of their
coupling signals. The dynamic characteristics of
unidirectionally entrained oscillators also apply to
mutually entrained oscillators (Buno & Fuentes, 1984;
Jalife, 1984; Pearce & Friesen, 1985).

IS THE INSPIRATION-RELATED SYMPATHETIC DISCHARGE GENERATED
BY AN INDEPENDENT SYMPATHETIC OSCILLATOR?

We have examined the periodic burst of SPN firing
which previous work has defined as inspiration-related on
the basis of its timing in the respiratory cycle and of
similarities of properties with the phrenic nerve burst
(Preiss et al., 1975; Gerber & Polosa, 1978, 1979). The
purpose of the study was to see whether the relation of
this component of sympathetic discharge to the phrenic
nerve burst would show the properties expected of a system
of coupled oscillators. A detailed description of these
experiments is presented elsewhere (Bachoo & Polosa, in
press). A brief summary of the relevant experiments is
presented here.

i)   Phase-Response Curve to Superior Laryngeal Nerve
Stimulation.

One way of characterizing the properties of an
oscillator is by describing the phase-dependent effects
(phase response curve described above) produced by brief
stimulation of an input. Stimulation of low threshold
afferents in the superior laryngeal nerve (SLN) was used
to perturb the cycle of the respiratory oscillator. Its
output, measured as the phrenic nerve burst, could be
phase-advanced or delayed, with respect to its free-run
period, by a stimulus train applied to the SLN (Bachoo &
Polosa, 1985). The phase response curve was identical for
the rhythm of both phrenic and sympathetic burst,
suggesting that the stimulus was acting on a common
oscillator mechanism. If sympathetic bursting activity
was indepently rhythmic, as the respiratory oscillator
cycle was phase-advanced or phase-delayed by the stimulus,
the respiratory oscillator input would occur at a
different phase of the hypothetical sympathetic oscillator
cycle and therefore, according to the behaviour of coupled
oscillators, the two waveforms would have to change their
time relation to each other. The assumption here is that
the SLN stimulus perturbs the respiratory oscillator and
that the latter then perturbs the sympathetic oscillator.
Thus, the SLN stimulus would not be expected to have the
same effect on the respiratory and sympathetic oscillator
cycles.

ii)   Entrainment of the Phrenic and Inspiration Related
Sympathetic Burst to the Mechanical Ventilator.

We modified the respiratory frequency, in cats with
intact cervical vagus, by changing the ventilation pump
frequency. The prediction here was that if the
sympathetic, inspiration-related, burst was generated by
an independent sympathetic oscillator which was entrained
to the respiratory oscillator, the relation between
phrenic and inspiration-related sympathetic burst would be
expected to display the behaviour observed in coupled
oscillator systems when the frequency of the driver
oscillator is changed. Namely, a limited 1:1 range and,
within this range, a different phase-relation at each
frequency. The results show instead an unlimited 1:1
range, i.e. whatever frequency the respiratory oscillator
was forced to adopt by the mechanical ventilator, so did

the sympathetic burst. Over the entire frequency range studied (10 to 40 cycles per min) the phase relation between the phrenic and inspiration-related sympathetic burst remained essentially constant. This constrasts with the phase relation of the phrenic burst to the inflation cycle, which was different at each frequency, as expected of an oscillator driven by a rhythmic input (Petrillo et al., 1983).

iii) Hypocapnic-Hyperthermic Polypnea and the Inspiration-Related Sympathetic Burst.

In vagotomized cats, raising the core temperature from 37 to 42°C by means of radiant heat increased the frequency of the phrenic and inspiration-related sympathetic burst from 15 to 36 bursts/min. Subsequent hyperventilation (lowering end-tidal pCO_2 to 10 mm Hg from a control of 35 mmHg) produced a very marked increase in the frequency of both bursts, which reached a maximum value of approximately 300 bursts/min (Cohen, 1964; Monteau et al., 1974). Over this entire range of frequencies, from 15 to 300 cycles/min, phrenic and sympathetic bursts maintained a 1:1 relation and a phase-relation which was essentially constant.

The fact that the phrenic and inspiration-related sympathetic burst maintained a one to one relation with essentially constant delay at all frequencies tested is inconsistent with the behaviour expected of coupled neural oscillators. Therefore, the equality of period of phrenic nerve burst and inspiration-related sympathetic burst is unlikely to result from the activity of an autonomous sympathetic oscillator coupled to the brainstem respiratory oscillator. Instead, these results are compatible with the hypothesis of a common oscillator which drives both the phrenic and the sympathetic discharges.

THE CARDIAC MODULATION OF SYMPATHETIC DISCHARGES

Modulation of sympathetic discharge at the frequency of the heart beat has been described by a number of investigators (Adrian et al., 1932; Downing & Siegel, 1963; Cohen & Gootman, 1970). The first detailed analysis

was presented by Green & Heffron (1968). The cardiac
modulation of sypathetic discharge was considered to be
the consequence of the sympatho-inhibitory baroreceptor
reflex: the arterial pressure increment associated with
systolic ejection produces an increment in the level of
sympathetic inhibition above that which exists at
diastolic levels of arterial pressure. Thus, the
records show bursts of spikes occurring between the
phases of depression produced by consecutive heart beats
(Green & Heffron, 1968). The bursting, however,
persists, at a mean frequency similar to that of the
heart beat, in barodenervated cats (Taylor & Gebber,
1975; Gebber 1976). In low-pass filtered records these
bursts appear as a series of irregular slow waves.
Based on these observations on barodenervated animals, the
hypothesis proposed by Gebber (1976) is that the slow wave
activity is the result of the activity of an independent
sympathetic oscillator which, in the presence of arterial
baroreceptor input, is entrained to the rhythm of the
heart beat. The published records (Gebber, 1976) show
that this slow wave activity is characterized, in
barodenervated cats, by waves of variable shape occurring
at irregular intervals. Statistical analysis of this
aperiodic burst discharge reveals a broad power spectrum
(2-6 Hz) without preferred frequencies and a flat
autocorrelogram. We are unaware of any previous
description of a biological oscillator with such aperiodic
characteristics. It is possible for an oscillator to show
aperiodic (chaotic) behaviour in particular conditions
associated with a forcing input (Guevara & Glass, 1982;
Olsen & Degan, 1985) and this could be a possible
explanation for lack of periodicity of the 2-6 Hz wave
activity. However, the lack of periodicity of this
signal, whether resulting from absence of intrinsic
rhythmicity in the generator or from chaotic behaviour of
an intrinsically rhythmic generator, precludes a search
for properties of coupled oscillator systems because such
an analysis presupposes a constant period of the signals
as a starting condition. Published records of this
activity in real time (Gebber, 1976) permit the additional
observation that in the presence of arterial baroreceptor
input the phase-relation between peaks of individual waves
and the cardiac cycle, at constant heart rate, is
variable. Averaged records are not useful in this context
because they give no information on the variability of the
signal and hence of the phase-relation. Since entrainment

of oscillators (see above) requires fixed phase-relation, this observation suggests that there is no entrainment of the 2-6 Hz waves to the cardiac cycle when the baroreceptor input is intact. Thus, the lack of evidence that the 2-6 Hz wave activity is rhythmic in barodenervated animals and the lack of evidence that the 2-6 Hz wave activity is locked to the cardiac cycle when baroreceptor input is intact precludes the possibility of applying the coupled oscillator hypothesis to the cardiac rhythm of sympathetic discharge. As a corollary, described phenomenology concerning the interaction of baroreceptor inhibition with the 2-6 Hz wave activity is not interpretable in terms of the properties of coupled oscillators.

CONCLUSION

This paper has attempted to identify the criteria that can be used to define a biological system as a system of two coupled oscillators. The approach is empirical, using criteria based on common features which underly the behaviour of known cases of coupled biological oscillators. When the respiratory and cardiac periodicities of sympathetic discharge are tested with such criteria, neither periodicity shows properties consistent with the hypothesis that it is generated by a system of coupled oscillators.

ACKNOWLEDGEMENT

The experimental work by the authors was supported by the Medical Research Council of Canada and the Quebec Heart Foundation.

REFERENCES

Adrian ED, Bronk DW, Phillips G (1932). Discharges in mammalian sympathetic nerves. J Physiol 74: 115-133.
Ayers AL, Selverston AI (1979). Monosynaptic entrainment of an endogenous pacemaker network: a cellular mechanism for von Holst's magnet effect. J Comp Physiol 129: 5-17.

Bachoo M, Polosa C (1985). Properties of a sympatho-inhibitory and vasodilator reflex evoked by superior laryngeal nerve afferents in the cat. J Physiol 364: 183-198.

Bachoo M, Polosa C. Properties of the inspiration-related activity of sympathetic preganglionic neurones of the cervical trunk in the cat. J Physiol. In press.

Barman SM, Gebber GL (1976). Basis for synchronization of sympathetic and phrenic nerve discharges. Am J Physiol 231: 1601-1607.

Buno W, Fuentes J (1984). Coupled oscillators in an isolated pacemaker neuron? Brain Res 303: 101-107.

Cohen MI (1964). Respiratory periodicity in the paralyzed vagotomized cat: hypocapnic polypnea. Am J Physiol 206: 847-864.

Cohen MI, Gootman PM (1970). Periodicities in efferent discharge of splanchnic nerve of the cat. Am J Physiol 218: 1092-1101.

Downing SE, Siegel H (1963). Baroreceptor and chemoreceptor influences on sympathetic discharge to the heart. Am J Physiol 204: 471-479.

Enright JT (1965). Synchronization and ranges of entrainment. In Aschoff J (ed): "Circadian Clocks", Amsterdam: North-Holland, pp. 112-124.

Gebber GL (1976). Basis for phase relations between baroreceptor and sympathetic nerve discharge. Am J Physiol 230: 263-270.

Gebber GL (1980). Central oscillators responsible for sympathetic nerve discharge. Am J Physiol 239: H143-H155.

Gerber U, Polosa C (1978). Effects of pulmonary stretch receptor afferent stimulation on sympathetic preganglionic neuron firing. Can J Physiol Pharmacol 56: 191-198.

Gerber U, Polosa C (1979). Some effects of superior laryngeal nerve stimulation on sympathetic preganglionic neuron firing. Can J Physiol Pharmacol 57: 1073-1081.

Glass L, Mackey M (1979). A simple model for phase-locking of biological oscillators. J Math Biol. 7: 339-352.

Green JH, Heffron PF (1968). Studies upon the relationship between baroreceptor and sympathetic activity. Quart J Exp Physiol 53: 23-32.

Guevara M, Glass L, Shrier A (1981). Phase locking, period-doubling bifurcations and irregular dynamics in periodically stimulated cardiac cells. Science 214: 1350-1353.

Guevara M, Glass L (1982). Phase locking, period doubling bifurcations and chaos in a mathematical model of a periodically driven oscillator: A theory for entrainment of biological oscillators and the generation of cardiac dysrhythmias. J Math Biol 14: 1-23.

Holst E. von (1939). Die relative koordination als phänomen und als methode zentral-nervose funktionanalyse. Erg Physiol Biol Chem u exp Pharmakol 42: 228-306.

Jalife J (1984). Mutual entrainment and electrical coupling as mechanisms for synchronous firing of rabbit sino-atrial pace-maker cells. J Physiol 356: 221-243.

Koepchen HP (1962). "Die Blutdruckrhythmik". Darmstadt, D. Steinkopff Verlag.

Levy MN, Iano T, Zieske H (1972). Effects of repetitive bursts of vagal stimulation on heart rate. Circ Res 30: 186-195.

Michaels DC, Matyas EP, Jalife J (1984). A mathematical model of the effects of acetylcholine pulses on sinoatrial pacemaker activity. Circ Res 55: 89-101.

Monteau R, Hilaire G, Ouedraogo C (1974). Contribution à l'étude de la fonction ventilatoire au cours de la polypnée thermique ou hypocapnique. J de Physiol 68: 97-120.

Moore-Ede MC, Sulzman FM, Fuller CA (1982). "The clocks that time us: Physiology of the circadian timing system". Cambridge Ma Harvard U Press.

Olsen LF, Degan M (1985). Chaos in biological systems. Quart Rev Biophys 18: 165-225.

Pavlidis T (1973). "Biological oscillators. Their mathematical analysis". New York Academic.

Pearce RA, Friesen WO (1985). Intersegmental coordination of the leech swimming rhythm. I. Role of cycle period gradient and coupling strength. J Neurophysiol 54: 1444-1459.

Perkel DM, Schulman J, Bullock TH, Moore GP, Segundo JP (1964). Pacemaker neurons: effects of regularly spaced synaptic input. Science 145: 61-63.

Petrillo GA, Glass L, Trippenbach T (1983). Phase-locking of the respiratory rhythm in cats to a mechanical

ventilator. Can J Physiol Pharmacol 61: 599-607.
Petrillo GA, Glass L (1984). A theory for phase locking of respiration in cats to a mechanical ventilator. Am J Physiol 246: R311-R320.
Pham Dinh T, Demongest J, Baconnier P, Benchetrit G (1983). Simulation of a biological oscillator: the respiratory system. J Theor Biol 103: 113-132.
Pinsker HM (1977a). Aplysia bursting neurons as endogenous oscillators. II. Synchronization and entrainment by pulsed inhibitory synaptic input. J Neurophysiol 40: 544-556.
Pinsker HM (1977b). Synaptic modulation of endogenous oscillators. Fed Proc 36: 2045-2049.
Pinsker HM, Ayers J (1983). Neuronal oscillators. In Rosenberg RN (ed.): "The Clinical Neurosciences", New York: Churchill Livingstone, vol. 5 pp 203-266.
Preiss G, Kirchner F, Polosa C (1975). Patterning of preganglionic neuron firing by the central respiratory drive. Brain Res 87: 363-374.
Segundo JP, Kohn AF (1981). A model of excitatory synaptic interactions between pacemakers. Its reality, its generality and the principles involved. Biol Cybern 40: 113-126.
Selverston AI, Moulins M (1985). Oscillatory neural networks. Ann Rev Physiol 47: 29-48.
Slenter VAJ, Salata JJ, Jalife J (1984). Vagal control of pacemaker periodicity and intranodal conduction in the rabbit sinoatrial node. Circ Res 54: 436-446.
Stein PSG (1976). Mechanisms of interlimb phase control. In Herman R, Grillner S, Stein PSG, Stuart DG (eds): "Neural Control of Locomotion", New York, Plenum pp 465-498.
Stein PSG (1977). Application of the mathematics of coupled oscillator systems to the analysis of the neural control of locomotion. Fed Proc 36: 2056-2059.
Taylor DG, Gebber GL (1975). Baroreceptor mechanisms controlling sympathetic nervous rhythms of central origin. Am J Physiol 228: 1002-1013.
Turek FW (1985). Circadian neural rhythms in mammals. Ann Rev Physiol 47: 49-64.
Vibert JF, Caille D, Segundo JP (1981). Respiratory oscillator entrained by periodic vagal afferents: An

experimental test of a model. Biol Cybern 41:
119-130.
Winfree AT (1980). "The geometry of biological time".
New York, Springer Verlag.

Organization of the Autonomic Nervous System:
Central and Peripheral Mechanisms, pages 203–212
© 1987 Alan R. Liss, Inc.

THE MEDIAL THALAMUS AS A POTENTIAL GENERATOR OF SYMPATHETIC TONE

Kurt J. Varner, Gerard L. Gebber, Susan M. Barman and Zhong-Sun Huang
Departments of Pharmacology/Toxicology and of Physiology, Michigan State University, East Lansing, MI 48824, U.S.A.

INTRODUCTION

Sympathetic nerve discharge (SND) contains a 2- to 6-Hz rhythmic component in anesthetized animals (Gebber, 1980). Although this rhythm persists in SND after midcollicular decerebration (Barman and Gebber, 1980), 2- to 6-Hz SND is locked to frontal-parietal cortical activity in some CNS-intact preparations. Synchronization of the 2- to 6-Hz components in SND and cortical activity has been observed in chloralose (Barman and Gebber, 1980) and diallylbarbiturate-urethan (Gebber and Barman, 1981) anesthetized cats and in chloralose anesthetized dogs (Camerer et al., 1977). These reports raise the possibility that the forebrain plays a role in setting the level of basal SND in the anesthetized animal. This paper summarizes work performed in our laboratory on this subject. We were particularly interested in testing the hypothesis that thalamic rhythm generators are involved in controlling SND. This hypothesis was considered since there is reason to believe that the 2- to 6-Hz rhythm in cortical activity of anesthetized animals (to which a component of SND can be locked) is generated in the thalamus. Regarding this point, Jahnsen and Llinas (1984) recorded 5-Hz rhythmic acivity from single thalamic neurons in in vitro guinea pig slice preparations. Moreover, Andersson and Manson (1971) recorded 6-Hz rhythmic activity in the deafferentated cat thalamus (decortication and decerebration were performed).

SYNCHRONIZATION OF SND AND THALAMIC ACTIVITY

Crosscorrelation analysis was used to study the temporal relationships between SND and multiunit thalamic activity in chloralose anesthetized cats. Activity was recorded from the postganglionic inferior cardiac sympathetic nerve, medial thalamus (0 to 3 mm lateral to midline) and lateral thalamus. Capacity-coupled preamplification with a bandpass of 1-1000 Hz was used to display multiunit activity in the form of slow waves. Thalamic activity was recorded between stereotaxic planes A7 and A11.

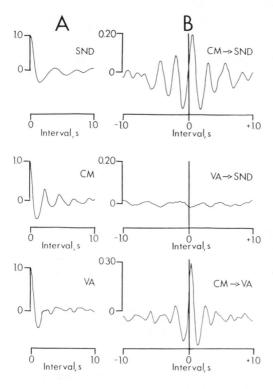

Fig. 1. Selective relationship between sympathetic nerve discharge (SND) and medial thalamic activity. A, autocorrelograms of SND and of activity recorded from nuclei centrum medianum (CM) and ventralis anterior (VA) of medial and lateral thalamus, respectively. B, crosscorrelograms. CM → SND crosscorrelogram shows SND relative to CM activity at zero lag. VA → SND crosscorrelogram shows SND relative to VA activity at zero lag. CM → VA crosscorrelogram shows VA activity relative to CM activity at zero lag. Analysis time for correlograms was 40 s. Bin width was 10 ms.

Crosscorrelation analysis revealed two patterns of relationship between SND and thalamic activity in both baroreceptor-innervated and -denervated cats. Inferior cardiac SND was related to both medial and lateral thalamic activity in 10 CNS-intact cats whereas SND was related only to medial thalamic activity in 7 other cats. A detailed description of the differential pattern of relationship follows. Figure 1 shows an example of this pattern in a baroreceptor-denervated cat with an intact neuraxis. The CM → SND crosscorrelogram (Fig. 1B) shows inferior cardiac nerve activity that preceded (left of zero lag) and followed (right of zero lag) activity recorded from the nucleus centrum medianum of the medial thalamus. The crosscorrelogram contains a sharp peak near zero lag. This peak indicates that a component of SND and CM activity were temporally related. The crosscorrelation function (rho value) at the peak was 0.2. A value of 1.0 signifies a perfect relationship. A rhythm with a period of approximately 240 ms appears in both the autocorrelogram of CM activity (Fig. 1A) and the CM → SND crosscorrelogram. Thus, the component common to SND and medial thalamic activity was in the 2- to 6-Hz range. In contrast, the VA → SND crosscorrelogram (Fig. 1B) was flat, indicating that SND was unrelated to activity recorded from the nucleus ventralis anterior of the lateral thalamus. The CM → VA crosscorrelogram in Fig. 1B shows a sharp peak near zero lag indicating that medial and lateral thalamic activity contained a common component. This component apparently was not responsible for the relationship between medial thalamic activity and SND.

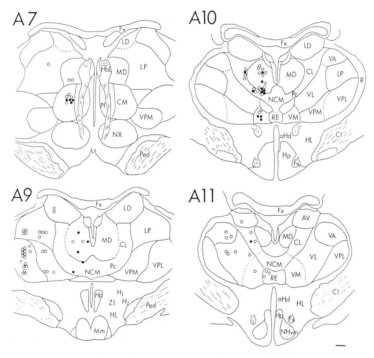

Fig. 2.   Distribution of recording sites in experiments in which sympathetic nerve discharge (SND) was related only to medial thalamic activity. Closed circles show thalamic sites with activity related to SND, as demonstrated with crosscorrelation analysis. Open circles show thalamic sites with activity unrelated to SND. Calibration is 1 mm. Abbreviations on frontal sections are those of

Jasper and Ajmone-Marsan (1954). aHd, area hypothalamica dorsalis; AV, N. anterior ventralis; CL, N. centralis lateralis; CM, N. centrum medianum; F_x, fornix; H_1, H_2, Forel's fields; HbL, N. habenularis lateralis; HL, hypothalamus lateralis; Hp, hypothalamus posterior; LD, N. lateralis dorsalis; LP, N. lateralis posterior; MD, N. medialis dorsalis; Mm, corpus mamillare; NR, N. ruber; NCM; N. centralis medialis; NHvm, N. hypothalami ventromedialis; Pc, N. paracentralis; Ped, pedunculus cerebralis; Pf, N. parafascicularis; R, N. reticularis; RE, N. reuniens; VA, N. ventralis anterior; VL, N. ventralis lateralis; VM, N. ventralis medialis; VPL, N. ventralis posterolateralis; VPM, N. ventralis posteromedialis; ZI, zona incerta.

Recordings were made from 53 medial thalamic and 40 lateral thalamic sites in the 7 experiments in which SND was temporally related only to medial thalamic activity. The distribution of thalamic recording sites in these experiments is shown in Fig. 2. Twenty-one of the medial thalamic sites had activity related to SND. The mean interval between zero lag and the first peak to the right of zero lag in the medial thalamic → SND crosscorrelograms for these 21 sites was 73+10 ms. Two of the cats in which SND was related only to medial thalamic activity were decorticate [see Andersson and Manson (1971) for procedure]. Thus, the integrity of connections between the thalamus and cerebral cortex was not essential for the synchronization of SND and medial thalamic activity.

ELECTRICAL AND CHEMICAL STIMULATION OF MEDIAL THALAMUS

The selective relationship between SND and medial thalamic activity in some experiments raises the question whether medial thalamic circuits are involved in the control of sympathetic tone. Two lines of evidence support this possibility. First, increases in SND were elicited by 10-ms trains of three pulses applied to medial thalamic sites in 17 cats, three of which were decorticate. The onset latencies of the sympathetic nerve responses elicited from different medial thalamic nuclei including centralis lateralis (CL), CM, medialis dorsalis (MD), paracentralis (Pc) and ventralis medialis (VM) were statistically indistinguishable. However, the mean onset latency of the increases in SND produced by medial thalamic stimulation was significantly longer than that for sympathetic nerve excitation elicited by posterior or lateral hypothalamic stimulation (Table 1). This was the case even when stimuli of supramaximal intensity (1 mA) were used. Moreover, increases in SND were elicited by medial thalamic stimulation with currents as

TABLE 1.   Mean onset latencies of inferior cardiac sympathetic nerve excitation produced by diencephalic stimulation with 10-ms trains of three pulses of supramaximal intensity (1 mA).

A. Cats with intact neuraxis (n=14)

	No. of Sites	Mean Onset $\pm$ S.E.
MTh	78	69 $+$ 1 ms*
HTh	27	60 $\pm$ 2 ms

B. Decorticate cats (n=3)

	No. of Sites	Mean Onset $\pm$ S.E.
MTh	7	64 $+$ 3 ms*
HTh	5	52 $\pm$ 2 ms

MTh and HTh are medial thalamus and hypothalamus, respectively.   * indicates that mean onset latency of responses elicited by MTh stimulation was significantly ($P < 0.05$) longer than that of the responses evoked by HTh stimulation.

low as or lower than that required to elicit shorter latency responses from the underlying hypothalamus and midbrain. Representative depth-threshold curves illustrating this point are shown in Fig. 3. Taken together, these results indicate that the sympathetic nerve responses evoked by medial thalamic stimulation were not the consequence of either current spread to the hypothalamus or activation of the axons of hypothalamic neurons coursing through the thalamus.   Rather, these responses may have involved the activation of neurons whose cell bodies were located in the medial thalamus.   Regarding this possibility, microinjection of picrotoxin into the medial thalamus increased SND and blood pressure. Experiments of this type provided the second line of evidence that supports the view that medial thalamic neurons are involved in the control of SND. Picrotoxin, a CNS stimulant with GABA antagonistic properties is believed to exert its actions by altering transmission in synaptic networks (Johnston, 1976). We chose to microinject this agent into the medial thalamus since this region receives GABAergic input (see review by Steriade et al., 1986).

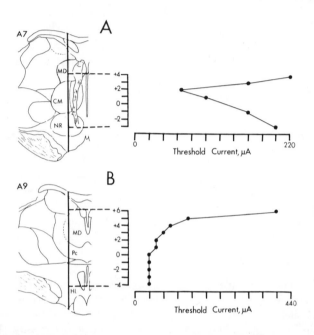

Fig. 3. Depth-threshold curves for sympathetic nerve excitation elicited by medial thalamic, hypothalamic and midbrain stimulation with 10-ms trains of three pulses. Stereotaxic horizontal plane (H) is plotted against threshold current (μA) for eliciting a response. Nuclei are labelled as in Fig. 2. Data in A and B are from different experiments.

One or two series of bilateral injections (5 μg picrotoxin in 0.5 μl) were made between stereotaxic planes A9 and A11, 0.5 to 1.5 mm lateral to the midline at H+1 or H+2. Fast green FCF dye injected at these sites at the end of each experiment spread to portions of CL, MD, Pc, and nuclei reuniens and centralis medialis of the medial thalamus. No dye was observed in the ventricular system, lateral thalamus (> 3 mm lateral to midline) or the hypothalamus. The changes in SND that became evident approximately 10 min after picrotoxin was injected are illustrated in Fig. 4. In this representative experiment, microinjection of picrotoxin led to an increase in the amplitude of the 2- to 6-Hz sympathetic nerve slow wave and a decrease in the variability of inter-slow wave intervals. The latter effect indicates that SND became more rhythmic in nature. The reduction in the variability of inter-slow wave intervals after picrotoxin administration is reflected by the sharp peak at 2.2 Hz in the power spectra of SND in Fig. 4 IIB. Sharp peaks were not observed in power spectra of SND constructed from data collected before picrotoxin was injected (Fig. 4 IB). The changes in SND produced by injection of picrotoxin into the medial thalamus were accompanied by a rise in blood pressure. Mean blood pressure was elevated approximately 30 mmHg in the experiment illustrated in Fig. 4. Recovery of SND and blood pressure to near control levels occurred between 1 and 1 1/2 hr after the local administration of picrotoxin (Fig. 4 III).

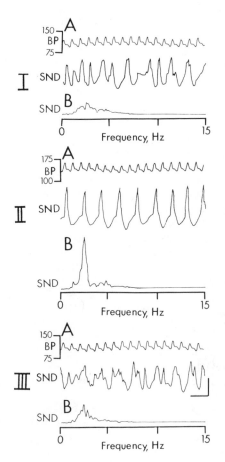

Fig. 4. Changes in sympathetic nerve discharge (SND) produced by microinjection of picrotoxin into medial thalamus. I, control. II, 10 min after bilateral injection of picrotoxin (total dose, 10 µg) into medial thalamus at stereotaxic plane A10. III, recovery approximately 1 hr after picrotoxin. Traces in IA, IIA and IIIA are oscillographic records of blood pressure (BP, mm Hg) and SND. Vertical calibration is 100 µV for SND. Horizontal calibration is 500 ms. Traces in IB, IIB and IIIB are power spectra of SND. Each spectrum is the average of twelve 8-s data blocks. Frequency resolution is 0.06 Hz. Vertical range of power (voltage squared) is same in all traces.

The pathways over which medial thalamic neurons influence SND remain to be elucidated. To our knowledge, there are no direct projections from the medial thalamus to caudal brain stem regions involved in sympathetic control. However, a pathway from the medial thalamus to the lateral hypothalamus has been described (Brutus et al., 1984). Interestingly, we found that inferior cardiac SND was temporally related to multiunit lateral hypothalamic activity in experiments in which SND and medial thalamic activity were synchronized. The mean interval (59+13 ms; n=19) between zero lag and the first peak to the right of zero lag in the hypothalamic → SND crosscorrelograms was shorter than that (73+10 ms; n=21) in the medial thalamic → SND crosscorrelograms. Thus, the sympathetic nerve-related component of hypothalamic activity lagged that in medial thalamic activity. These data are consistent with the possibility that medial thalamic influences on SND are mediated via circuits of hypothalamic neurons. This hypothesis, however, has not yet been directly tested.

DECEREBRATION EXPERIMENTS

Decerebration should reduce sympathetic nerve activity and blood pressure if the diencephalon is involved in setting the level of basal SND. Regarding this point, it has been the experience of several laboratories (Wang and Chai, 1962; Reis and Cuenod, 1964; Peiss, 1965) that midcollicular transection acutely lowers the blood pressure of anesthetized animals. These studies, however, did not determine whether the fall in blood pressure reflected the loss of forebrain control or a nonphysiological effect of the transection such as mechanical stimulation of descending sympathoinhibitory tracts. Experiments were performed by us to distinguish between these potential mechanisms. For this purpose, blood pressure and integrated inferior cardiac SND were measured in baroreceptor-denervated cats anesthetized with chloralose before and after serial transections of the midbrain at stereotaxic planes A3 and AP0. A3 transection produced a 38+7% decrease in SND and a concomitant fall in blood pressure that averaged 34+5 mm Hg (17 cats). SND and blood pressure returned to near control levels within 30 min after A3 transection. Importantly, subsequent transection of the midbrain at AP0 failed to affect SND or blood pressure. This observation argues against the possibility that the reductions in SND and blood pressure produced by A3 transection were due to mechanical stimulation of descending sympathoinhibitory tracts. Rather, these results suggest that the forebrain participates in generating basal SND. The loss of forebrain involvement, however, is partially compensated for within a short period of time. The effects produced by A3 transection were dependent upon the integrity of diencephalic structures. Regarding this point, midbrain transection at this level had little effect on SND and bood pressure in 11 cats in which the medial thalamus and hypothalamus were previously removed by suction. Finally, participation of the forebrain in the generation of basal SND was not attributable to the use of a cataleptic anesthetic (i.e., chloralose) since similar effects of A3 transection were observed in cats anesthetized with diallylbarbiturate-urethan.

SUMMARY

SND was temporally related to medial but not lateral thalamic activity in some CNS-intact and in decorticate cats. Three observations suggest that the temporal relationship reflects a role of medial thalamic neurons in generating a component of basal SND. First, electrical stimulation of the medial thalamus elicited an increase in SND that could not be attributed to activation of the underlying hypothalamus. Second, microinjection of picrotoxin into the medial thalamus increased SND. This agent is believed to act selectively on synaptic networks. Third, midbrain transection led to a 38% decrease in SND that was prevented by prior removal of the medial diencephalon. Indirect evidence is presented that medial thalamic influences on SND are mediated via hypothalamic neurons. Finally, it is unclear why SND was synchronized to activity recorded from the lateral thalamus (including specific sensory relay nuclei) in some experiments. Perhaps such occurrences were related to the level of cataleptic anesthesia produced by chloralose, an agent known to hypersynchronize activity in different thalamic nuclei and cortical regions (Winters and Spooner, 1966).

REFERENCES

Andersson SA, Manson JR (1971). Rhythmic activity in the thalamus of the unanesthetized decorticate cat. Electroenceph clin Neurophysiol 31:21-34.
Barman SM, Gebber GL (1980). Sympathetic nerve rhythm of brain stem origin. Am J Physiol 239:R42-R47.
Brutus M, Watson RE Jr, Shaikh MB, Siegel HE, Weiner S, Siegel A (1984). A [^{14}C]2-deoxyglucose analysis of the functional neural pathways of the limbic forebrain in the rat. IV. A pathway from the prefrontal cortical-medial thalamic system to the hypothalamus. Brain Research 310:279-293.
Camerer H, Stroh-Werz M, Kreinke B, Langhorst P (1977). Postganglionic sympathetic activity with correlation to heart rhythm and central cortical rhythms. Pfluegers Arch 370: 221-225.

Gebber GL (1980). Central oscillators responsible for sympathetic nerve discharge. Am J Physiol 239:H143-H155.

Gebber GL, Barman SM (1981). Sympathetic-related activity of brain stem neurons in baroreceptor-denervated cats. Am J Physiol 240:R348-R355.

Jahnsen H, Llinas R (1984). Ionic basis for the electroresponsiveness and oscillatory properties of guinea-pig thalamic neurons in vitro. J Physiol London 349:227-247.

Jasper HH, Ajmone-Marsan C (1954). "A Stereotaxic Atlas of the Diencephalon of the Cat." Ottawa: National Research Council Canada, p 70.

Johnston GAR (1976). Physiologic pharmacology of GABA and its antagonists in the vertebrate nervous system. In Roberts E, Chase TN, Tower DB (eds): "GABA in Nervous System Function," New York: Raven, p 395.

Peiss CN (1965). Concepts of cardiovascular regulation: Past, present and future. In Randall WC (ed): "Nervous Control of the Heart," Baltimore: Williams and Wilkins, p 154.

Reis DJ, Cuenod M (1964). Tonic influence of rostral brain structures on pressure regulatory mechanisms in the cat. Science 145:64-65.

Steriade M, Domich L, Oakson G (1986). Reticularis thalamic neurons revisited: Activity changes during shifts in states of vigilance. J Neurosci 6:68-81.

Wang SC, Chai CY (1962). Central control of sympathetic cardio-acceleration in medulla oblongata of the cat. Am J Physiol 202:31-34.

Winters WD, Spooner CE (1966). A neurophysiological comparison of alpha-chloralose with gamma-hydroxybutyrate in cats. Electroenceph clin Neurophysiol 20:83-90.

ACKNOWLEDGEMENTS

The authors are grateful to Mr. William Cook for technical assistance and to Ms. Diane Hummel for typing the manuscript. This study was supported by National Institutes of Health grants HL-13187 and HL-33266.

SECTION IV: Ventrolateral Medulla and Cardiovascular Regulation

One of the most exciting aspects of research in the central control of the circulation to emerge within the last few years has been the elucidation of neural circuits specifically responsible for generating tonic sympathetic nervous discharge. Although it has been generally thought that these neural circuits were widely distributed in the central nervous system, a considerable amount of new physiological and neuroanatomical data suggest that some of these circuits involve neurons found on or near the ventral surface of the medulla. The contributions to follow are representative of the very active research in the area.

The paper by Guyenet, Sun and Brown, briefly reviews the experimental evidence for different transmitters mediating sympatho-excitatory effects on sympathetic preganglionic neurons. In addition, it presents data suggesting that glutamatergic neurons are involved in the mediation of baroreflex effects on vagal cardiomotor and presumed sympatho-excitatory bulbo-spinal neurons, of hypothalamic excitation of nucleus paragigantocellularis lateralis cells, and of sympathetic preganglionic neuron excitation by bulbo-spinal neurons.

The paper by Caverson and Ciriello described anatomical and physiological properties of neurons near the ventral surface of the medulla which project directly to the intermediolateral nucleus of the thoracolumbar cord and that receive baroreceptor and peripheral chemoreceptor afferent inputs.

The paper by Barman presents an electrophysiological analysis of the pattern of axonal branching within the spinal cord and medulla, of axons of ventrolateral medullary neurons. The paper also presents evidence that these neurons are involved in relaying input from lateral tegmental field neurons to sympathetic preganglionic neurons.

The paper by McAllen, Dampney and Goodchild concerns the mechanism of the vasomotor responses evoked by electrical and chemical activation of the ventrolateral medulla. Their data suggests that a collection of bulbo-spinal neurons, within a region labelled the retrofacial, is essential in mediating these responses.

Organization of the Autonomic Nervous System:
Central and Peripheral Mechanisms, pages 215–225
© 1987 Alan R. Liss, Inc.

Role of GABA and excitatory aminoacids in medullary
baroreflex pathways.

Patrice G. Guyenet, Miao–Kun Sun,
and D. Les Brown.
University of Virginia, Dept. of Pharmacology
Charlottesville, VA 22908.

Introduction.

Two main points will be made in this brief review.
First, the processing of cardiovascular information
appears highly concentrated within a few specialized
neuronal clusters of the nucleus of the solitary tract
(NTS) and ventrolateral medulla (VLM). Second, the
hardwiring of medullary baroreflexes consists of neurons
which use either glutamate or GABA but not monoamines as
primary transmitters. In this paper the word glutamate
will be used generically in the sense of excitatory
aminoacid neurotransmitter.

Nuc. PGCL reticulospinal sympathoexcitatory neurons and
the origin of the sympathetic tone

In the rat, the most rostral portion of the VLM
(retrofacial portion of nuc. paragigantocellularis
lateralis, henceforth called retrofacial PGCL, after
Andrezik et al. 1981 a,b; Fig. 1) contains a population of
cells which provide a tonic excitatory drive to vasomotor
preganglionic neurons and function as the descending limb
of the sympathetic baroreflex (Brown and Guyenet 1984,
1985, Guyenet and Brown 1986). These neurons are
concentrated within 400 μm of the base of the medulla,
between 0-400 μm posterior to the caudal end of the facial
motor nucleus and between 1.7 and 2 mm lateral to the
midline. Iontophoretic deposits of the anterograde

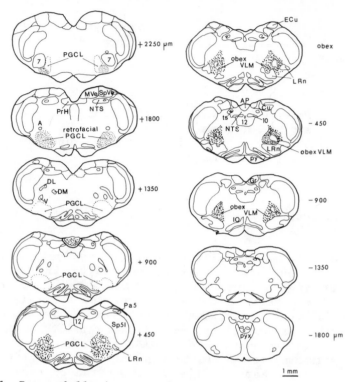

Fig. 1 Rat medulla in coronal sections.
Retrofacial PGCL (finely stippled) represents location
of electrophysiological identified medullospinal sympathoexcitatory neurons (PGCL: nuc. paragigantocellularis
lateralis after Andrezik et al.)
Obex-VLM (heavily stripped) represents general area of
ventrolateral medulla containing third-order, presumably
GABAergic, neurons of sympathetic baroreflex pathway.
Other abbreviations: A nuc. ambiguus, Ecu external
cuneate, DL dorsolateral subnuc. of A, DM dorsomedian
subnuc. of A, Gr nuc. graclilis, IO inferior olive LRn lat.
retic. nuc., MVe medial vestibular nuc., NTS nuc. tractus
solitarius, 7 facial nuc., 10 dorsal nuc. of vagus, 12
hypoglossal nuc.

tracer Phaseolus lectin (PhaL) into this site produces
terminal labelling in the following areas:
intermediolateral cell column (IML), lamina X and nuc.
intercalatus, NTS complex around obex (including area
postrema, motor nuc. of X and hypoglossal nuc.), lateral
parabrachial nuc., locus coeruleus and subcoeruleus area
(Guyenet and Young, unpublished). The ventral horn at
thoracic level is involved when injections include more
dorsal aspects of nuc. PGCL. This and other evidence
(Amendt et al. 1978, Ross et al. 1984) indicates that the
spinal projections of retrofacial PGCL are targeted to
where the soma or dendrites of sympathetic preganglionic
neurons are located as well as to the thoracic ventral
horn. However the latter projection probably consists of
fast conducting cells without detectable role in
sympathetic vasomotor function (Barman and Gebber, 1985).
In the rat, the predominant type of tonically active
medullospinal cell found in nuc. PGCL consists of slow
conducting neurons with high level of spontaneous firing
(5-40 spike/sec) and a pulse-synchronous activity due to a
powerful baroreceptor inhibitory input (Brown and Guyenet
1984, 1985 Guyenet and Brown 1986). These cells can be
further subdivided into very slow conducting clonidine
sensitive ones (0.6 m/sec, the minority) and a predominant
group of slow-conducting (3.5 m/sec) clonidine-insensitive
ones (Sun and Guyenet, 1986a). The relationship between
the firing rate of these cells and mean AP is identical to
that existing between lumbar SND and MAP during
experimental perturbations of the latter produced by
increasing afterload, reducing preload or administering
pressor or depressor agents. This observation holds true
for WKY normotensive, spontaneously hypertensive and
Sprague-Dawley rats (Sun et al. 1986b). Also the pulse
synchronous inhibition of peripheral SND (L_4) lags 100
msec. behind that of these PGCL neurons, a latency which
is identical to that of the predominant peak of
sympathoactivation produced by nuc. PGCL stimulation
(Guyenet and Brown 1986). These data and those of Barman
and Gebber (1985) in the cat support the notion that the
sympathetic vasomotor tone of anesthetized animals is due
largely to the tonic discharge of these excitatory
medullospinal PGCL units and that the baroreflex results
from their inhibition. Two plausible hypothesis could
explain the high level of activity of these cells, namely
synaptic driving by neurons located elsewhere in the
medulla (cf Gebber and Barman 1985) or pace-maker
discharge.

Hypothalamic glutamatergic input to PGCL sympathetic
neurons. Selectivity of kynurenate as a
glutamate-receptor antagonist.

Iontophoretic application of kynurenate (KYN) blocks
the excitatory effect of glutamate on the discharges of
PGCL sympathetic neurons without affecting their
spontaneous firing rate nor their response to
iontophoretic ACh (Sun and Guyenet 1986c). KYN affects
neither the inhibitory effect of iontophoretically applied
GABA nor the GABA-mediated baroreceptor feedback
inhibition of these cells (Sun and Guyenet 1986c). 8-OH
kynurenate (xanthurenate, XAN) is uniformly ineffective in
all these tests. Thus KYN is a specific
glutamate-receptor antagonist in nuc. PGCL as it is
elsewhere in the brain (Stone and Connick 1985).
Bilateral injections of KYN (5 nanomoles, 100 nl) into
nuc. PGCL block the sympathoactivation (L_3-L_4) and
arterial pressure elevation produced by electrically
stimulating the perifornical area of the lateral
hypothalamus but do not alter basal SND nor baroreflex
inhibition (Sun and Guyenet 1986c). Bilateral injections
of 5 nmoles XAN into nuc. PGCL are uniformly ineffective
in all regards. Moreover, the vast majority (> 80 %) of
nuc. PGCL sympathoexcitatory neurons are excited by
perifornical area stimulation and microinjections of l-glu
into the lateral hypothalamus increases AP and excites 40%
of these neurons. These results confirm Hilton's
hypothesis that sympathetic activation of hypothalamic
origin is relayed synaptically in the anterior VLM (Hilton
et al. 1983). Our data further indicate that these
hypothalamic sympathoexcitatory inputs excite PGCL
sympathoexcitatory neurons by releasing glu.

Is an aminoacid the transmitter released in the cord by
sympathoexcitatory neurons of nuc. PGCL?

Epinephrine (EPI), substance P (sP) and serotonin
(5HT) have all been previously proposed as possible
candidates for the main excitatory neurotransmitter
released in the IML by sympathoexcitatory neurons of the
VLM. The case for EPI is inferential and based on the
anatomical observation that the C_1 group of
PNMT-immunoreactive cells group projects to the IML and
and that the distribution of these cells overlaps the
pressor area of the VLM (Ruggiero et al. 1985, Ross et al.

1984c). Using a retrograde labelling technique (rhodamine-tagged microbeads) in combination with the immunohistochemical localization of PNMT-containing neurons (Guyenet and Young, unpublished), we have recently found that the same group of C_1 cells massively innervates the somata of the NE neurons of the locus coeruleus. It is well known that the application of EPI on locus coeruleus NE cells produces an α_2-mediated hyperpolarization, and that EPI also inhibits sympathetic preganglionic neurons by the same mechanism (Guyenet and Cabot, 1981). Therefore EPI is very unlikely to be the sympathoexcitatory transmitter released in the IML by PGCL sympathexcitatory neurons and it is possible that the adrenergic neurons of the VLM may even represent an inhibitory system which turns off the central release of NE (via its action on the locus coeruleus) as well as that of peripheral catecholamines (via its inhibitory effect on sympathetic preganglionic neurons). The hypothesis that 5HT is an excitatory transmitter released by some raphe projections to the IML is supported by the work of McCall, 1984, Morrison and Gebber 1984 and Chalmers group (Howe et al. 1983). Yet it is also clear that methysergide, the antagonist which blocks the excitatory effect of 5HT on preganglionic neurons doesnot significantly affect resting SND or baroreflexes, therefore 5HT cannot be the main transmitter released by sympathoexcitatory neurons of the VLM. A somewhat stronger case has been made for substance P since it increases SND when applied intrathecally at spinal levels and a few substance P antagonists decrease resting SND when administered via the same route (Loewy and Sawyer 1982, Yashpal et al. 1985). Yet the hypothesis has been weakened considerably by reports that sP antagonists produce powerful local anesthetic actions (Post et al. 1985).

On the other hand we recently found that intrathecal (T_{10}) administration of the glutamate-receptor antagonist kynurenic acid (5 µmoles) abolishes resting SND and the sympathoactivation produced by stimulation of nuc. PGCL. Yet SND can be restored to prekynurenate levels and beyond by subsequent intrathecal injections of the glutamate agonist kainic acid (30 nmoles) indicating that the blockade by KYN can be overcome and therefore is not due to local anesthetic effects. In fact after SND is restored to control levels with kainic acid, nuc. PGCL stimulation results in sympathoinhibition which could conceivably be due to the release of EPI from C_1 adrenergic neurons although this fact remains to be established. This evidence suggests that glutamate could be the main excitatory transmitter released by PGCL sympathoexcitatoryneurons. It remains to be determined whether or not this glutamate-like transmitter could be released by PNMT-immunoreactive cells.

Role of glutamate in cardiac parasympathetic baroreflexes.

Bilateral injections (2.5 nanomoles) of the glutamate-receptor antagonist kynurenic acid (KYN) into the VLM at the level of the obex (henceforth called obex-VLM see Fig. 1) blocks the cardioinhibition produced by elevating arterial pressure in nadolol-pretreated rats (Guyenet, Filtz and Donaldson unpublished). Because of the β_1-adrenergic antagonist activity of nadolol, cardioinhibition in this preparation is totally atropine-sensitive and therefore solely due to vagal activation. Similar administrations of KYN 1.5 mm away from obex-VLM are ineffective and injections of 2.5 nanomoles of the inactive analog of KYN, xanthurenic acid (XAN) in obex-VLM are also ineffective. Thus vagal motoneuron activation seems to be prevented by antagonizing glutamate receptors in obex-VLM. It is therefore possible that glu is released by second order neurons of the baroreflex arc; the somata of these cells are located in the dorsomedial NTS and they may project monosynaptically to the cardiac vagal motorneurons of nuc. ambiguus (Meeley et al. 1985).

Role of glutamate in sympathetic baroreflexes.

Bilateral injections of KYN (2.5 nanomoles) into obex-VLM also abolish the sympathoinhibition produced by increasing arterial pressure via gradual aortic constriction (Guyenet et al., unpublished). This effect is fully reversible and not produced when XAN is injected into obex-VLM or when KYN is injected outside obex-VLM (1.5 mm away including most notably nuc. PGCL). It is therefore probable that second-order baroreceptor neurons involved in baroreflex inhibition of SND release a glutamate-like substance into obex-VLM which excites third-order GABA-ergic baroreceptor neurons. The latter are presumably responsible for inhibiting sympathoexcitatory neurons of nuc. PGCL (vide infra). The presence in the intermediate portion of the VLM of a synaptic relay for sympathetic baroreflexes is compatible with data of Blessing et al. in the rabbit (1981) and of

Willette et al. in the rat (1983b, 1984a and b).

GABA is the inhibitory transmitter responsible for the baroreflex inhibition of sympathoexcitatory neurons of nuc. PGCL.

Intraparenchymal injections of the GABA-A receptor antagonist bicuculline (Bic) into retrofacial PGCL completely block baroreflex inhibition of lumbar SND (Sun and Guyenet, unpublished, Willette et al. 1984a). Injections of the same amount in a variety of other medullary areas are ineffective. Microinjections of bicuculline into PGCL also block the sympathoinhibition produced by low-frequency (5 cps) stimulation of the central end of the vagus (cardiopulmonary afferents) in rats with aortic depressor nerve, cervical sympathetic chain and superior laryngeal nerves cut (Sun and Guyenet, unpublished). These result confirm and extend previous data by Loewy's group who showed that surface applications of BIC on the rostral VLM of cats impairs sympathetic baroreflexes (Yamada et al. 1984).
Iontophoretic applications of BIC also block the inhibition of PGCL sympathoexcitatory neurons produced by activation of either arterial baroreceptors (Sun and Guyenet 1985) or vagal afferents (Sun and Guyenet, unpublished). Thus both types of sympathetic baroreflexes appear to result from the GABA-mediated inhibition of PGCL sympathoexcitatory neurons.

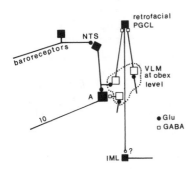

Fig. 2 Medullary Baroreflex Pathways.
A nuc. ambiguus, NTS nuc. solitary tract, PGCL nuc. paragigantocellularis lateralis, VLM ventrolateral medulla.

Conclusion.

Three areas of the medulla (Fig. 2) appear to be of critical importance for baroreflexes and their modulation by somatosensory and hypothalamic inputs, namely the dorsomedial NTS, the ventrolateral medulla at the level of the obex (obex-VLM) and the anterior tip of the VLM (rostral part of RVL of Ross et al. 1985, VLM pressor area of Sapru et al., retrofacial portion of nuc. PGCL after Andrezik et al. 1981 a and b). The putative role of these three areas is as follows. Glutamatergic arterial baroreceptors (Talman et al. 1982) excite second order glutamatergic neurons located in the dorsomedial NTS which project to obex-VLM. Second order neurons excite cardiac vagal motoneurons as well as third order GABA-ergic neurons. The latter project to nuc. PGCL and inhibit medullospinal sympathoexcitatory neurons with direct projections to sympathetic preganglionic neurons. The medullospinal projection consists of spontaneously active perhaps pacemaker cells responsible for the basal vasomotor tone. Their major transmitter may be an excitatory amino acid. These cells receive glutamatergic inputs from the lateral hypothalamus and are also involved in long-loop somatosympathetic reflexes (Guyenet and Brown 1986). The "A_1 area" (obex-VLM) is also involved in the baroreflex control of the release of argininvasopressin and probably contains other active and non baroreceptor-related systems which tonically decrease both vagal and sympathetic outflows (Blessing et al. 1981, Willette et al. 1984 a and b). This scheme is still based on relatively indirect evidence since only the sympathoexcitatory neurons of nuc. PGCL and the raphe have been unambiguously characterized with electrophysiological techniques. The monosynaptic nature of the postulated connections is still not demonstrated in a single case. Monoaminergic neurons (NE neurons of the A_1, A_2, A_5, A_6, A_7 groups, and raphe 5HT neurons) are not represented in this scheme.

References

Amendt K, Czachurski J, Dembowsky K, Seller H (1978) Neurones within the "chemosensitive area" on the ventral surface of the brainstem which project to the intermediolateral cell column. Pflugers Arch. ges. Physiol. 375:289-292.

Andrezik JA, Chan-Palay V (1981a) The nucleus paragigantocellularis lateralis in the rat conformation and cytology. Anal. Embryol. 161:355-371.

Andrezik JA, Chan-Palay V (1981b) The nucleus paragigantocellularis lateralis: demonstration of afferents by the retrograde transport of HRP. Anat. Embryol. 161:373-390.

Barman SM, Gebber GL (1985) Axonal projection patterns of ventrolateral medullospinal sympathoexcitatory neurons. J. Neurophysiol. 53:1567-1582.

Blessing WW, Reis DJ (1982) Inhibitory cardiovascular funtion of neurons in the caudal ventrolateral medulla of the rabbit. Relationship to the area containing A_1 NE neurons. Brain Research 253:161-172.

Blessing WW, West MJ, Chalmers J (1981) Hypertension, bradycardia and pulmonary edema in the conscious rabbit after brainstem lesions coinciding with the A_1 group fo catecholamine neurons. Circ. Res. 49:449-958.

Brown DL, Guyenet PG (1984) Cardiovascular neurons of the brain stem with projections to spinal cord. Am. J. Physiol. 247:R1009-R1016.

Brown DL, Guyenet PG (1985) Electrophysiological study of cardiovascular neurons in the rostral ventrolateral medulla in rats. Circ. Research 56:359-369.

Day TA, Ro A, Renaud LP (1983) Depressor area within caudal ventrolateral mmedulla of the rat does not correspond to the A_1 catecholamine cell group. Brain Res. 279:299-302.

Gebber GL, Barman SM (1985) Lateral tegmental field neurons of cat medulla: a potential source of basal sympathetic nerve discharge. J. Neurophysiology 54:1498-1512.

Guertzenstein PG, Silver A (1974) Fall in blood pressure produced from discrete regions of the ventral surface of the medulla by glycine and lesions. J. Physiol. 242:489-503.

Guyenet PG, Brown DL (1986) Nucleus paragigantocellularis lateralis and lumbar sympathetic discharge in the rat. Am. J. Physiol. (in press).

Guyenet PG, Cabot JB (1981) Inhibition of sympathetic preganglionic neurons by catecholamines and clonidine. J. Neurosci. 1:908-917.

Hilton SM, Marshall JM, Timms RJ (1983) Ventral medullary relay neurons in the pathway from the defence areas of the cat and their effect on blood pressure. J. Physiol. (Lond.) 345:149-166.

Howe PRC, Kuhn DM, Minson JB, Stead BH, Chalmers P (1983) Evidence for a bulbospinal serotoninergic pressor pathway in the rat brain. Brain Res. 270:29-36.

Loewy AD, Sawyer WB (1982) SP antagonist inhibits vasomotor responses elicited from ventral medulla in rat. Brain Research 245:379-383.
Loewy AD, Wallach JH, McKellar S (1981) Efferent connections of the ventral medulla oblongata in the rat. Brain Res. Reviews 3:63-80.
McCall RB (1984) Evidence for a serotonergically mediated sympathoexcitatory response to stimulation of medullary raphe nuclei. Brain Res. 311:131-140.
Meeley MP, Ruggiero DA, Ishitsuka T, Reis DJ (1985) Intrinsic -aminobutyric acid neurons in the nucleus of the solitary tract and the rostral ventrolateral medulla of the rat: an immunohistochemical and biochemical study. NS Letters 58:83-89.
Morrison SF, Gebber GL (1984) Raphe neurons with sympathetic related activity: baroreceptor responses and spinal connections. Amer. J. Physiol. 246:R338-R348.
Post C, Butterworth JF, Strichartz GR, Karlsson JA, Persson CGA (1985) Tachykinin antagonists have potent local anesthetic actions. E.J. Pharmacol. 117:347-354.
Ross CA, Ruggiero DA, Joh TH, Park DH, Reis DJ (1984b) Rostral ventrolateral medulla: selective projecions to the thoracic autonomic cell column from the region containing C_1 adrenaline neurons. J. Comp. Neurol. 228:168-185.
Ross CA, Ruggiero DA, Park PH, Joh TH, Sved AF, Fernandez-Pardal J, Saavedra JM, Reis DJ (1984b) Tonic vasomotor contol by the rostral ventrolateral medulla, effect of electrical on chemical stimulation of the area containing C_1 adrenaline neurons on arterial pressure, heart rate and plasma catecholamines and vasopressin. J. Neurosci. 4:474-494.
Ross CA, Ruggiero DA, Reis DJ (1985) Projections from the nucleus tractus solitarii to the rostral ventrolateral medulla. JCN 242:511-534.
Ruggiero DA, Meeley MP, Anwar M, Reis DJ (1985) Newly identified GABAergic neurons in regions of the ventrolateral medulla which regulate blood pressure. Brain Research 339:171-178.
Ruggiero DA, Ross CA, Anwar M, Park DA, Joh TH, Reis DJ (1985) Distribution of neurons containing phenylethanolamine N-methyltransferase in medulla and hypothelamus of rat. JCN 239:127-154.
Stone TW, Connick JH (1985) Quinolinic acid and other kynurenines in the central nervous system. Neuroscience 15:597-618.

Sun M-K, Guyenet PG (1985) GABA-mediated baroreceptor inhibition of reticulospinal neurons. Am. J. Physiol. 249:R672-R680.

Sun M-K, Guyenet PG (1986a) Effect of clonidine and GABA on the discharges of medullospinal sympathoexcitatory neruons in the rat. Brain Research 368:1-17.

Sun M-K, Guyenet PG (1986b) Medullospinal sympathoexcitatory neurons in normotensive and spontaneously hypertensive rats. Am. J. Physiol. 250 (Regul. Int. Comp. Physiol. 19):R910-R917.

Sun M-K, Guyenet PG (1986c) Hypothalamic glutamatergic input to medullary sypathoexcitatory neurons in rat. Am. J. Physiol. (in press).

Talman WT, Perrone MH, Reis DJ (1980) Evidence for l-glutamate as the neurotransmitter of baroreceptor afferent nerve fibers. Science 209:813-815.

West MJ, Blessing WW, Chalmers J (1981) Arterial baroreceptor reflex function in the conscious rabbit after brainstem lesions coinciding with the A_1 group of CA neurons. Circ. Res. 49:959-970.

Willette RN, Barcas PP, Krieger AJ, Sapru HN (1983a) Vasopressor and depressor areas in the rat medulla identification by microinjection of glutamate. Neuropharmacology 22:1071-1080.

Willette RN, Krieger AJ, Barcas PP, Sapru HN (1983b) Medullary -aminobutyric acid receptors and the regulation of blood pressure in the rat. J.P.E.T. 226:893-899.

Willette RN, Barcas PP, Krieger AJ, Sapru HN (1984a) Endogenous GABAergic mechanisms in the medulla and the regulation of blood pressure. J.P.E.T. 230:34-39.

Willette RN, Punnen S, Krieger AJ, Sapru HN (1984b) Interdependance of costral and caudal ventrolateral medullary areas in the control of blood pressure. Brain Research 321:169-174.

Yamada K, McAllan RM, Loewy AD (1984) GABA antagonists applied to the ventral surface of the medulla oblongata block the baroreceptor reflex. Brain Research 297:175-180.

Yashpal K, Gauthier SG, Henry JL (1985) Substance P given intrathecally at the spinal T9 level increases adrenal output of adrenaline and noradrenaline in the rat. Neuroscience 15:529-536.

Organization of the Autonomic Nervous System:
Central and Peripheral Mechanisms, pages 227–237
© 1987 Alan R. Liss, Inc.

VENTROLATERAL MEDULLOSPINAL NEURONS INVOLVED IN THE CONTROL
OF THE CIRCULATION

Monica M. Caverson and John Ciriello

Department of Physiology, Health Sciences Centre,
University of Western Ontario, London, Ontario,
Canada   N6A 5C1

INTRODUCTION

For over a century evidence has been available which
suggests that the neurons responsible for the maintenance of
vasomotor tone are found in the medulla oblongata (Dittmar,
1870, 1873; Owsjannikow, 1871). These neurons are thought
to be located in the region of the medullary reticular formation recently termed the ventrolateral medulla (VLM;
Alexander, 1946; Amendt et al., 1979; Dampney and Moon, 1980;
Dampney et al., 1982; Dembowsky et al., 1981; Feldberg, 1976;
Guertzenstein and Silver, 1974; Loewy et al., 1981; McAllen
et al., 1982; Miura et al., 1983; Ross et al., 1984a,b;
Schlaefke, 1981). However, the precise anatomical location
and function of neurons in the VLM which may be involved in
relaying cardiovascular afferent information directly to
sympathetic areas of the thoracolumbar spinal cord remain
equivocal.

The present experiments, therefore, were done to functionally and histologically establish the location of neurons
in the region of the VLM which may be involved in altering
sympathetic outflow to the heart and blood vessels through
direct connections with spinal preganglionic cardioacceleratory and vasoconstrictor neurons or antecedent interneurons.
In addition, some of the peripheral and central cardiovascular
afferent inputs which are received by these neurons and relayed to spinal sympathetic areas were investigated.

This report presents a summary of three series of experiments. First, the location of pressor sites in the VLM

was investigated using electrical stimulation. These pressor
responses were subsequently shown to be due to the activation
of cell bodies in the VLM as microinjections of L-glutamate
elicited similar responses. The second series involved using
the autoradiographic tract tracing technique to identify the
sites of termination of VLM neurons within spinal sympathetic
areas. Conversely, the horseradish peroxidase technique was
used to map the precise distribution in the VLM of neurons
which send axons directly to spinal sympathetic areas. In
the final series, extracellular single unit recording experiments were done to investigate some of the electrophysiological characteristics of VLM neurons antidromically activated
from spinal sympathetic areas and the synaptic responses of
these units to cardiovascular afferent inputs of peripheral
and central origin.

ELECTRICAL AND L-GLUTAMATE STIMULATION OF THE VLM

To determine the location of pressor sites in the region
of the VLM, experiments were done in alpha-chloralose anesthetized, paralyzed and artificially ventilated cats. Arterial pressure (AP) and heart rate (HR) were continuously recorded and all animals had the carotid sinus (CSN), aortic
depressor (ADN), vagus and cervical sympathetic nerves cut
bilaterally.

Unipolar stainless steel electrodes were used to electrically stimulate the VLM; the stimulus consisted of a 10s
train of rectangular pulses (50 µA, 100 Hz, 0.2 ms pulse
duration). L-glutamate (L-glu) injections (0.5 M; pH, 7.8)
were made into regions of the VLM from which pressor responses were elicited during electrical stimulation. All stimulation sites were histologically verified at the completion
of each experiment. Sites from which pressor responses were
elicited during electrical stimulation were found from approximately the level of the obex to 5 mm rostral to the obex.
In the caudal VLM, these pressor sites were located in the
region extending from just lateral to the inferior olivary
nucleus (ION), around the exiting intramedullary rootlets of
the hypoglossal nerve (12N), to immediately ventral to the
spinal trigeminal nucleus. In the rostral VLM, pressor sites
were found throughout the nucleus paragigantocellularis lateralis (PGL) from the rostral extent of the lateral reticular
nucleus (LRN) to approximately the level of the facial nucleus.
The largest pressor responses (+50-80 mmHg) were elicited

from sites in the PGL near the ventral surface of the medulla
(Fig. 1A).

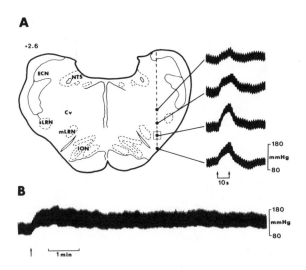

Figure 1. A, transverse section of the cat medulla showing
the location of sites in the rostral VLM from which pressor
responses were elicited by electrical or L-glutamate stimulation. Each dot (●) represents a site which was electrically stimulated with a 10 s train of pulses of 50 μA, 0.2 ms
pulse duration, at 100 Hz. Stimulus applied between arrows.
B, response to microinjection of 50 nl of L-glutamate at the
site marked by a dot within a square (◙). Injections made
at arrow. Cv, nucleus medullae oblongatae centralis subnucleus ventralis; ECN, external cuneate nucleus; ION, inferior olivary nucleus; mLRN, magnocellular component of lateral
reticular nucleus; NTS, nucleus of the solitary tract; sLRN,
subtrigeminal component of lateral reticular nucleus.

Characteristic pressor responses are shown in Figure 1A.
The AP response consisted of an increase both in diastolic
and systolic pressure immediately at the onset of stimulation,
was sustained during stimulation, and returned to baseline
after the stimulus was discontinued. The pressor response
was usually accompanied by a cardioacceleration of 5 to 15

beats/min, although stimulation of any one site did not necessarily elicit changes in both variables. L-glu injections into regions of the VLM which elicited large pressor responses during electrical stimulation consistently elicited increases in AP which occurred immediately after the injection, usually reached a peak within 5 sec, and gradually returned to baseline within 3-7 min (Fig. 1B). In the majority of cases the rise in AP was not accompanied by changes in HR.

TRITIATED-AMINO ACID AND HORSERADISH PEROXIDASE TRANSPORT STUDIES

Projections from pressor regions in the VLM, to spinal sympathetic areas were identified using the autoradiographic technique (Cowan et al., 1972). In brief, a small volume (20-50 nl) of a solution containing equal parts of tritiated proline and leucine (100 μCi/μl) was injected into pressor regions of the VLM (Fig. 2A), identified in the previous study, in cats anesthetized with pentobarbital. After a survival period of 14-28 days the animals were perfused and sections of the medulla containing the injection site, and spinal segments T_1-L_6 were processed for autoradiography.

Anterograde labeling was observed throughout the thoracolumbar cord primarily in the region of the intermediolateral nucleus (IML), and to a lesser extent in the central autonomic area (CA), and nucleus intercalatus (IC),bilaterally, with an ipsilateral predominance (Fig. 2B-D). In addition, a small amount of labeling was observed along the ventrolateral aspect of the ventral horn in the region known to contain intercostal motorneurons. The descending fiber tracts from the VLM coursed mainly in the dorsolateral funiculus, bilaterally, with an ipsilateral predominance. A smaller number of labeled fibers were observed in the lateral and ventrolateral funiculi, bilaterally. Fiber and terminal labeling in the IML was most dense at the T_1-T_3, T_8-T_9, T_{12} and L_1 levels (Fig. 2B and D), whereas the greatest density of labeling in the CA was between T_2-T_5 (Fig. 2C). The labeling in IC was most dense at T_5, T_9-T_{10}, T_{12} and L_1 (Fig. 2C-D).

To identify the precise location in pressor regions of the VLM of neurons which projected to spinal sympathetic areas, injections of horseradish peroxidase (HRP; Sigma Type VI) were made into the regions of the IML and CA at different thoracic levels in cats under pentobarbital anesthesia.

After 2 to 6 days the animals were perfused and the brain
stem sections were processed according to the tetramethyl
benzidine procedure (Mesulam, 1978). Most of the retrogradely
labeled HRP cells were found in the rostral VLM (1 to 5 mm
rostral to obex) bilaterally, but with an ipsilateral predominance, in the regions in which microinjections of L-glu
elicited pressor responses and in which tritiated amino acid
injections resulted in anterograde labeling in spinal sympathetic areas. In the caudal VLM, the majority of the HRP
labeled cells were observed clustered in an area lateral to
the ION around the intramedullary rootlets of the 12N. In
the rostral VLM, labeled cells were found scattered along
the ventral surface of the medulla throughout the PGL.

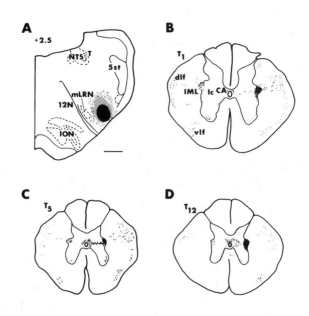

Figure 2. Schematic representation of a tritiated amino acid
injection (20 nl; stippling) into a pressor site in the rostral VLM (A) and the resulting fiber and terminal labeling
in the T_1 (B), T_5(C) and T_{12} (D) segments of the spinal cord.
Calibration mark in A, 1 mm. CA, central autonomic area;
dlf, dorsolateral funiculus; Ic, nucleus intercalatus; IML,
intermediolateral nucleus; T, tractus solitarius; vlf, ventrolateral funiculus; 5st, spinal trigeminal tract; 12N, hypoglossal nerve; See Fig. 1 for additional abbreviations.

SINGLE UNIT RECORDING STUDIES

Pressor regions in the VLM shown in the previous anatomical studies to contain neurons which projected directly to
spinal sympathetic areas were explored for single units which
were antidromically activated by electrical stimulation of
functionally and histologically verified sites in the region
of the upper thoracic IML and CA in alpha-chloralose anesthetized, paralyzed and artificially ventilated cats. These
units were further tested for their orthodromic response to
electrical stimulation of the CSN, ADN, and of pressor sites
in the paraventricular nucleus of the hypothalamus (PVH) and
lateral hypothalamus (Hla). In addition, some VLM antidromically activated units were tested for their orthodromic response to selective activation of peripheral chemoreceptors
by intraarterial injections of sodium cyanide (20-60 µg in
0.1-0.3 ml saline) via a cannula in the medial thyroid artery
and of baroreceptors by the intravenous infusion of phenylephrine (2 µg/kg) and by carotid occlusion (20 sec). The
results of these experiments have been presented in detail
elsewhere (Caverson et al., 1983a,b, 1984; Ciriello et al.,
1986).

A total of 266 single units in the VLM were antidromically activated by electrical stimulation of the region of
either the IML or CA. One hundred and eighty-five of these
units were tested for their orthodromic response to stimulation of the ADN and CSN and to stimulation of pressor sites
in either the PVH (n=137) or Hla (n=48). The remaining 81
units in the VLM excited antidromically by stimulation of the
IML were tested for their orthodromic responses to selective
activation of peripheral chemo- and baroreceptors. Of the
185 units tested for ADN and CSN inputs, 110 (60%) were found
to respond orthodromically to stimulation of the buffer nerves
with either excitation or inhibition. In addition, 38%
(52/137) were also excited by stimulation of the PVH and 31%
(15/48) were excited by stimulation of the Hla. Finally, of
the 81 units tested for their response to chemo- and baroreceptor activation 61% (49/81) were found to respond orthodromically
in various combinations. An example of a single unit in the
VLM antidromically activated by stimulation of the IML which
was inhibited by baroreceptor activation and excited by chemoreceptor activation is shown in Figure 3.

The latencies of only those antidromic units in the VLM
which responded orthodromically to stimulation of cardiovascu-

lar afferent inputs and which had clear two component spikes
(IS-SD components) were re-examined since the possibility
cannot be completely excluded that the electrical activity
recorded from units without IS-SD components originated in
axons. These antidromic units were found to respond with
latencies corresponding to conduction velocities ranging
between 2.0 and 28.1 m/s (mean, 13.3 ± 0.8 m/s).

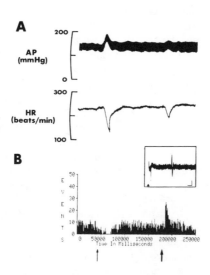

Figure 3. Cardiovascular responses (A) and firing frequency
of antidromically identified single unit in VLM to stimulation
of ipsilateral IML (B) during selective activation of baroreceptors (thin arrow) and of chemoreceptors (thick arrow).
A, arterial pressure (AP) and heart rate (HR). Thin arrow
in B corresponds to time of intravenous injection of phenylephrine and injection of sodium cyanide. B, continuous frequency histogram of single unit; 2 s bins. Inset in B, 5
superimposed oscilloscope tracings of antidromic response of
unit; arrow head, time of stimulation, 5 ms and 50 μV.

The anatomical distribution of the antidromically activated single units in this study was similar to that observed
for retrogradely labeled cells following injections of HRP
into the IML. Although single units were recorded from sites

0.5 mm caudal to 4.5 mm rostral to the obex, most were found between 1 and 3 mm rostral to the obex, in a region lateral to the ION, near the intramedullary rootlets of the 12N, and extending rostrally into the PGL.

CONCLUSIONS

On the basis of the combined neuroanatomical and neurophysiological data presented it is concluded that neurons in the VLM are components of descending sympatho-excitatory or -inhibitory pathways that receive cardiovascular afferent information and in turn alter the discharge rate of vasoconstrictor and cardioacceleratory neurons in the region of the IML and CA either directly or through antecedent interneurons. This conclusion is based on the following observations. First, activation of cell bodies in the rostral VLM was shown to elicit increases in AP. This finding is supported by similar observations in several different species (Dampney et al., 1982; McAllen et al., 1982; Ross et al., 1984b; Schlaefke, 1981). Second, cell bodies in pressor regions of the VLM had axons which presumably terminated at all segmental levels of the thoracolumbar cord. The pattern of anterograde fiber and terminal labeling in the thoracolumbar cord following an injection of tritiated amino acids into pressor sites in the VLM was almost exclusively localized to the regions of the IML, CA and IC where sympathetic preganglionic neurons are located (Oldfield and McLachlan, 1981). This finding is supported by similar observations in the rat (Loewy et al., 1981; Ross et al., 1984a). Third, retrogradely labeled cells following injections of HRP into the IML were found in regions of the VLM from which pressor responses were elicited. Finally, single units antidromically activated by stimulation of spinal sympathetic areas and responding orthodromically to activation of peripheral cardiovascular receptors and central pressor sites were also found in pressor regions of the VLM. The finding that a large number (60%) of VLM units received converging inputs from more than one site suggests that VLM neurons may integrate peripheral and central cardiovascular afferent information before sending a command signal directly to spinal sympathetic areas. In addition, it was apparent from the anatomical distribution of these units that most were localized to an area of the VLM between 1 and 3 mm rostral to the obex. This area overlaps with the region originally described by Feldberg and colleagues as the "glycine" sensitive area (Feldberg, 1976). Bilateral topical application of glycine or electrolytic lesions of this VLM region have been shown to result in a pronounced fall in AP (Guertzenstein and Silver, 1974), suggesting that some of the units recorded in this study likely functioned in the maintenance of vasomotor tone.

The axons of VLM units which responded orthodromically to cardiovascular afferent inputs had an estimated conduction velocity of 13.3 ± 0.8 m/s (range 2.0-28.1 m/s). This is an interesting observation as several recent studies have described units in the VLM involved in the control of the circulation with axons that conduct within a similar range (Barman and Gebber, 1985; Lovick et al., 1985). Furthermore, Dembowsky et al. (1985) have reported EPSP's evoked in sympathetic preganglionic neurons to stimulation of the dorsolateral funiculus with latencies corresponding to conduction velocities ranging from 2.6 to 25 m/s. Taken together, this evidence suggests that neurons located in pressor regions of the VLM which relay cardiovascular afferent information directly to spinal sympathetic areas conduct over a wider range of velocities that was previously thought (Gebber et al., 1973; Gootman and Cohen, 1971).

ACKNOWLEDGEMENTS

This work was supported by the Heart and Stroke Foundation of Ontario. J. Ciriello is a Canadian Heart Foundation Scholar and M. M. Caverson is a Canadian Heart Foundation Fellow. The authors would like to acknowledge the involvement of F. R. Calaresu in some of these studies.

REFERENCES

Alexander RS (1946). Tonic and reflex functions of medullary sympathetic cardiovascular centers. J Neurophysiol 9:205-217.
Amendt K, Czachurski J, Dembowsky K, Seller H (1979). Bulbospinal projections to the intermediolateral cell column; a neuroanatomical study. J Autonom Nerv Syst 1:103-117.
Barman SM, Gebber GL (1985). Axonal projection patterns of ventrolateral medullospinal sympathoexcitatory neurons. J Neurophysiol 53:1551-1566.
Caverson MM, Ciriello J, Calaresu FR (1983a). Direct pathway from cardiovascular neurons in the ventrolateral medulla to

the region of the intermediolateral nucleus of the upper thoracic cord: an anatomical and electrophysiological investigation in the cat. J Autonom Nerv Syst 9:451-475.

Caverson MM, Ciriello J, Calaresu FR (1983b). Cardiovascular afferent inputs to neurons in the ventrolateral medulla projecting directly to the central autonomic area of the thoracic cord in the cat. Brain Res 274:354-358.

Caverson MM, Ciriello J, Calaresu FR (1984). Chemoreceptor and baroreceptor inputs to ventrolateral medullary neurons. Amer J Physiol 247:R872-R879.

Ciriello J, Caverson MM, Calaresu FR (1986). Lateral hypothalamic and peripheral cardiovascular afferent inputs to ventrolateral medullary neurons. Brain Res 347:173-176.

Cowan WM, Gottlieb DI, Hendrickson AE, Price JL, Woolsey TA (1972). The autoradiographic demonstration of axonal connections in the central nervous system. Brain Res 37:21-51.

Dampney RAL, Goodchild AK, Robertson LG, Montgomery W (1982). Role of ventrolateral medulla in vasomotor regulation: a correlative anatomical and physiological study. Brain Res 249:223-235.

Dampney RAL, Moon EA (1980). Role of ventrolateral medulla in vasomotor response to cerebral ischemia. Amer J Physiol 239:H349-H358.

Dembowsky K, Czachurski J, Seller H (1985). An intracellular study of the synaptic input to sympathetic preganglionic neurones of the third thoracic segment of the cat. J Autonom Nerv Syst 13:201-244.

Dembowsky K, Lackner K, Czachurski J, Seller H (1981). Tonic catecholaminergic inhibition of the spinal somatosympathetic reflexes originating in the ventrolateral medulla oblongata. J Autonom Nerv Syst 3:277-290.

Dittmar C (1870). Ein neuer beweis die Reizbarkeit der centripetalen Endfasern des Ruckenmarks. Akademic der Wissenschaften Leipzig Mathematisch-physische Klasse Berichte 22:18-45.

Dittmar C (1873). Uber die Hage des sogenannten Gefasscentrums in der Medulla oblongata. Ber Sachs Akad Wiss 25:449-469.

Feldberg W (1976). The ventral surface of the brainstem: A scarcely explored region of pharmacological sensitivity. Neuroscience 1:427-441.

Gebber GL, Taylor DG, Weaver LC (1973). Electrophysiological studies on organization of central vasopressor pathways. Amer J Physiol 224:470-481.

Gootman PM, Cohen MI (1971). Evoked splanchnic potentials produced by electrical stimulation of medullary vasomotor regions. Exp Brain Res 13:1-14.

Guertzenstein PG, Silver A (1974). Fall in blood pressure produced from discrete regions of the ventral surface of the medulla by glycine and lesions. J Physiol (Lond) 242: 489-503.

Loewy AD, Wallach JH, McKellar S (1981). Efferent connections of the ventral medulla oblongata in the rat. Brain Res Rev 3:63-80.

Lovick TA, Smith RR, Hilton SM (1984). Spinally projecting neurones near the ventral surface of the medulla in the cat. J Autonom Nerv Syst 11:27-33.

McAllen RM, Neil JJ, Loewy AD (1982). Effects of kainic acid applied to the ventral surface of the medulla oblongata on vasomotor tone, the baroreceptor reflex and hypothalamic autonomic responses. Brain Res 238:65-76.

Mesulam M-M (1978). Tetramethyl benzidine for horseradish peroxidase neurochemistry: a non-carcinogenic blue reaction product with superior sensitivity for visualizing neural afferents and efferents. J Histochem Cytochem 26: 106-117.

Miura M, Onai T, Takayama K (1983). Projections of upper structure to the spinal cardioacceleratory center in cats: an HRP study using a new microinjection method. J Autonom Nerv Syst 7:119-139.

Oldfield BJ, McLachlan EM (1981). An analysis of the sympathetic preganglionic neurons projecting from the upper thoracic spinal roots of the cat. J Comp Neurol 196:329-345.

Owsjanikow PH (1871). Die tonischen und reflectorischen Centren der Gefassnerven. Ber Sachs Akad Wiss 23:135-147.

Ross CA, Ruggiero DA, Joh TH, Park DH, Reis DJ (1984a). Rostral ventrolateral medulla: selective projections to the thoracic autonomic cell column from the region containing C1 adrenaline neurons. J Comp Neurol 228:168-185.

Ross CA, Ruggiero DA, Park DH, Joh TH, Sved AF, Fernandez-Pardal J, Saavedra JM, Reis DJ (1984b). Tonic vasomotor control by the rostral ventrolateral medulla: effect of electrical or chemical stimulation of the area containing C1 adrenaline neurons on arterial pressure, heart rate and plasma catecholamines and vasopressin. J Neurosci 4:474-494.

Schlaefke ME (1981). Central chemosensitivity: a respiratory drive. Rev Physiol Biochem Pharmacol 90:171-244.

Organization of the Autonomic Nervous System:
Central and Peripheral Mechanisms, pages 239–249
© 1987 Alan R. Liss, Inc.

ELECTROPHYSIOLOGICAL ANALYSIS OF THE VENTROLATERAL MEDULLOSPINAL SYMPATHOEXCITATORY PATHWAY

Susan M. Barman
Department of Pharmacology and Toxicology, Michigan
State University, East Lansing, Michigan 48824, U.S.A.

INTRODUCTION

A great deal of evidence indicates that rostral ventrolateral medullospinal (VLM-spinal) neurons play a major role in the control of sympathetic nerve discharge (SND) and blood pressure. First, electrical or L-glutamate-induced stimulation of the rostral VLM increases blood pressure and SND (Dampney and Moon, 1980; Dampney et al., 1982; Goodchild et al., 1982; McAllen et al., 1982; Ross et al., 1984), whereas its destruction decreases blood pressure (Dampney and Moon, 1980; McAllen et al., 1982). Second, a pathway from the rostral VLM to the sympathetic intermediolateral nucleus (IML) of the thoracolumbar spinal cord has been demonstrated with anterograde and retrograde transport techniques (Amendt et al., 1978; Loewy et al., 1981; Caverson et al., 1983). Third, the spontaneous activity of some rostral VLM neurons is temporally related to that in sympathetic nerves (Barman and Gebber, 1983, 1985). This report summarizes some recent work from this laboratory on VLM sympathoexcitatory neurons (Barman and Gebber, 1985; Gebber and Barman, 1985). Specifically, I will describe the spinal and medullary axonal branching patterns of these neurons, and I will provide data suggesting that adjacent VLM neurons may be synaptically coupled. Moreover, I will describe data supporting the view that more caudally located lateral tegmental field (LTF) neurons influence SND by affecting VLM-spinal sympathoexcitatory neurons.

METHODS

Details of experimental conditions and protocols can be found in earlier reports from this laboratory (Barman and Gebber, 1985;

Gebber and Barman, 1985). Briefly, experiments were performed on Dial-urethane anesthetized cats that were paralyzed, pneumo-thoracotomized, and artificially respired. End-tidal CO_2 and body temperature were kept within physiological ranges. Standard procedures were used to record systemic arterial blood pressure and lead II of the electrocardiogram. The dorsal surface of the medulla was exposed and recording microelectrodes were positioned into the rostral VLM or medullary LTF. Unitary action potentials were recorded extracellularly with either a tungsten microelectrode (1-μm tip diam; 2-4 MΩ impedance) or one barrel of a three-barrel glass micropipette (4-6 μm composite tip diam) filled with 2 M NaCl. The recording electrode impedance was 3-6 MΩ measured at 1,000 Hz in saline. The distribution of recording sites in the rostral VLM and LTF can be found in earlier reports (Barman and Gebber, 1985; Gebber and Barman, 1985). The second and third barrels of the glass micropipette were used for the iontophoresis of L-glutamate (1 M, pH 8) and for current balancing. Recordings were made from the left inferior cardiac postganglionic sympathetic nerve. The amplifier bandpass was set at 1-1,000 Hz to display the synchronized discharges of the sympathetic nerve in the form of slow waves (i.e., envelopes of spikes).

Laminectomy was completed to allow placement of stimulating microelectrodes in the intermediolateral nucleus (IML) of the second thoracic spinal segment (T2) and in the gray or white matter of T6 and T11. In some experiments a stimulating microelectrode was also positioned into either the rostral VLM or the LTF. The stimulating microelectrodes were electrolytically etched in potassium nitrate to provide a tip impedance of 10-30 KΩ. Stimulus current was measured by monitoring the voltage drop across a 100Ω resistor in series with the anode (an alligator clip on back muscle).

RESULTS AND DISCUSSION

Identification of VLM-spinal Sympathoexcitatory Neurons

Time-controlled collision of spontaneous (or L-glutamate-induced) and antidromic action potentials was routinely used to identify VLM neurons with sympathetic nerve-related activity whose axons projected to the T2 IML region. Antidromic activation is indicated if the minimum interval between a spontaneous spike and a stimulus that elicits a response at the recording site is the sum of the response latency plus the axonal refractory period (Lipski, 1981). Axonal refractory period is estimated by determining the minimum interval between paired stimuli (1.5X threshold)

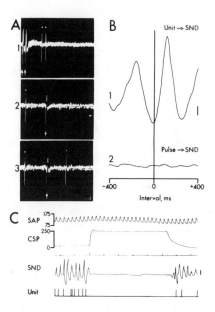

Fig. 1. Characteristics of a VLM-spinal sympathoexcitatory neuron. A: antidromic activation by T2 IML stimulation (4 superimposed traces in each panel). Dots, spontaneous and stimulus-induced action potentials; arrows, stimuli. See text for details. B: normalized midsignal spike-triggered (1) and "dummy" (2) averages of SND (700 trials each). Bin width, 0.8 ms; vertical calibration, 30 μV. C: baroreceptor reflex responses. Traces show systemic arterial pressure (mm Hg), carotid sinus pressure (mm Hg), time base (1 s/division), SND and standardized pulses coincident with unitary action potentials. Vertical calibration, 100 μV. (Reprinted from Barman and Gebber, 1985, with the permission of The American Physiological Society.)

that elicit two action potentials 100% of the time. In the example illustrated in Fig. 1A, the VLM neuron was antidromically activated with an onset latency of 26 ms, and the axonal refractory period was 3.8 ms (A1). A response was not recorded when the interval between a spontaneous action potential and the spinal stimulus was 28 ms (A2), but an antidromic response was always recorded when the interval was 30 ms (A3). Although not shown here, post-R wave analysis revealed that the spontaneous activity of both the VLM-spinal unit and inferior cardiac sympathetic nerve contained a prominent cardiac-related component. Spike-triggered averaging was used to determine the temporal relationship between the cardiac-related VLM neuronal activity and SND. The average in Fig. 1B1 shows inferior cardiac SND that preceded (left of time 0) and followed (right of time 0) unit spike occurrence. The interval between unit spike occurrence and the peak of the cardiac-related slow wave in inferior cardiac SND was 125 ms. As shown by the distribution in Fig. 2B, the mean interval between VLM unit spike occurrence and peak SND was 81+3 ms (n=87). Since the firing rate of VLM-spinal neurons with sympathetic nerve-related activity decreased in parallel to SND during baroreceptor reflex activation (Fig. 1C), these neurons likely subserved a sympathoexcitatory function. The firing rate of these neurons increased during the iontophoresis of L-glutamate, an amino acid that selectively depolarizes neuronal cell bodies (Goodchild et al., 1982; Fries and Zieglgansberger, 1974). This observation supports the view that recordings were made from the cell bodies of VLM-spinal sympathoexcitatory neurons.

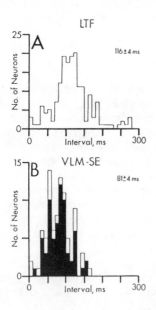

Fig. 2. Comparison of firing times of LTF and VLM neurons with sympathetic nerve-related activity. Interval refers to lag between unit spike occurrence and peak of the cardiac-related sympathetic nerve slow waves. Solid bars, VLM sympathoexcitatory neurons antidromically activated by microstimulation of T2 IML. (Modified from Gebber and Barman, 1985, with the permission of The American Physiological Society.)

Antidromic mapping in T2 revealed that the axons of these VLM sympathoexcitatory neurons coursed through the dorsolateral or ventrolateral funiculus to innervate the T2 IML. This conclusion was based on the observation that sites in these regions required the least stimulus current to elicit the shortest and longest latency antidromic responses, respectively. Mean spinal axonal conduction velocity of these VLM sympathoexcitatory neurons was 3.5 ± 0.2 m/s (n=67).

Axonal Branching Patterns of VLM-spinal Sympathoexcitatory Neurons

One of the most interesting aspects of the study by Barman and Gebber (1985) was the marked differences in the axonal branching patterns among these VLM-spinal sympathoexcitatory neurons. The axons of 50% of the neurons that branched to innervate the T2 IML region extended at least as far caudal as T11. Moreover, the axons of these same neurons also branched to innervate the gray matter in T6. Branching in T2 and T6 was clearly indicated by the results of two tests. First, raising the stimulus current applied in the T2 and T6 gray matter above threshold for antidromic activation decreased (3.3 ± 0.4 ms and 4.1 ± 1.5 ms, respectively) the antidromic response latency. The longer latency response elicited with thresold stimulus current likely reflects slowed conduction velocity in axonal branches (Jankowska and Roberts, 1972; Lipski, 1981). The second test for axonal branching involved time-controlled collision of the action potentials initiated by stimulation in T2 or T6 and in T11 (Shinoda et al., 1976). Specifically, we determined the maximum interval (collision interval; CI) after a threshold T2 (or T6) stimulus at which a T11 stimulus failed to elicit an antidromic response at the recording site. If an axonal branch is activated, then CI is greater than the difference between the onset latency of the antidromic responses elicited by caudal and rostral spinal stimulation (L_c-L_r) plus the axonal refractory period (R). This test allows one to calculate conduction time from the branch point on the main axon to the point of activation in the gray matter. The conduction time in the axonal branch (t_B) is calculated using the formula: $t_B = 1/2(CI - L_c + L_r - R)$. This formula is modified from the one derived by Shinoda et al. (1976). The conduction time in T2 axonal branches was 5.7 ± 0.9 ms. The corresponding value in T6 was 7.0 ± 2.9 ms. These data are the first to show that an individual VLM-spinal sympathoexcitatory neuron can influence sympathetic outflow at widely separated spinal segments. In contrast, the axons of one-third of the VLM-spinal sympathoexcitatory neurons that innervated the T2 IML did not extend beyond the upper thoracic spinal cord. This was indicated by the failure to antidromically activate these neurons by stimulation of T5, T6, and T11, despite an extensive search in the gray and white matter at each of these levels. Thus, some VLM-spinal neurons may be in pathways that exert regional control over SND. Morrison and Gebber (1985) reported similar differences in the axonal branching patterns among raphespinal sympathoinhibitory neurons that innervated the thoracic IML.

Regarding the possible functional implications of these findings, it is known that the discharges of sympathetic nerves innervating different organs can be changed uniformly or nonuniformly depending on the experimental conditions (Futuro-Neto and Coote, 1982; Hilton, 1982). Future studies should entertain the possibility that uniform responses are mediated by medullospinal neurons whose axons branch to innervate widely separated spinal segments. Likewise, nonuniform responses may result form the differential activation of subsets of medullospinal neurons that innervate different pools of spinal sympathetic neurons.

Recent studies from this laboratory (Barman and Gebber, unpublished observations) showed for the first time that the axons of some VLM-spinal sympathoexcitatory neurons branched in the medulla. The main axon and axonal branches were activated by microstimulation of the LTF. It was not surprising to activate the main axons of VLM-spinal neurons since anatomical studies (Ross et al., 1984; Ruggiero et al., 1985) show that the axons of at least the epinephrine-containing rostral VLM neurons in the rat course through this region enroute to the spinal cord. Activation of intramedullary axonal branches was indicated by the decrease in antidromic response latency produced by raising stimulus current above threshold and by the results of time-controlled collision of the action potentials initiated by T2 IML and LTF stimulation. The brain stem has not yet been extensively mapped to locate the precise trajectory and termination sites of these branches. Nonetheless, these data raise the possibility that some VLM neurons can influence SND by actions mediated at both spinal and supraspinal levels.

Short Time Scale Interactions of VLM Sympathoexcitatory Neurons

Crosscorrelation analysis is used to determine whether the spontaneous discharges of two neurons are synchronized on the time scale of a few milliseconds (Moore et al., 1970). This analysis was performed in 17 instances in which two VLM sympathoexcitatory neurons were identified in the same recording field. The details of this methodology are described by Barman et al. (1982) in a study of the interactions of LTF and of raphe neurons with sympathetic nerve-related activity. Figure 3 shows crosscorrelograms for two pairs of VLM sympathoexcitatory neurons. The unit 1 → unit 2 crosscorrelogram depicts the firing times of unit 2 relative to spike occurrence of unit 1 at zero lag. The presence of

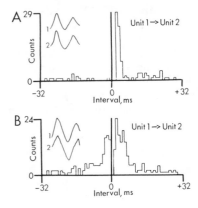

Fig. 3. Crosscorrelograms of two pairs of adjacent VLM sympathoexcitatory neurons. Bin width, 1 ms. Sampling time was 11.2 min for A and 16.1 min for B. Insets show normalized spike-triggered averages of SND for each VLM neuron (500 trials). Trigger occurred at start of each trace; sweep time was 400 ms.

distinct peaks in such histograms indicates that the probability of firing of unit 2 relative to the timing of activity of unit 1 is greater than that expected by chance. The crosscorrelograms constructed on a time scale of +32 ms for five VLM sympathoexcitatory neuronal pairs contained a sharp paracentral peak to the right of zero lag. In the example shown in Fig. 3A, the distinct peak in the crosscorrelogram indicates that the probability of discharge of unit 2 was markedly increased 2-5 ms after unit 1 spike occurrence. The paracentral peak may indicate that the two neurons were directly connected. That is, an axonal branch of unit 1 may have synapsed on unit 2. Alternatively, units 1 and 2 may have received input from a common source over pathways with slightly different conduction velocities. Independent of the mechanisms involved, it is clear that the discharges of the two neurons were synchronized on the time scale of a few milliseconds. The crosscorrelograms for six VLM neuronal pairs contained a dispersed pericentral peak (i.e., around time zero) that likely reflects shared input to the two neurons. In the example shown in Fig. 3B, the probability of discharge of unit 2 was increased above background from 5 ms before to 8 ms after unit 1 spike occurrence. The absence of counts in the first bin to the right of zero lag is due to the "dead time" problem inherent to the single microelectrode recording technique (see Barman et al., 1982). The crosscorrelograms of six VLM sympathoexcitatory neuronal pairs were flat, indicating that the discharges of the two neurons were not synchronized on the time scale of a few milliseconds.

Comparison of Firing Times of VLM and LTF Neurons with Sympathetic Nerve-Related Activity

In addition to the rostral VLM, the medullary LTF also plays a role in the control of SND. Lesions of the LTF (Kumada et al., 1979; Dampney and Moon, 1980) decreases blood pressure, whereas electrical or chemical stimulation of this region can increase SND and blood pressure (Dampney and Moon, 1980; Gebber and Barman, 1985; Goodchild and Dampney, 1985). This region contains the cell bodies of neurons with sympathetic nerve-related activity (Gebber and Barman, 1985). This contention is based on the responsiveness of LTF neurons to the microiontophoresis of L-glutamate. Some LTF neurons with sympathetic nerve-related activity may subserve a sympathoexcitatory function since their firing rate decreases during baroreceptor reflex activation. Goodchild and Dampney (1985) provided additional evidence indicating that LTF neurons exert excitatory effects on SND. They reported that microinjection of L-glutamate into this region in the rabbit increases blood pressure.

Gebber and Barman (1985) made three observations that support the view that LTF neurons influence SND by affecting VLM-spinal sympathoexcitatory neurons. First, by comparing the firing times of the two groups of neurons relative to the peak of the cardiac-related slow wave in inferior cardiac SND, they found that LTF neurons fire significantly earlier (35 ms on the average) than VLM neurons (Fig. 2). Second, the onset latency of the excitatory sympathetic nerve response elicited by electrical stimulation of the LTF is significantly longer (34 ms on the average) than the corresponding value for VLM stimulation. Third, the axons of LTF neurons do not project to the thoracic spinal cord. Recent data from this laboratory support the view that LTF neurons project to VLM-spinal neurons (Barman and Gebber, unpublished observations). LTF neurons with sympathetic nerve-related activity were antidromically activated by microstimulation of the VLM. In addition, VLM-spinal sympathoexcitatory neurons were synaptically activated by microstimulation of the LTF. This latter observation indirectly supports the view that the axons of LTF neurons terminate in the rostral VLM. Importantly, the onset latencies of synaptic activation of VLM neurons and antidromic activation of LTF neurons were long enough to account for the difference in firing times of neurons in the two regions. These data suggest that LTF neurons are a source of background activity in VLM-spinal sympathoexcitatory neurons.

SUMMARY

The data summarized in this report describe several major new findings regarding VLM sympathoexcitatory neurons. First, whereas some of these neurons can influence sympathetic outflow at widely separated spinal segments, the spinal axons of other VLM neurons innervate restricted portions of the IML. Second, since the axons of some VLM-spinal sympathoexcitatory neurons branch in the medulla, it is probable that an individual VLM neuron influences SND by actions mediated at both spinal and supraspinal levels. Third, the discharges of pairs of VLM sympathoexcitatory neurons are synchronized on the time scale of a few milliseconds. Paracentral peaks in crosscorrelograms may reflect the activation of one VLM sympathoexcitatory neuron by an axonal branch of an adjacent neuron. Fourth, LTF neurons appear to influence SND by exciting VLM-spinal sympathoexcitatory neurons.

ACKNOWLEDGEMENTS

The author is grateful to Dr. Gerard L. Gebber for his critical review of the manuscript and to Ms. Diane Hummel for typing the manuscript. This study was supported by National Institutes of Health grants HL-33266 and HL-13187.

REFERENCES

Amendt K, Czachurski J, Dembowsky K, Seller H (1978). Neurons within the 'chemosensitive area' on the ventral surface of the brainstem which project to the intermediolateral column. Pfluegers Arch 375:289-292.

Barker JL, Crayton JW, Nicoll RA (1971). Antidromic and orthodromic responses of paraventricular and supraoptic neurosecretory cells. Brain Res 33:353-366.

Barman SM, Gebber GL (1983). Sequence of activation of ventrolateral and dorsal medullary sympathetic neurons. Am J Physiol 245 (Regulatory Integrative Comp Physiol 14): R438-R447.

Barman SM, Gebber GL (1985). Axonal projection patterns of ventrolateral medullospinal sympathoexcitatory neurons. J Neurophysiol 53:1551-1566.

Barman SM, Morrison SF, Gebber GL (1982). Short time scale interactions between brain stem neurons with sympathetic nerve-related activity. Brain Res 250:173-177.

Caverson MM, Ciriello J, Calaresu FR (1983). Direct pathway from cardiovascular neurons in the ventrolateral medulla to the region of the intermediolateral nucleus of the upper thoracic cord: An anatomical and electrophysiological investigation in the cat. J Auton Nerv Syst 9:451-475.

Dampney RAL, Goodchild AK, Robertson LG, Montgomery W (1982). Role of ventrolateral medulla in vasomotor regulation: A correlative anatomical and physiological study. Brain Res 249:223-235.

Dampney RAL, Moon EA (1980). Role of the ventrolateral medulla in vasomotor response to cerebral ischemia. Am J Physiol 239 (Heart Circ Physiol 8): H349-H358.

Fries W, Zieglgansberger W (1974). A method to discriminate axonal from cell body activity and to analyze "silent" cells. Exp Brain Res 21:441-445.

Futuro-Neto HA, Coote JH (1982). Changes in sympathetic activity to the heart and blood vessels during desynchronized sleep. Brain Res 252:259-268.

Gebber GL, Barman SM (1985). Lateral tegmental field neurons of cat medulla: A potential source of basal sympathetic nerve discharge. J Neurophysiol 54:1498-1512.

Goodchild AK, Dampney RAL (1985). A vasopressor cell group in the rostral dorsomedial medulla of the rabbit. Brain Res 360:24-32.

Goodchild AK, Dampney RAL, Bandler R (1982). A method for evoking physiological responses by stimulation of cell bodies, but not axons of passage, within localized regions of the central nervous system. J Neurosci Meth 6:351-363.

Hilton SM (1982). The defence-arousal system and its relevance for circulatory and respiratory control. J Exp Biol 100:159-174.

Jankowska E, Roberts WJ (1972). An electrophysiological demonstration of the axonal projections of single spinal interneurons in the cat. J Physiol London 222:597-622.

Kumada M, Dampney RAL, Reis DJ (1979). Profound hypotension and abolition of the vasomotor component of the cerebral ischemic response produced by restricted lesions of medulla oblongata in rabbit. Circ Res 44:63-70.

Lipski J (1981). Antidromic activation of neurones as an analytic tool in the study of the central nervous system. J Neurosci Meth 4:1-32.

Loewy AD, Wallach JH, McKellar J (1981). Efferent connections of the ventral medulla oblongata in the rat. Brain Res Rev 3:63-80.

McAllen RM, Neil JJ, Loewy, AD (1982). Effects of kainic acid applied to the ventral surface of the medulla oblongata on vasomotor tone, the baroreceptor reflex, and hypothalamic autonomic responses. Brain Res 238:65-76.

Moore GP, Segundo JP, Perkel DH, Levitan H (1970). Statistical signs of synaptic interaction in neurons. Biophysical J 10:876–900.

Morrison SM, Gebber GL (1985). Axonal branching and funicular trajectories of raphespinal sympathoinhibitory neurons. J Neurophysiol 53:759–772.

Ross CA, Ruggiero DA, Park DH, Joh TH, Sved AF, Fernandez-Pardal J, Saavedra JM, Reis DJ (1984). Tonic vasomotor control by the rostral ventrolateral medulla: Effect of electrical or chemical stimulation of the area containing C1 adrenaline neurons on arterial pressure, heart rate, and plasma catecholamines and vasopressin. J Neurosci 4:474–494.

Ruggiero DA, Ross CA, Anwar M, Park DH, Joh TH, Reis DJ (1985). Distribution of neurons containing phenylethanolamine N-methyltransferase in medulla and hypothalamus of rat. J Comp Neurol 239:127–154.

Shinoda Y, Arnold AP, Asanuma H (1976). Spinal branching of corticospinal axons in the cat. Exp Brain Res 26:215–234.

Organization of the Autonomic Nervous System:
Central and Peripheral Mechanisms, pages 251–263
© **1987 Alan R. Liss, Inc.**

THE SUB-RETROFACIAL NUCLEUS AND CARDIOVASCULAR CONTROL

R. M. McAllen, R. A. L. Dampney* and A. K. Goodchild*

Department of Physiology, University of Bristol, Bristol BS8 1TD, U.K. and *University of Sydney, N.S.W. 2006, Australia

INTRODUCTION

A number of recent studies have emphasized the importance of neurons in the rostral ventrolateral medulla for the control of the cardiovascular system in mammals (e.g. Dampney et al., 1985b; Guertzenstein and Silver, 1974; Hilton et al., 1983; McAllen, 1985; McAllen et al., 1982). The present article reviews some relevant work from other laboratories and reports on recent experiments from our own, in which we have attempted to define their role in cats. We will argue the case that a compact group of bulbospinal neurons, which we now call the sub-retrofacial nucleus (SRF), mediate vasomotor actions attributable to the region. Five sections will discuss the following questions: 1) How important are rostral ventrolateral medullary neurons for cardiovascular control? 2) How localized are these 'cardiovascular' neurons? 3) Do they have the right connections? 4) How specific are their actions? 5) Do they have the right properties?

1) IMPORTANCE OF ROSTRAL VENTROLATERAL MEDULLARY NEURONS FOR CVS CONTROL

In 1974, Guertzenstein and Silver demonstrated that in anesthetized cats, inactivation of neurons in a small area close to the ventral surface of the rostral medulla caused arterial pressure to fall to low levels. Neurons had to be disabled on both sides of the medulla for such an effect, but this could be achieved by either electrolytic lesions, topical application of the inhibitory amino acid glycine or combinations of the two. Since glycine is not believed to interrupt traffic in axons, it was inferred that cell bodies crucial for the maintenance of vasomotor tone are to be found beneath this 'glycine-sensitive area'. This basic observation has been confirmed many times by other workers.

Besides 'resting' arterial pressure, it has since become clear that a number of reflex and centrally evoked vasomotor responses are dependent on neurons in this same area. Chemical inhibition or lesions there can also block or severely reduce pressor responses to stimulation of the hypothalamus, (Hilton et al., 1983; McAllen et al., 1982) midbrain (Hilton et al., 1983) and cerebellum (McAllen, 1985), as well as the cerebral ischemic response (Dampney and Moon, 1980), baroreceptor (McAllen et al., 1982) and long-circuited somatosympathetic reflexes (McAllen, 1985). McAllen, Neil and Loewy (McAllen et al., 1982) further showed that while hypothalamic effects on sympathetic vasomotor activity were blocked after kainic acid application to the ventral medulla, those on the pupils and nictitating membranes were spared.

The evidence above could be interpreted as indicating that much, or perhaps even all sympathetic vasomotor drive from the brain under the conditions of the experiment, depends on the activity of a small group of neurons close to the ventrolateral medullary surface. A note of caution, however: topically applied drugs can spread, and lesions may have effects (by for example destruction of blood vessels) beyond the region of apparent damage. It is therefore prudent to use additional methods to try and localize the neurons responsible. Moreover, even at face value, such results do not deny the potential importance of descending pathways with sympatho-inhibitory actions, and there might be others which need a degree of background 'tone' to be seen. Nor is it yet known whether ventro-lateral medullary neurons generate or simply transmit resting vasomotor tone.

2) LOCALIZATION OF VENTRAL MEDULLARY VASOPRESSOR NEURONS

As an alternative means of localizing medullary vasomotor neurons, we have microinjected excitant amino acids into the ventral medullary surface. This technique is believed to activate virtually all neuronal cell bodies, but not passing axons (Goodchild et al., 1982). It therefore has the advantage over electrical stimulation which activates both. The resultant maps reflect this difference: chemical stimulation shows up a discrete, well-defined pressor region, while as one would expect of a stimulus acting on fibers of passage, electrical stimulation over wide areas of medulla stimulates sympathetic vasomotor nerves and usually a number of other features as well (Alexander, 1946; Hilton et al., 1983). We believe the former method gives a truer picture of where vaso-pressor neurons are to be found, even though it has poorer temporal and spatial resolution.

In a recent study (McAllen, 1986a) injections of 30-50 nl of either 0.2M DL homocysteic acid or 0.5M sodium glutamate were used to map pressor neurons. Points from which arterial pressure rises of 50 mmHg or more were obtained had a striking agreement with Guertzenstein and Silver's localization of the 'glycine-sensitive area'. A more recent study (Goodchild et al., 1986) has used smaller injections (15-30 nl) of glutamate with a small admixture of horseradish peroxidase (HRP), to map these vasopressor neurons more precisely and localize them on histological sections. Figure 1 shows the results of this more refined study: points from which moderate or large pressor responses can be evoked are found in a highly restricted region, corresponding to a compact column of cells we now call the sub-retrofacial nucleus (SRF, see below).

3) ANATOMICAL CONNECTIONS

In 1978, Amendt and colleagues first injected HRP into the region of the intermediolateral horn (IML) of the thoracic cord in cats and subsequently noted retrograde labelling of neurons in the ventrolateral medulla. Their major concentration was found in the very region to which pressor neurons were localized by the methods described above. Labelled cells were mostly between 450 and 1150 μm of the brain surface, and their spinal projection was strongly ipsilateral (Alexander, 1946).

These experiments have now been repeated with spinal injections of wheatgerm agglutinin-conjugated HRP (WGA-HRP) centered at (though not confined to) IML, and a more

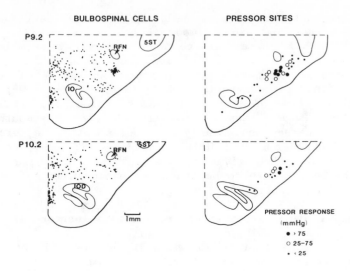

Figure 1. The right hand pictures show points which 15-30 nl injections of glutamate evoked pressor responses plotted on cross hemisections of the ventral medulla at the stereotaxic levels indicated. The left hand pictures show the locations of cell bodies retrogradely labelled by retrograde transport of WGA-HRP previously injected at T1, centered on IML. IO = inferior olive, IOD = dorsal accessory olive, RFN = retrofacial nucleus, 5ST = spinal trigeminal tract. (Data from reference Goodchild et al., 1986).

detailed analysis of retrogradely labelled cells in the ventrolateral medulla (Goodchild et al., 1986). A dense group of spinally-projecting cells was found ventral to the retrofacial nucleus, in exactly the site from which glutamate injections evoked maximal pressor responses (Fig. 1). We have named this group the sub-retrofacial nucleus (SRF). SRF cells are histochemically as well as anatomically distinct from their neighbors, including other spinally-projecting cells, in that they stain histochemically for tyrosine hydroxylase and neuropeptide Y. They are thus probably part of the 'C1' adrenaline-containing cell group, as has been suggested for the pressor neurons of the homologous region in rabbits and rats (Dampney et al., 1985a; Ross et al., 1984). They do not appear to contain substance P.

The anatomical connections of SRF have also been studied by observing both retrograde and orthograde transport of WGA-HRP injected directly into this nucleus (localized by the pressor response to glutamate injection, Dampney et al., 1985a). Orthograde transport of the lectin labelled spinally-projecting axons that appeared to terminate exclusively within IML (Dampney et al., 1985a). Retrograde transport revealed major inputs to SRF from several 'central autonomic nuclei' including the para-ventricular nucleus, lateral hypothalamic area, para-brachial nucleus and nucleus of tractus solitarius (Dampney et al., 1985a).

4) SPECIFICITY OF ACTION OF SRF NEURONS

The discussion so far has assumed that the primary actions of SRF cells are to drive vasomotor neurons, but is this really so? We can investigate this question by observing the range of responses produced when SRF cells are activated. Because many different fiber types pass through the area, electrical stimulation for this purpose would be inappropriate and potentially misleading, so microinjection of excitant amino acids is again the method of choice. Figure 2 summarizes the results of such a study (McAllen, 1986b).

Injection of amino acids into the SRF region increased the activity in all sympathetic nerves studied. The renal nerve and filaments supplying hindlimb muscle and skin were probably vasoconstrictor in function, while the cervical and splanchnic nerves, though of mixed composition, also contain many vasoconstrictor fibers. Vasoconstriction was confirmed directly by perfusion in the case of the femoral, superior- and inferior mesenteric vascular beds. Cardiac sympathetic activity increased and, though often masked if the vagi were intact, tachycardia was also seen. Activating SRF neurons also caused a large increase in circulating catecholamine levels (McAllen, 1986b).

By contrast, activating SRF neurons had little effect on 'non-cardiovascular' sympathetic activity. Piloerection

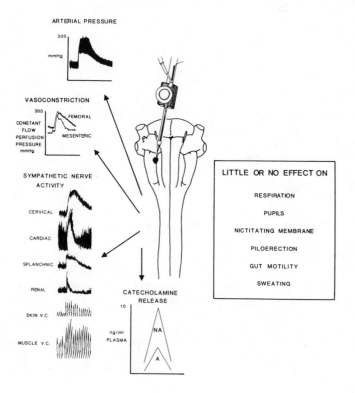

EFFECTS OF ACTIVATING SRF
NEURONES WITH AMINO ACIDS

Figure 2. Schematic summary of the effects of excitant amino acid injections into the sub-retrofacial nucleus (data from references Dampney and McAllen, 1986; McAllen, 1986a; McAllen, 1986b). Skin, muscle V.C refers to activity in vasoconstrictor fibers supplying these tissues. NA and A are noradrenaline and adrenaline.

and retraction of the nictitating membrane were never seen, and slight mydriasis was only noted in under 1% of cases, when it was probably related to damage caused by the injection (McAllen, 1986b). Electrical stimulation, however, was very effective, suggesting that a pupillo-

dilator pathway passes through the region without synapsing. Only small, inconsistent effects on intestinal
motility followed amino acid injections among the SRF
pressor neurons, and little effect noted on sweating,
measured as the electrodermal response at the paw (McAllen,
1986b). It was striking, though, that injections as little
as 1 mm away from SRF could produce large electrodermal
responses, without affecting blood pressure. A similar
spatial separation was also noted between points that
stimulated respiration and the SRF vasopressor region
(McAllen, 1986a).

It would thus seem that SRF neurons drive sympathetic
nerves supplying blood vessels, heart and adrenal medulla,
but have little action on 'non-cardiovascular' end organs.
It may be no accident that the same selectivity is shown by
the baroreceptor reflex.

Recent experiments (Dampney and McAllen, 1986) have
now provided evidence that within SRF there may be subpopulations of neurons with even greater specificity. Injections of 5-10 nl glutamate into different parts of SRF can
differentially activate postganglionic vasoconstrictor
fibers which supply cutaneous or skeletal muscle vasculature in the hindlimb (identified following Janig, 1985).
Thus SRF may be topographically organized in terms of the
end organs it affects.

5)   ELECTROPHYSIOLOGY OF SRF NEURONS

Spinally-projecting neurons have been identified in
electrophysiological recordings from SRF region of chloralose-anesthetized, paralyzed cats. Neurons were recorded
extracellularly and identified by their antidromic response
to electrical stimulation of the ipsilateral dorsolateral
funiculus at C5-6 or IML at T1. The use of 'tungsten plus
glass' multibarrel recording electrodes (McAllen and
Woollard, 1985) enabled excitation by iontophoresis of
homocysteic acid to be used as a test that recordings came
from the soma region (they did) and recording sites to be
marked with pontamine blue dye.

These experiments identified a population of bulbospinal cells whose properties make them strong candidates
for the proposed role of descending vasomotor pathway

(McAllen, 1986c; McAllen, 1986d). The neurons in question had axonal conduction velocities between 2 and 9 m/sec (Fig. 4, left), corresponding almost exactly to estimates for the descending vasomotor tract in the cat (Coote and Macleod, 1984). Their cardial feature was a profound inhibition of activity when baroreceptors were stimulated by carotid sinus inflation. Figure 3 illustrates an example of one such neuron firing with the moderately slow spontaneous activity typical of this population (McAllen, 1986d) and how baroreceptor stimuli silence it. Also shown is how that cell's activity could be raised several fold by iontophoresis of homocysteic acid, yet baroreceptors were still able to silence this additional discharge. Such behavior strongly suggests direct postsynaptic inhibition by baroreceptor signals.

Baroreceptor-sensitive bulbospinal neurons were usually found between 0.5 and 1 mm from the ventral medullary surface, in a closely packed group approximately 250 μm thick. Marked recording sites were all located ventral to the retrofacial nucleus, and the compact cell group of SRF was usually apparent in Nissl counterstained sections in their immediate vicinity. The locations of 19 baroreceptor-sensitive bulbospinal neurons are shown in Figure 4 (right). It is hard to doubt that they belong to the same population as those identified by anatomical methods (Fig. 1).

6) DISCUSSION AND CONCLUSIONS

This article has assembled evidence from four different experimental approaches - ablation, chemical stimulation, anatomical tracing and electrophysiological recording - to try and define medullary neurons that control the cardiovascular system. Although studies using ablation methods suffer from poor resolution or specificity, they do indicate that neurons in the rostral ventrolateral medullary region have an overriding importance for cardiovascular control. On the other hand, the localization of pressor neurons by microinjections, spinally-projecting neurons by retrograde transport, and baroreceptor-sensitive bulbospinal neurons by electrophysiology, all to SRF makes a strong case that it functions as a descending vasomotor pathway. Whether SRF is the only such pathway cannot be said at present, though the evidence noted above suggests

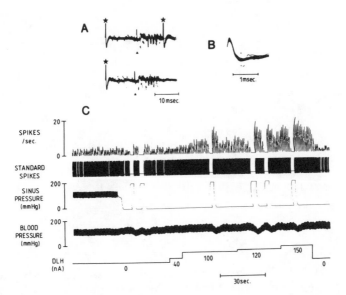

Figure 3.   Identification and properties of an SRF bulbo-spinal neuron (Taken from reference McAllen, 1986d).

A: collision test.   Each trace shows 5 superimposed oscilloscope sweeps, triggered by a spontaneous spike of the neuron under study (starred).   After a set delay a suprathreshold stimulus was applied (at arrowhead) to its axon in the spinal cord.   If this was done just after the critical delay (upper trace) a constant-latency antidromic spike always resulted; if just before the critical time, the antidromic spike was always cancelled by collision with the spontaneous (orthodromic) action potential (c.f. reference Lipski, 1981).   Note also downward-going spikes activated synaptically by the stimulus.

B: discrimination.   Superimposed oscilloscope sweeps triggered by the unit studied.   Constancy of size and shape are used to check that a single unit is discriminated and counted.   Dots show the time window through which potentials must pass to be counted.   C: Continuous record showing the response of the unit identified above (shown as discriminated standard pulses and rate recording) to baroreceptor stimulation (inflation of carotid sinus blind sac) and iontophoresis of D. L. Homocysteic acid (DLH) at the currents indicated below.   The common carotid was initially open, but occluded during baroreceptor tests.

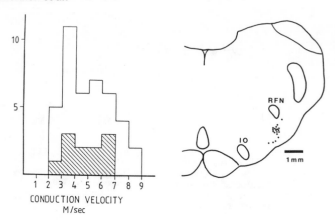

Figure 4. Left: histogram of axonal conduction velocities of baroreceptor-sensitive SRF bulbospinal neurons. Hatched columns indicate those identified by antidromic activation from IML, open columns those activated from the dorso-lateral funiculus (Taken from reference McAllen, 1986d).

Right: Location of 19 SRF baroreceptor-sensitive bulbo-spinal neurons reconstructed from dye marks and plotted on a cross section of medulla at the rostral pole of the inferior olive (IO). RFN = retrofacial nucleus.

that cells in this part of the brainstem are the most important source of descending vasomotor drive, at least in anesthetized animals. Possibly SRF represents the nuclear core, but some outlying cells also belong to the same functional group. However, the scarcity of significant pressor responses from amino acid injections away form SRF suggests that such outliers are few and/or sparse.

Our experiments have also shown that when activated, SRF neurons drive sympathetic nerves to the heart, blood vessels and adrenal medulla but apparently not those supplying other organs. Individual SRF cells probably have an even more precise 'address' for their actions. Finally, electrophysiological identification and study of these cells has added evidence for a supraspinal site of action (probably directly on SRF cells) for the inhibition of vasomotor tone by baroreceptors. A summary diagram is shown in Figure 5.

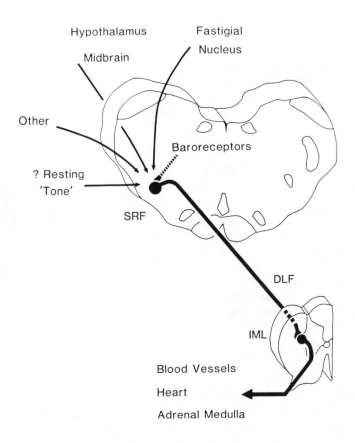

Figure 5. Summary diagram of the connections of SRF neurons.

ACKNOWLEDGEMENTS

This work was supported by the (British) Medical Research Council and (Australian) National Health and Medical Research Council. R. M. McAllen is British Heart Foundation senior research fellow. We also thank Sue

Woollard for excellent technical assistance, Perry Robbins for photography and Sue Maskell for help in preparing the manuscripts.

REFERENCES

Alexander RS (1946). Tonic and reflex functions of the medullary sympathetic cardiovascular centers. J Neurophysiol 9:205-217.

Amendt K, Czachurski J, Dembowsky K, Seller H (1978) Neurones within the 'Chemosensitive area' on the ventral surface of the brainstem which project to the intermediolateral column. Pfluger's Arch 375: 289-292.

Coote JH, Macleod VH (1984). Estimation of conduction velocity in bulbospinal excitatory pathways to sympathetic outflows in cat spinal cord. Brain Res 311:97-107.

Dampney RAL, Czachurski J, Dembowsky K, Seller H (1985a). Afferent and efferent connections of the rostral ventrolateral pressor region in the medulla oblongata of the cat. Pfluger's Arch 403:R51.

Dampney RAL, Goodchild AK, Tan E (1985b). Vasopressor neurons in the rostral ventrolateral medulla of the rabbit. J Auton Nerv Syst 14:239-254.

Dampney RAL, McAllen RM (1986). Specificity of presympathetic neurones in the ventral medulla of the cat. J Physiol (Abstr) (In press).

Dampney RAL, Moon EA (1980). Role of the ventrolateral medulla in vasomotor response to cerebral ischaemia. Am J Physiol 239:H349-358.

Goodchild AK, Cao K-Y, Dampney RAL (1986). The subretrofacial nucleus in the medulla of the cat: anatomical and histochemical properties and cardiovascular function. Proc Aust Physiol Pharmacol Soc.

Goodchild AK, Dampney RAL, Bandler R (1982). A method for evoking physiological responses by stimulation of cell bodies, but not axons of passage, within localized regions of the central nervous system. J Neurosci Meth 6:351-363.

Guertzenstein PG, Silver A (1974). Fall in blood pressure produced from discrete regions of the ventral surface of the medulla by glycine and lesions. J Physiol 242:489-503.

Hilton SM, Marshall JM, Timms RJ (1983). Ventral medullary relay neurones in the pathway from the defence areas of the cat and their effect on blood pressure. J Physiol

345:149-166.

Janig W (1985). Organization of the lumbar sympathetic outflow to skeletal muscle and skin of the cat hindlimb and tail. Rev Physiol Biochem Pharmacol 102:119-213.

Lipski J (1981). Antidromic activation of neurones as an analytical tool in the study of the central nervous system. J Neurosci Meth 4:1-32.

McAllen RM (1985). Mediation of fastigial pressor response and a somatosympathetic reflex by ventral medullary neurones in the cat. J Physiol 368:423-433.

McAllen RM (1986a). Location of neurones with cardio-vascular and respiratory actions, at the ventral surface of the cat's medulla. Neuroscience 18:43-49.

McAllen RM (1986b). Action and specificity of ventral medullary vasopressor neurones in the cat. Neuroscience 18:51-59.

McAllen RM (1986c). Subretrofacial bulbospinal neurones: identification of a putative descending vasomotor pathway in the cat. In: Cardiogenic Reflexes. Ed. Hainsworth R, Linden RJ, McWilliam PW, Mary DASG. Oxford Univ. Press (In press).

McAllen RM (1986d). Identification and properties of sub-retrofacial bulbospinal neurones: a descending cardio-vascular pathway in the cat. J Auton Nerv Syst (In press).

McAllen RM, Neil JJ, Loewy AD (1982). Effects of kainic acid applied to the ventral medullary surface on vasomotor tone, the baroreceptor reflex and hypothalamic autonomic responses. Brain Res 238:65-76.

McAllen RM, Woollard S (1985). 'Tungsten plus glass' multibarrel electrodes. J Physiol 364:9.

Ross CA, Ruggiero DA, Park DH, Joh TH, Sved AF, Fernandez-Pardal J, Saavedra JM, Reis DJ (1984). Tonic vasomotor control by the rostral ventrolateral medulla: effect of electrical or chemical stimulation of the area containing C.1. adrenaline neurons on arterial pressure, heart rate and plasma catecholamines and vasopressin. J Neurosci 4:274-294.

SECTION V: Supraspinal Mechanisms in the Control of the Circulation

This section illustrates well the necessity for using many techniques to approach the problem of dynamic interactions and the hierarchical organization of central structures involved in the control of the circulation. The nine contributors have used a variety of new techniques from microinjections of excitatory substances to 2-deoxyglucose autoradiography as well as more established approaches such as electrical stimulation and recording from single units. Because of this diversity of technical approaches it will be obvious to the reader that it has been difficult to place the contributions to this section in a logical order.

The first paper by Sawchenko, Cunningham and Levin presents recent information on the anatomical organization and chemical composition of three well established central autonomic pathways using very elegant tracing and immunohistochemical techniques. As the authors suggest our hopes for the future are to investigate the "degree of convergence in these various anatomically and chemically defined subpopulations" of central autonomic neurons.

McCall in the second paper presents experiments attempting to identify neurotransmitters mediating cardiovascular effects elicited by activation of a bulbo-spinal pathway.

Erdélyi, Simon and Tóth in the third paper present the hypothesis that spinal cord, brain stem and cerebellum together constitute a very powerful integrating system "assuring smooth changes in the output variables instead of potentially harmful sudden jumps". To be sure, the problem of integration is the central focus of any attempts at studying interactions of the different neuronal components affecting the cardiovascular system.

In the fourth paper Spyer, Mifflin and Withington-Ray present intracellular recordings of post-synaptic inhibition of second-order neurons that receive baroreceptor information elicited by hypothalamic stimulation. This is an elegant demonstration of the cellular mechanism responsible for the suppression of the baroreceptor reflex during the defense reaction.

The fifth paper by Hilton and Redfern presents recent evidence obtained by pressure microinjection of excitatory aminoacids into the "defence area" of the hypothalamus that this area as previously outlined by electrical stimulation probably consists of axons of passage. This finding raises the issue of the validity of observations made using electrical stimulation of the central nervous system.

In the sixth paper Pittman, Riphagen and Martin report some interesting experiments suggesting a physiological role as a synaptic transmitter for the hormone arginine vasopressin. Their findings add to the excitement generated recently by the role of peptides in synaptic transmission.

Harris, Banks, Stokes and Jamieson in the seventh paper present a study using 2-DG as a marker of metabolic activity of neurons and electrophysiological techniques to investigate central sites receiving information from arterial chemoreceptors. An exciting new finding is that the arcuate nucleus of the hypothalamus appears to be involved in receiving chemoreceptor information.

The eighth paper by Langhorst, Lambertz, Schulz and Stock reviews extensive statistical studies of firing patterns of single units in the lower brain stem and in the amygdala to propose that functional interactions between these two areas of the central nervous system are based on feedback loops.

Finally, the last paper reviews recent results from Calaresu's laboratory using single unit recording and microinjection techniques in limbic structures and suggests the existence of long-loop reflexes controlling the cardiovascular system during complex behavioral and physiological responses.

Organization of the Autonomic Nervous System:
Central and Peripheral Mechanisms, pages 267–281
© 1987 Alan R. Liss, Inc.

ANATOMIC AND BIOCHEMICAL SPECIFICITY IN CENTRAL AUTONOMIC PATHWAYS

P.E. Sawchenko, E.T. Cunningham, Jr. & M.C. Levin

The Salk Institute for Biological Studies and the Clayton Foundation for Research--California Division and Department of Neuroscience, University of California at San Diego, La Jolla, CA 92037

INTRODUCTION

Over the past decade, anatomical studies have defined a circuitry that may be viewed as constituting a "core" of the central representation of the autonomic nervous system. This comprises not only the cell groups that provide the final common (preganglionic) outflow, but also those involved in receiving and processing of visceral afferent information and those that mediate complementary neuroendocrine and behavioral responses to perturbations in the internal environment. Figure 1 illustrates a substantial portion of this circuitry, specifically that subserving vagal nerve function. The cell groups that constitute this system are distributed throughout the neuraxis and are extensively interconnected. Moreover, they are characterized by the presence of an impressive diversity of neuropeptides, which, along with certain catecholamines, present themselves as candidates for mediating information transfer between its components.

The purpose of the present paper is to summarize recent studies from our laboratory that bear on the anatomy and/or biochemical makeup of three distinct, yet interrelated, components of central autonomic circuitry: (1) some local projections of the nucleus of the solitary tract (NTS), the principal recipient of primary visceral afferent information carried via the vagus and glossopharyngeal nerves, (2) projections to the hypothalamus from brainstem catecholamine cell groups that are thought to play a role in the dispersal of visceral sensory information, and (3) vagal motor neurons.

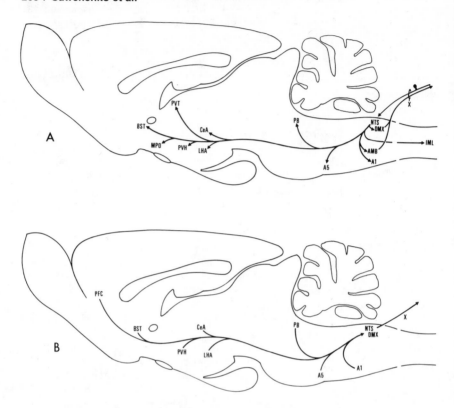

Figure 1. Schematic drawings of a sagittal section of a rat
brain to show (A) the organization of efferent projections
from the nucleus of the solitary tract (NTS) and (B)
projections to the dorsal vagal complex (NTS and dorsal
motor nucleus of the vagus, DMX). These are shown to
illustrate the interconnectedness of some key components of
the central autonomic system under consideration here.
Other abbreviations: A1, A5, catecholamine cell groups;
AMB, nucleus ambiguus; BST, bed nucleus of the stria
terminalis; CeA, central nucleus of the amygdala; IML,
intermediolateral column of the spinal cord; LHA, lateral
hypothalamic area, MPO, medial preoptic area; PB, parabrachial nucleus; PFC, prefrontal cortex; PVH, paraventricular nucleus of the hypothalamus; PVT, paraventricular nucleus of the thalamus. Modified from Sawchenko,
1983a.

BRAINSTEM PROJECTIONS OF THE NTS

A precise delineation of the organization of the efferent projections of the NTS is of obvious and fundamental importance in understanding how visceral sensory information is distributed and processed throughout the central nervous system. Several now classic studies employed the autoradiographic method to describe a widespread set of projections that include pathways that are in a position to mediate short-loop autonomic reflexes involving both vagal and sympathetic mechanisms, a pathway involving a relay in the parabrachial nucleus by which this class of sensory information may reach the ventrobasal complex of the thalamus and cortex, and a surprisingly widespread set of inputs to limbic forebrain and hypothalamic structures that have been implicated in a variety of regulatory responses involving various admixtures of neuroendocrine, autonomic and behavioral mechanisms (Ricardo and Koh, 1978; Norgren, 1978; Loewy and Burton, 1978). We (Cunningham and Sawchenko, 1986b) have begun a reexamination of the projections of the NTS using an axonally transported plant lectin (Phaseolus vulgaris--leucoagglutinin, or PHA-L) as an anterograde tracer (see Gerfen and Sawchenko, 1984). The resolution and sensitivity afforded by this method make it particularly well-suited for studies of the topographic organization of the intramedullary projections of a structure as discrete and internally complex as the NTS.

Previous studies suggested the existence of a rather extensive set of NTS outputs that remain within the confines of the dorsal vagal complex (i.e., the NTS and dorsal motor nucleus of the vagus), though the distribution and extent of these pathways proved resistant to detailed characterization with the autoradiographic method. In addition, these analyses consistently described ventrolaterally directed pathways that appeared to terminate, among other regions, in the nucleus ambiguus. These latter pathways have recently attracted considerable interest in light of a recent retrograde transport study that has challenged the prominence of a substantial NTS - nucleus ambiguus projection (Travers and Norgren, 1984), and in light of indications of the key roles played by catecholaminergic neurons in the ventral medulla in specific aspects of central autonomic function. Thus, the more caudally situated A1 (noradrenergic) cell group is now thought to serve as the principal source of aminergic inputs to the magnocellular neurosecretory system of the hypothalamus and has been implicated in anatomic and physiologic studies as comprising an essential relay in the route by which afferent information from the cardiovascular system may influence vasopressin secretion (Sawchenko and Swanson, 1982; Day et al., 1984). The more rostrally situated C1 (adrenergic) cell group, in contrast, has been proposed on the basis of anatomic and physiologic evidence as comprising the source of inputs to the intermediolateral cell column of the spinal cord that is responsible for the maintenance of basal sympathetic tone (Reis et al., 1984). Clearly then, a more precise delineation of the projections of the NTS upon key cell groups in both the dorsomedial and ventrolateral portions of the medulla is critical to achieving a better appreciation of the manner by which sensory information from the viscera is distributed to various pools of effector neurons.

The most widespread set of projections in our studies was found after deposits of PHA-L centered in the medial part of the NTS at the level of the area postrema. Such placements labeled heavy projections to both the dorsal motor nucleus of the vagus and to portions of the medial solitary nucleus throughout their longitudinal extents. These projections, like most of those seen in these experiments were predominantly ipsilateral, though prominent contralateral components of similar distribution were evident. In addition, injections at this level of the NTS labeled prominent ventrolaterally-directed pathways throughout much of the medulla whose topography suggested possible interactions with both the A1 and C1 catecholamine cell groups; only very sparse inputs to the nucleus ambiguus were evident in these experiments.

In contrast, deposits centered in the medial NTS at a level just rostral to the area postrema labeled an extremely heavy and discrete input to the nucleus ambiguus, with considerably fewer fibers apparent in the dorsal vagal complex or the A1 and C1 regions. Injections placed caudal to the level of the area postrema, in the commissural part of the NTS, labeled fibers restricted primarily to the commissural and subpostrema regions of the NTS and to the area postrema itself (Cunningham and Sawchenko, 1986b).

Collectively, these results indicate the existence of a

considerable degree of topographic order in the local projections of the NTS and suggest possible routes by which visceral afferent information may be directed to various pools of effector neurons. For example, the apparent existence of a prominent input to the nucleus ambiguus, which is generally acknowledged to provide the bulk of the vagal preganglionic supply to the heart (e.g., Geis and Wurster, 1980; Stuesse, 1982), from a circumscribed part of the NTS makes accessible to detailed anatomic and physiologic investigation a potential substrate mediating the vagal component of the baroreceptor reflex. Further study will be required to confirm the existence of such pathways at the ultrastructural level and to identify agents that may serve as neurotransmitters or modulators in these projections.

BRAINSTEM CATECHOLAMINERGIC PROJECTIONS TO THE HYPOTHALAMUS

As noted above, specific groupings of catecholamine-containing neurons in the brainstem have been implicated as playing major roles in conveying visceroceptive information to the forebrain, including the hypothalamus. Much of the work in this area has focussed specifically on one particularly well-characterized and representative cell group in the hypothalamus, the paraventricular nucleus (PVH). The PVH is now known to contain separate and topographically organized populations of cells that participate quite directly in three quintessentially hypothalamic functions. These include (1) magnocellular neurosecretory neurons responsible for the synthesis of the peptide hormones oxytocin and vasopressin and their delivery to the posterior pituitary for release into the general circulation, (2) parvocellular neurosecretory neurons that produce one or another of the releasing- or release-inhibiting peptides of the hypothalamus and deliver them to the hypophyseal portal circulation for the control of trophic hormone secretion from the anterior pituitary, and (3) neurons that project directly to a number of brainstem and spinal components of the central autonomic system, including preganglionic cell groups subserving both vagal and sympathetic function (see Swanson and Sawchenko, 1983).

Earlier studies identified three regions of the brainstem as potential sources of catecholaminergic inputs to the PVH; the A1/C1 region of the ventral medulla, the A2/C2 region of the NTS, and the A6 (locus coeruleus) cell group (Sawchenko and Swanson, 1981; 1982). Complementary autoradiographic studies showed the outputs of these regions to be differentially distributed within the PVH. Thus, the A1/C1 projection provided a broadly distributed projection that included most parts of the parvocellular divison and those regions of the magnocellular division in which vasopressinergic neurons are concentrated. The input from the NTS also terminated throughout much of the parvocellular division, while that from the locus coeruleus impinged primarily on a restricted, periventricular, zone; neither the NTS nor the locus coeruleus was found to provide detectable inputs to the magnocellular neurosecretory system (Jones and Moore, 1978; Loewy et al., 1981; McKellar and Loewy, 1981; Sawchenko and Swanson, 1981; 1982).

To provide additional details on the distribution within the PVH of inputs from brainstem catecholaminergic neurons, we have again employed the PHA-L method, focussing initially on noradrenergic cell groups (Cunningham and Sawchenko, 1986a). The principal new finding of this analysis was that after some deposits in the A1 region of the ventral medulla, the distribution of labeled fibers in the PVH was almost exclusively restricted to those parts of the magnocellular division in which vasopressinergic neurons are most heavily concentrated. Other, ostensibly similar,deposits gave rise to somewhat more widespread labeling of fibers and terminals in the parvocellular division in addition to a principal plexus in the magnocellular division. These results suggest the existence of a heterogeneity in the A1 input to the PVH, in which some neurons, or pools of neurons, appear to project exclusively to the magnocellular neurosecretory system. Any topographic ordering of cells that provide more restricted as opposed to more exuberant projections was not evident in our studies.

Deposits of PHA-L in the A2 region of the NTS or in the locus coeruleus labeled projections to the PVH that were essentially comparable to those described in autoradiographic studies alluded to above. One significant exception was that in addition to a prominent projection to much of the parvocellular division of the PVH, deposits in the A2 region also consistently labeled inputs to the magnocellular division of the PVH and to associated magnocellular neurosecretory neurons in the supraoptic nucleus.

This aspect of the A2 projection, first described by Tribollet et al. (1985), was sparse, relative to that provided by A1 neurons, and its distribution in the magnocellular neurosecretory system failed to suggest any preferential interaction with oxytocinergic versus vasopressinergic neurons.

In addition to these newly found complexities in the anatomic organization of catecholaminergic inputs to the hypothalamus, it is also clear that the cells that give rise to these pathways are less biochemically homogeneous than had previously been appreciated. Recent combined retrograde transport-double immunohistochemical labeling studies have provided evidence for the presence of at least two peptides in subsets of aminergic neurons that project to the PVH (Sawchenko et al.,1985; Levin and Sawchenko, 1986). The results are summarized in Figure 2.

Earlier reports of the localization of an avian pancreatic polypeptide-like molecule in certain brainstem aminergic neurons have been supported by the demonstration of the recently isolated peptide, neuropeptide Y (NPY), in the mammalian brain where it has been extensively co-localized with various amines in specific cell groups (Everitt et al., 1984). Using antisera against enzyme markers specific for adrenergic and/or noradrenergic neurons we have shown that virtually all of the adrenergic neurons in both the C1 and C2 regions that project to the PVH also contain NPY. Of the noradrenergic neurons that contribute to these pathways, only a subset of cells in the A1 region also stained positively for NPY (Sawchenko et al., 1985).

Similar studies have been carried using antisera against galanin, a 29 amino acid peptide recently isolated from porcine intestine, whose distribution in the central nervous system suggests a rather extensive colocalization in some aminergic cell groups (Skofitsch and Jacobowitz, 1985). Of the cells that we were able to label retrogradely after tracer injections into the PVH and that stained positively for dopamine-beta-hydroxylase (DBH; a marker for adrenergic and noradrenergic neurons), only those in the locus coeruleus and a small fraction (<15%) of those in the A1 region also stained positively for galanin. None of the retrogradely labeled neurons in the regions of adrenergic cell groups were galanin positive (Levin and Sawchenko,

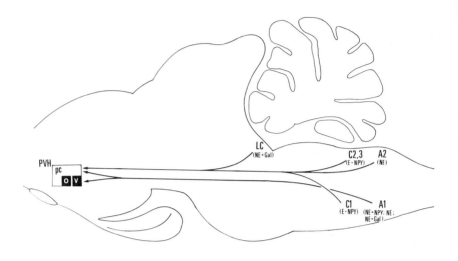

Figure 2. Schematic drawing of a sagittal section through the rat brain to show the organization and co-existing neuropeptides in ascending catecholaminergic inputs to the paraventricular nucleus (PVH). Ascending epinephrine (E) containing pathways innervate primarily the parvocellular (pc) division of the PVH and arise from the C1, C2 and C3 cell groups, each of which also expresses neuropeptide Y- (NPY) immunoreactivity. Norepinephrine containing projections arise from the A1, A2 and locus coeruleus (LC) cell groups; of these, only the A1 group provides a substantial input to the magnocellular division of the PVH. Subpopulations of neurons in the A1 group express either NE alone, NE and NPY, or NE and galanin (Gal). Cells in the LC are predominantly also Gal-immunoreactive, while those in the A2 group express neither peptide.

1986).

It is worthy of note that additional, non-aminergic,

sources of both NPY- and galanin-immunoreactive inputs to the PVH have been described (Bai et al., 1985, Levin and Sawchenko, 1986), and that the distributions of galanin-, NPY-, and DBH-immunoreactive fibers in the PVH are all distinctive with respect to the functional subpopulations of the PVH described above. The picture that has emerged from these analyses is one in which individual cell groups that contribute to the aminergic inputs to the PVH may be further differentiated by the presence of one or more coexisting neuropeptides. While the functional consequences of such colocalization have not yet been investigated, the potential for elaborate sculpting of responses based on differential neuronal and/or hormonal regulation of individual cell groups or participating neuroactive agents seems limitless.

BIOCHEMICAL HETEROGENEITY IN VAGAL MOTOR NEURONS

Ever since the pronouncement by Dale (1933) that all autonomic preganglionic neurons employ acetylcholine as a neurotransmitter, considerable pharmacological, histo-chemical and immunohistochemical evidence has been mar-shalled to support this view. Vagal motor neurons are certainly no exception, though from time to time since the advent of modern immunohistochemical technology several indirect lines of evidence have suggested the presence of additional neuroactive agents within these cells. More direct evidence has been provided by studies in which subpopulations of cells in the dorsal motor nucleus that were retrogradely labeled after tracer injections in the cervical vagus have been shown to express one or another of the enzymes involved in catecholamine biosynthesis (Ritchie et al., 1982; Sawchenko, 1983; Kalia et al., 1984; see Leslie, 1985 for a review). Others have recently reported a failure to confirm aspects of these results (Blessing et al., 1985). This controversy, coupled with the demon-stration of presence of the novel neuropeptide, calcitonin gene-related peptide (CGRP), in a substantial subset of neurons in the nucleus ambiguus (Rosenfeld et al., 1983), has prompted us to survey a number of candidate amines and peptides for their presence in identified vagal motor neurons.

Near the rostral pole of the dorsal motor nucleus, a substantial number of neurons that were retrogradely labeled after tracer deposits in the cervical vagus were found to stain positively for DBH. Because aminergic cells in this region are generally thought to be adrenergic, and because we consistently failed to identify any retrogradely labeled neurons at this level with antisera against either tyrosine hydroxylase (TH; a marker for all catecholaminergic neurons) or phenylethanolamine-N-methyltransferase (PNMT; a marker specific for adrenergic neurons), we are led to question the authenticity of DBH staining in this region. Near the midextent of the dorsal motor nucleus, at the level of the caudal pole of the area postrema, a prominent population of retrogradely labeled cells stained for TH-, but not DBH- or PNMT-, immunoreactivity, suggesting the presence of vagal preganglionic neurons at this locus that may utilize either dopamine or DOPA as a transmitter, co-transmitter or modulator (see Figure 3). Finally, throughout the caudal third of the nucleus, cells doubly labeled with the tracer and either anti-TH or anti-DBH were evident, suggesting the presence of dopaminergic and/or noradrenergic vagal motor neurons at this level.

While several antisera against neuropeptides stained very small numbers of retrogradely labeled neurons in the dorsal motor nucleus, only anti-galanin identified a substantial population. Such doubly labeled cells were clustered primarily in the lateral aspect of the nucleus at, and just rostral to, the level of the area postrema, making their distribution distinct from that of TH-immunoreactive cells at this level.

In the nucleus ambiguus, retrogradely labeled neurons were never stained positively with antisera against the catecholamine-synthetic enzymes, but, as predicted, a majority were immunopositive for CGRP. Roughly two-thirds of all identified ambigual cells were CGRP-immunoreactive, and this correspondence was most pronounced rostrally within the compact part of the nucleus; a lesser proportion of retrogradely labeled cells in the more caudal aspects of the nucleus were immunostained. In addition to CGRP, it now appears that galanin is another marker for a substantial number of ambigual neurons. Although roughly equal numbers of CGRP- and galanin-immunoreactive cells have been detected in the nucleus ambiguus, those stained with anti-galanin appear more evenly distributed throughout the length of the nucleus. Neither antiserum stained effectively the scattered neurons found ventral to the compact column of the nucleus.

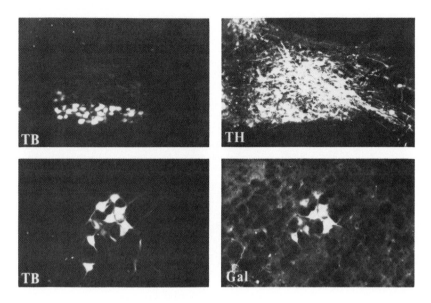

Figure 3. Pairs of fluorescence photomicrographs of the region of the dorsal motor nucleus of the vagus (top) and the nucleus ambiguus (bottom) to show cells retrogradely labeled after injections of the fluorescent tracer true blue (TB) into the cervical vagus and that express either tyrosine hydroxylase-(TH) or galanin- (Gal) immunoreactivity. A subset of cells in the medial aspect of the dorsal motor nucleus at this level are TH positive; the overlying A2 cell group of the NTS is also stained with anti-TH. A majority of the retrogradely labeled cells in the nucleus ambiguus are Gal-immunoreactive.

These results provide evidence for the existence of an unexpected degree of heterogeneity in the chemical makeup of vagal motor neurons. Thus, it would appear that the presence of a number of neuropeptides and amines define topographically distinct aspects of both of the principal motor nuclei of the vagus. Presumably these novel agents coexist with acetylcholine in individual vagal motor neurons, though this has thus far been demonstrated only for CGRP in the nucleus ambiguus (Takami et al., 1985; Stuesse and Sawchenko, 1986). The extent to which such biochemically defined subpopulations may correspond to functionally or anatomically defined groupings of vagal motor neurons is not yet clear.

CONCLUSIONS

The studies described here provide additional information on the anatomic organization and chemical makeup of some well-established central autonomic pathways. On the basis of these results, and other recent studies, several characterizing generalizations applicable to many components of the system may be offered. As more refined data are gathered, it becomes more and more clear that the central autonomic system is characterized by a high degree of topographic ordering and specificity in its component pathways. Superimposed upon this is the fact that most individual cell groups are composed of an elaborate patchwork of chemically specified neurons in which a high degree of colocalization of neuroactive substances is evident. One major task that remains is to sort out the degree of congruence in these various anatomically and chemically defined subpopulations.

ACKNOWLEDGMENTS

The studies from our laboratory described here were supported by grant HL-35137 from the NIH, a Grant-in-Aid from the American Heart Association--California Affiliate, and by a McKnight Foundation Scholar's Award. M.C.L. is the recipient of a Medical Student Research Fellowship from the American Heart Association. This work was conducted in part by the Clayton Foundation for Research--California Division. P.E.S. is a Clayton Foundation Investigator. We are grateful to Ms. P. Thomas and Mr. K. Trulock for their help in the preparation of this manuscript.

REFERENCES

Bai FL, Yamano M, Shiotani Y, Emson PC, Smith AD, Powell JF, Tohyama M (1985). An arcuato-paraventricular and - dorsomedial hypothalamic neuropeptide Y-containing system which lacks noradrenaline in the rat. Brain Res 331:172-175.
Blessing WW, Willoughby JO, Joh TH (1985). Evidence that catecholamine-synthesizing perikarya in the rat medulla oblongata doe not contribute axons to the vagus nerve. Brain Res 348:397-400.
Cunningham ET Jr, Sawchenko PE (1986a). Anatomical specifi-

city of noradrenergic inputs to the paraventricular and supraoptic nuclei of the rat hypothalamus. Anat Rec 214:27A.

Cunningham ET Jr, Sawchenko PE (1986b). Local projections from the medial part of the nucleus of the solitary tract in the rat. Soc Neurosci Abstr, in press.

Dale HH (1933). Nomenclature of fibers in the autonomic nervous system and their effects. J Physiol 80:10P-11P.

Day TA, Ferguson AV, Renaud LP (1984). Facilitatory influence of noradrenergic afferents on the excitability of rat paraventricular nucleus neurosecretory cells. J Physiol 355:237-249.

Everitt BJ, Hokfelt, T Terenius L, Tatemoto K, Mutt V, Goldstein M (1984). Differential co-existence of neuropeptide Y (NPY)-like immunoreactivity with catecholamines in the central nervous system of the rat. Neuroscience 11:443-462.

Geis GS, Wurster RD (1980). Horseradish peroxidase localization of cardiac vagal preganglionic neurons. Brain Res 182:19-30.

Gerfen CR, Sawchenko, PE (1984). An anterograde neuroanatomical tracing method that shows the detailed morphology of neurons their axons and terminals: Immunohistochemical localization of an axonally transported plant lectin, Phaseolus vulgaris-leucoagglutinin (PHA-L). Brain Res 90:219-238.

Jones BJ, Moore RY (1977). Ascending projections of the locus coeruleus in the rat. II. Autoradiographic study. Brain Res 127:23-53.

Kalia M, Fuxe K, Goldstein M, Harfstrand A, Agnati LF, Coyle JT (1984). Evidence for the existence of putative dopamine-, adrenaline-, and noradrenaline-containing vagal motor neurons in the brainstem of the rat. Neurosci Lett 50:57-62.

Leslie RA (1985). Neuroactive substances in the dorsal vagal complex of the medulla oblongata: Nucleus of the tractus solitarius and dorsal motor nucleus of the vagus. Neurochem Int 7:191-211.

Levin MC, Sawchenko PE (1986). The distribution and cells of origin of galanin-containing projections to the paraventricular and supraoptic nuclei of the rat. Soc Neurosci Abstr, in press.

Loewy AD, Burton H (1978). Nuclei of the solitary tract: efferent projections to lower brain stem and spinal cord of the cat. J Comp Neurol 181:421-450.

Loewy AD, Wallach JH, McKellar S (1981). Efferent connections of the ventral medulla oblongata in the rat. Brain Res Rev 3:63-80.

McKellar S, Loewy AD (1981). Organization of some brainstem afferents to the paraventricular nucleus of the hypothalamus in the rat. Brain Res 217:351-357.

Norgren R (1978). Projections from the nucleus of the solitary tract in the rat. Neuroscience 3:207-218.

Ricardo J, Koh ET (1978). Anatomical evidence of direct projections from the nucleus of the solitary tract to the hypothalamus, amygdala, and other forebrain structures in the rat. Brain Res 153:1-26.

Ritchie TC, Westlund KN, Bowker RM, Coulter JD, Leonard RB (1982). The relationship of the medullary catecholamine containing neurones to the vagal motor nuclei. Neuroscience 7:1471-1482.

Reis DJ, Granata AR, Joh TH, Ross CA, Ruggiero DA, Park DH (1984). Brain stem catecholamine mechanisms in tonic and reflex control of blood pressure. Hypertension 6 (Suppl 2):II-7-II-15.

Rosenfeld MG, Mermod J-J, Amara SG, Swanson LW, Sawchenko PE, Rivier J, Vale WW, Evans RM (1983). Production of a novel neuropeptide encoded by the calcitonin gene via tissue-specific RNA processing. Nature 304:129-135.

Sawchenko PE (1983a). Central connections of the sensory and motor nuclei of the vagus nerve. J Autonom Nerv Syst 9:13-26.

Sawchenko PE (1983b). Catecholamines and neuropeptides in the vagal motor nuclei: evidence for topographically organized subpopulations of chemically specified preganglionic neurons. Soc Neurosci Abstr 9:548.

Sawchenko PE, Swanson LW (1981). Central noradrenergic pathways for the integration of hypothalamic neuroendocrine and autonomic responses. Science 214:685-687.

Sawchenko PE, Swanson LW (1982). The organization of noradrenergic parthways from the brainstem to the paraventricular and supraoptic nuclei in the rat. Brain Res Rev 4:275-325.

Sawchenko PE, Swanson LW, Grzanna R, Howe PRC, Bloom SR, Polak JM (1985). Colocalization of neuropeptide Y immunoreactivity in brainstem catecholaminergic neurons that project to the paraventricular nucleus of the hypothalamus. J Comp Neurol 241:138-153.

Skofitsch G, Jacobowitz DM (1985). Immunohistochemical mapping of galanin-like neurons in the rat central nervous system. Peptides 6:509-546.

Stuesse SL (1982). Origins of cardiac vagal preganglionic

fibers: a retrograde transport study. Brain Res 236:15-25.

Stuesse SL, Sawchenko, PE (1986). Calcitonin gene-related peptide and choline acetyltransferase: co-distribution in visceral subpopulations within the nucleus ambiguus. Soc Neurosci Abstr, in press.

Swanson LW, Sawchenko PE (1983). Hypothalamic integration: organization of the paraventricular and supraoptic nuclei. Ann Rev Neurosci 6:269-324.

Takami K, Kawai Y, Shiosaka S, Lee Y, Girgis S, Hillyard CJ, MacIntyre I, Emson PC, Tohyama M (1985). Immuno-histochemical evidence for the coexistence of calci-tonin gene-related peptide and choline acetyltransfer-ase-like immunoreactivity in neurons of the rat hypo-glossal, facial and ambiguus nucleus. Brain Res 328:386-389.

Travers JB, Norgren R (1983). Afferent projections to the oral motor nuclei in the rat. J Comp Neurol 220:280-298.

Tribollet E, Armstrong WE, Dubois-Dauphin M, Dreifuss JJ (1985). Extra-hypothalamic afferent inputs to the supraoptic nucleus of the rat as determined by retro-grade and anterograde tracing techniques. Neuroscience 15:135-148.

Organization of the Autonomic Nervous System:
Central and Peripheral Mechanisms, pages 283–293
© **1987 Alan R. Liss, Inc.**

IDENTIFICATION OF NEUROTRANSMITTERS WHICH MEDIATE
CARDIOVASCULAR EFFECTS ELICITED FROM THE MIDLINE MEDULLA

Robert B. McCall

Cardiovascular Diseases Research
The Upjohn Company
Kalamazoo, MI 49001

INTRODUCTION

It is well established that the medullary raphe
complex plays an integral role in the sympathetic control of
the cardiovascular system. Wang and Ranson (1939)
originally reported that electrical stimulation of medial
medullary raphe nuclei elicits a marked decrease in blood
pressure. The decrease in blood pressure resulting from
stimulation of this "depressor zone" is accompanied by a
bradycardia and an inhibition of spontaneously occurring
sympathetic nervous discharge (SND). Serotonergic neurons
which descend to the intermediolateral cell column (i.e. the
main site of origin of sympathetic preganglionic neurons)
are located in the medullary raphe nuclei (Loewy and Neil,
1981). The association between serotonin (5-HT) neurons and
the midline depressor area coupled with the fact that 5-HT
precursors produce a depression of spinal sympathetic
reflexes (Franz et. al., 1982) have led several
investigators to suggest that medullo-spinal 5-HT neurons
inhibit the discharges of sympathetic preganglionic neurons.

In spite of the fact that the midline medulla is
generally thought to be involved in vasodepressor
mechanisms, Adair et. al., (1977) found that stimulation of
midline medullary raphe nuclei elicited pressor as well as
depressor responses. In addition, Morrison and Gebber,
(1982) have identified both sympathoexcitatory and
sympathoinhibitory neurons within medullary raphe nuclei.
The presence of two distinct types of sympathetic neurons
indicates that the midline medulla is heterogenous with

respect to autonomic function and suggests that 5-HT neurons may act as sympathoexcitatory rather than sympathoinhibitory neurons. In support of this, McCall and Humphrey (1982) found that compounds which block excitatory but not inhibitory effects of serotonin in the central nervous system (i.e. methysergide and metergoline) inhibit spontaneous SND. Therefore, the purpose of the present experiments was to determine the nature of the neurotransmitters which mediate sympathoexcitatory and sympathoinhibitory responses elicited from the midline medulla and to provide evidence for the functional importance of this area in cardiovascular regulation.

METHODS

The methods employed in this study have been previously described (McCall, 1983, 1984; McCall and Humphrey, 1985). Spontaneous SND was recorded from the left inferior cardiac nerve in dial-urethane anesthetized cats. Pneumothoracotomy was performed and the animals were paralyzed. Blood pressure, heart rate and SND were monitored throughout the experiment. Stimulating electrodes were stereotaxically positioned in the midline of the medulla 2-7mm rostral to the obex. Pressor and depressor sites were identified by high frequency electrical stimulation. The effects of single shock raphe stimulation (4-10V, 0.5 ms, 0.5 Hz) on SND were quantitated using computer summating techniques. Antidromically identified single sympathetic preganglionic neurons were recorded extracellularly from the central barrel of a 5-barrel micropipette. Stimulating and recording sites were histologically verified.

Results

High frequency electrical stimulation of medullary raphe nuclei elicited both depressor (Fig. 1A) and pressor (Fig. 1B) responses. The medullary raphe complex appeared to be a heterogeneous region yielding pressor and depressor responses in a single electrode track. Computer summating techniques were used to assess the sympatho-inhibitory and sympathoexcitatory effects of electrical stimulation. Inhibition of SND elicited by single shocks applied to depressor sites was displayed as a summated potential (i.e. downward curve in Fig. 1A, Panel 3) while

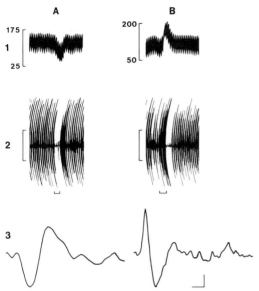

Fig. 1. Effects of stimulation of medullary raphe depressor (A) and pressor (B) sites. Panels 1 and 2: effect of high frequency stimulation on arterial blood pressure (panel 1) and SND (panel 2). Horizontal line represents stimulation duration. Vertical calibration is 50 µV. Panel 3: post-stimulus computer summed averages of SND evoked by single shocks. Trace triggered by stimulus. Vertical calibration is 30 µV. Horizontal calibration is 30 s for panels 1 and 2 and 100 ms for panel 3.

shocks applied to pressor sites resulted in an increase in SND which was displayed as an upward curve in the computer summated potential (Fig. 1B, Panel 3). The modal onset latency of sympathetic excitation occurred 98 ± 4 ms after the stimulus. Allowing for a 15 ms conduction time in the inferior cardiac nerve, the mean conduction velocity in the excitatory raphe-spinal pathway to sympathetic preganglionic neurons was 1.24 ± 0.06 ms.

Pharmacological agents were used to identify putative neurotransmitters which mediate sympathoexcitatory and sympathoinhibitory responses evoked by stimulation of the midline medulla. The 5-HT antagonists methysergide (0.2-0.8 mg/kg, i.v.) and metergoline (0.05-0.2 mg/kg, i.v.) produced a dose-related inhibition of the excitatory potential of SND elicited by single shock stimulation of the medullary raphe complex (Fig. 2, n=14). Methysergide failed to antagonize the sympathoinhibitory response produced by stimulation of raphe depressor sites (n=4). In fact, methysergide often converted a sympathoexcitatory response to raphe stimulation into a sympathoinhibitory response (Fig. 2, column 1). 5-HT antagonists failed to affect sympathoexcitatory responses evoked from pressor sites in the rostral ventrolateral

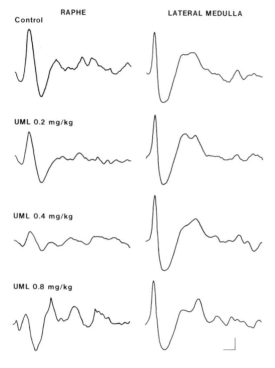

RAPHE   LATERAL MEDULLA

Control

UML 0.2 mg/kg

UML 0.4 mg/kg

UML 0.8 mg/kg

Fig. 2. Effect of methysergide (UML) on computer-summed evoked potentials of SND elicited from raphe and lateral medulla pressor sites (64 trials). Raphe stimulation parameters were 10 V/0.5 ms/0.5 Hz. Lateral medulla stimulation was 6 V/0.5 ms/0.5 Hz. Horizontal calibration is 100 ms. Vertical calibration is 30 µV for raphe and 20 µV for lateral medulla.

medulla (Fig. 2, column 2). These data indicate that the depressant effect of 5-HT antagonists on excitatory potentials is specific for those evoked from raphe nuclei and suggests that raphe sympathoexcitatory potentials may be mediated by 5-HT.

In order to provide further evidence that the sympathoexcitatory effects of raphe stimulation were mediated by 5-HT, we studied the effects of the 5-HT uptake inhibitor chlorimipramine on excitatory potentials evoked from the raphe and ventrolateral medulla pressor sites. Chlorimipramine (0.3-1.0 mg/kg, i.v., n=5) consistently increased the duration of the excitatory evoked potential elicited from the raphe (Fig. 3). In contrast, chlorimipramine failed to alter the duration of the excitatory potential evoked from the lateral medulla (Fig. 3, column 2).

In order to localize a possible site of interaction between 5-HT and sympathetic neurons, methysergide was

administered topically on the dorsal surface of the
medulla at the level of the obex and intrathecally into

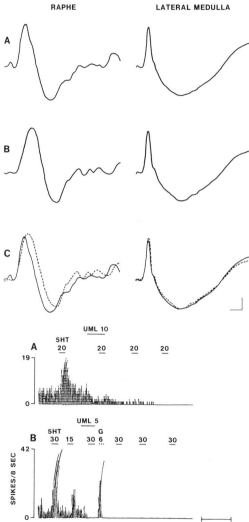

RAPHE   **LATERAL MEDULLA**

A

B

C

Fig. 3. Effect of chlorimipramine
(0.5 mg/kg, i.v.) on computer
summed (64 trials) excitatory
evoked potential of SND elicited
by stimulation of raphe (10 V/0.5
ms/0.5 Hz) and lateral medulla (5
V/0.5 ms/0.5 Hz) . A: before drug.
B: 15 min after drug. C: composite
of A & B. Solid line before drug,
dashed line after drug. Horizontal
calibration is 50 ms. Vertical
calibration is 25 µV.

UML 10

A 5HT 20   20   20   20
19 ─┐ 20

0 ─┘

UML 5

B 5HT   G
   30 15   30 6   30   30   30
42 ─┐

SPIKES/8 SEC

0 ─┘

Fig. 4. Iontophoretically applied
methysergide (UML) blocked the
excitatory effect of 5-HT on
sympathetic preganglionic
neurons in intact animals. Neurons
were excited by glutamate (G)
following antagonist
administration. Horizontal
calibration is 2 min.

the upper thoracic spinal cord (i.e. T_1). Topical
methysergide (50 µg) failed to alter the sympathoexcitatory response to electrical stimulation of the
midline medulla. In contrast, intrathecal methysergide
(50 µg) blocked the raphe evoked sympathoexcitation.
These data suggest that 5-HT neurons in the medullary
raphe nuclei project to the spinal cord to directly, or

indirectly, excite sympathetic preganglionic neurons. To further test this hypothesis, the effects of microiontophoretically applied 5-HT and 5-HT antagonists on antidromically identified sympathetic preganglionic neurons were determined. Iontophoretic 5-HT consistently excited sympathetic preganglionic neurons (Fig. 4, n=95 cells). In no case did 5-HT inhibit the discharges of sympathetic preganglionic neurons. Iontophoretic 5-HT antagonists blocked the excitatory effects of 5-HT but not those of glutamate. 5-HT antagonists decreased the spontaneous discharge rate of sympathetic preganglionic units (Fig. 4A, B).

The effects of iontophoretic and intravenous 5-HT antagonists were also tested in acute spinal animals (Fig. 5). Methysergide and metergoline consistently blocked the excitation of sympathetic preganglionic neurons produced by 5-HT. In contrast to intact animals, methysergide and metergoline failed to inhibit the spontaneous discharge rate of sympathetic preganglionic neurons (Fig. 5). No local anesthetic effects of the iontophoretically applied 5-HT antagonists were observed.

The data presented above strongly suggest that the sympathoexcitatory response to medullary raphe stimulation is mediated through a descending serotonergic pathway. Attempts were next made to determine the nature of the neurotransmitter mediating raphe-evoked sympathoinhibition. The depressor response to high frequency

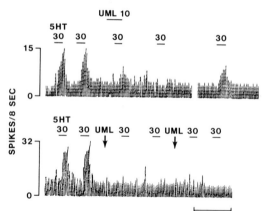

Fig. 5. Effect of methysergide (UML) in spinal transected animals. Iontophoretic methysergide (10 nA) blocked excitation of preganglionic neurons by 5-HT (30 nA) but failed to effect spontaneous firing rate. Neuron was recorded for 1 h (break in baseline). Intravenous methysergide (0.2 mg/kg/arrow) blocked excitatory effect of 5-HT but failed to effect spontaneous firing rate.

stimulation of the midline medulla was blunted, eliminated or reversed following the intravenous administration of the GABA antagonist picrotoxin (Fig. 6A). The inhibition of the depressor response did not result from any change in blood pressure or SND produced by picrotoxin, since these experiments were performed in midcollicularly transected animals. In this regard, picrotoxin fails to alter blood pressure or SND in midcollicularly transected animals (McCall, 1986). The computer summed sympatho-inhibitory response to single shock stimulation of the midline medulla was also blocked by picrotoxin (Fig. 6B) and by a second GABA antagonist bicuculline (Fig. 6C). In contrast, GABA antagonists failed to block baroreceptor mediated sympathoinhibition.

The loss of raphe-mediated inhibition with picrotoxin and bicuculline suggests that GABA may mediate this sympathoinhibitory process. Since benzodiazepines are known to enhance GABAergic neurotransmission by facilitating the interaction of this amino acid with its receptor, we examined the effects of diazepam on raphe elicited SND inhibition. Diazepam (0.3 mg/kg, i.v., n=4)

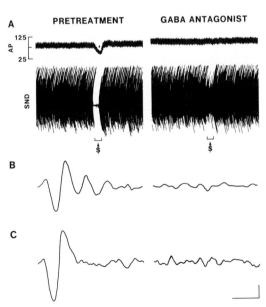

Fig. 6. Effects of GABA antagonists on sympathoinhibition evoked from stimulation of medullary raphe depressor site. A: arterial blood pressure (AP, mm Hg) and spontaneous SND before (left column) and after (right column) picrotoxin (1 mg/kg, i.v.) in midcollicular transected cat. S represents 15 s raphe stimulation (10 V, 0.5 ms, 20 Hz). B-C: computer summed traces of SND before (left column) and after (right column) picrotoxin (1.0 mg/kg, i.v., B) or bicuculline (1 mg/kg, i.v., C). Computer sweep triggered by stimulus applied to raphe, 64 trials, 4 ms bins. B: 8 V, 0.5 ms, 0.5 Hz. C: 6 V, 0.5 ms, 0.5 Hz. Horizontal scale: A = 1 min, B-C = 256 ms. Vertical scale: A = 80 μV, B-C = 512 μV.

consistently increased the duration (i.e. 175 ± 9 ms to 315 ± 12 ms) of the SND inhibitory response evoked by raphe stimulation (Fig. 7A). Higher doses of picrotoxin (1.0-2.0 mg/kg, i.v.) were required to abolish the sympathoinhibition following diazepam (Fig. 7A3). Picrotoxin often reversed the sympathoinhibitory response to midline medullary stimulation into an excitatory response. The sympathoexcitatory responses following picrotoxin could be blocked by 5-HT antagonists (Fig. 7B).

The functional significance of the midline medulla with respect to cardiovascular function was determined by lesioning the midline medulla from 2 to 7 mm rostral to the obex. This lesion failed to alter arterial blood pressure or heart rate but resulted in a marked increase in SND (+163%). Baroreceptor and somatosympathetic reflexes were unaltered by the lesion. In addition, the effects of stimulation of vagal afferents and hypothalamic pressor sites were not changed following the lesion. Interestingly, however, the vasodepressor responses evoked by electrical stimulation of trigeminal tract or hypothalamic depressor sites were completely blocked by midline medullary lesions.

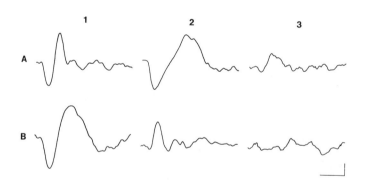

Fig. 7. Computer summed traces (64 trials) triggered by stimulus applied to raphe depressor site. A1: pretreatment sympathoinhibition (6 V, 0.5 ms, 0.5 Hz). A2: sympathoinhibition potentiated after diazepam (0.3 mg/kg, i.v.). A3: picrotoxin (2 mg/kg, i.v.) blocks sympathoinhibition. B1: pretreatment sympathoinhibition (8 V, 0.5 ms, 0.5 Hz). B2: picrotoxin (1 mg/kg, i.v.) converted sympathoinhibitory response into sympathoexcitatory response. B3: methysergide (0.8 mg/kg, i.v.) blocks sympathoexcitatory response to raphe stimulation. Horizontal scale = 256 ms. Vertical scale = 512 µV.

DISCUSSION

This study was designed to determine the nature of the neurotransmitters which mediate the cardiovascular effects of electrical stimulation of the midline medullary raphe nuclei. High frequency electrical stimulation of medullary raphe nuclei produced both pressor and depressor responses. Several observations indicate that the sympathoexcitatory response to stimulation was mediated by serotonergic neurons. First, sites which yielded sympathoexcitatory responses were contained within the B1-B3 5-HT cell groups. Second, the mean conduction velocity in the raphe-spinal sympathoexcitatory pathway to preganglionic neurons was 1.24 m/s. This is consistent with it being mediated by unmyelinated fibers such as 5-HT containing axons. Third, 5-HT antagonists blocked the sympathoexcitatory but not the sympathoinhibitory effects of raphe stimulation. The effect of the 5-HT antagonists was specific in that they blocked the sympathoexcitatory response elicited from the raphe but not from the ventrolateral medulla. Fourth, the 5-HT uptake inhibitor chlorimipramine increased the duration of the sympatho-excitatory potential evoked from the raphe but not from the ventrolateral medulla. These observations provide strong evidence that 5-HT neurons in medullary raphe nuclei provide an excitatory input to central sympathetic neurons.

Several observations indicate that the excitatory interaction between 5-HT and sympathetic neurons occurs at the level of the preganglionic neuron in the intermedio-lateral cell column of the spinal cord. First, medullary 5-HT neurons project to the intermediolateral cell column (Loewy and Neil, 1981). Second, methysergide given intrathecally, but not topically to the dorsal surface of the medulla, blocked the sympathoexcitatory response to raphe stimulation. Third, iontophoretically applied 5-HT consistently increased the discharge rate of sympathetic preganglionic neurons. These observations suggest that serotonergic neurons excite sympathetic preganglionic neurons. The fact that 5-HT antagonists depressed the spontaneous discharges rate of preganglionic neurons in intact but not spinal animals suggests that sympathetic preganglionic neurons receive a tonic excitatory input from 5-HT neurons located in the brain stem.

The data also indicate that GABA is involved in the sympathoinhibitory response to raphe stimulation. Picrotoxin, an agent that blocks the Cl⁻ channel associated in GABA receptor activation, abolished the sympathoinhibitory response to raphe stimulation. Similar effects were seen with bicuculline, a direct GABA receptor antagonist. GABA antagonists also blocked the raphe elicited sympathoinhibition in midcollicularly transected animals but failed to increase blood pressure or sympathetic activity. Thus, the elimination of the sympathoinhibitory period did not result from changes in blood pressure or SND. In addition, picrotoxin selectively inhibited raphe-mediated sympathoinhibition as opposed to non-specifically antagonizing all sympatho-inhibitory processes since GABA antagonists failed to block baroreceptor-mediated sympathoinhibition. Thus, it is unlikely that picrotoxin acted to simply depolarize central sympathetic neurons, therefore making them less responsive to non-GABAergic inhibition. The fact that diazepam potentiated the sympathoinhibition supports the contention that raphe-evoked inhibition is mediated specifically by GABA.

Lesions of the midline medullary nuclei eliminated the sympathoinhibitory responses evoked from the hypothalamus and the trigeminal tract but failed to alter sympathoexcitatory responses to stimulation of pressor sites in the hypothalamus or somatosympathetic afferents. These data suggest that neuronal elements within the medullary raphe mediate vasodepressor responses elicited in other areas of the central nervous system. This statement cannot be generalized to all sympathoinhibitory processes, since baroreceptor and vagal afferent mediated sympathoinhibition was not altered by the lesion. The midline medulla does not appear to be involved in sympathetic slow wave generation, since lesions did not alter the periodicity of sympathetic slow waves.

In conclusion, this study indicates that the midline medullary raphe nuclei are heterogenous with respect to autonomic function. Serotonergic neurons provide a tonic excitatory input to sympathetic preganglionic neurons. The sympathoinhibitory responses elicited from medullary raphe nuclei are mediated by GABA. The reversability of raphe-evoked sympathoexcitatory and inhibitory responses following pharmacological antagonism indicates that the net effect of raphe stimulation is a summation of activation and inhibition of sympathetic elements.

REFERENCES

Adair JR, Hamilton BL, Scappaticci KA, Helke CJ, Gillis RA (1977). Cardiovascular responses to electrical stimulation of the medullary raphe area of the cat. Brain Research 128: 141-145.

Franz DN, Madsen PW, Peterson RG, Sangdee C (1982). Functional roles of monoaminergic pathways to sympathetic preganglionic neurons. Clin Exp Hypertension A4:543-562.

Loewy AD, Neil JJ (1981). The role of descending monoaminergic systems in central control of blood pressure. Fed Proc 40:2778-2785.

McCall RB (1983). Serotonergic excitation of sympathetic preganglionic neurons: a microiontophoretic study. Brain Research 289:121-127.

McCall RB (1984). Evidence for a serotonergically mediated sympathoexcitatory response to stimulation of medullary raphe nuclei. Brain Research 311:131-139.

McCall RB (1986). Lack of involvement of GABA in baroreceptor-mediated sympathoinhibition. Amer J Physiol 250:R1065-R1073.

McCall RB, Humphrey SJ (;1982). Involvement of serotonin in the regulation of blood pressure: Evidence for a facilitating effect on sympathetic nerve activity. J Pharmacol Exp Therap 222:94-102.

McCall RB, Humphrey SJ (1985). Evidence for GABA mediation of sympathetic inhibition evoked from midline medullary depressor sites. Brain Research 339:356-360.

Morrison SF, Gebber GL (1982). Classification of raphe neurons with cardiac-related activity. Amer J Physiol 243:R49-R59.

Wang SC, Ranson SW (1939). Autonomic responses to electrical stimulation of the lower brain stem. J Comp Neurol 71:437-455.

**Organization of the Autonomic Nervous System:
Central and Peripheral Mechanisms, pages 295–306**
© **1987 Alan R. Liss, Inc.**

Possible Cerebello-Vestibulo-Spinal Interactions in the
Organization of Sympathetic Activity

András Erdélyi, László Simon[+], Tibor Tóth
Natl. Inst. Occup. Hlth., Dept. Physiol. and
[+]1st Inst. of Anatomy, Semmelweis Univ. Med.
Sch., Budapest, Hungary

INTRODUCTION

The presently available body of knowledge concerning
the role of spinal systems in the integration of sympathetic activity has been recently summarized by Koizumi and
Brooks (1984). Their review lends considerable support to
the notion that the spinal cord is much more than merely a
bundle of passive ascending and descending conducting
cables between the periphery and the higher levels of
central nervous integration. Yet, quite a few questions
have been left open. We are going to deal with two of
them only: 1) Is it really true that "the spinal cord is
less of an integrating center than it is a transporter of
incoming signals to and of outgoing signals from the
hierarchy of higher centers" (Koizumi & Brooks, 1984). 2)
If the reverse can be proven to be true, i.e. if the
spinal cord is less of a transporter of signals than it is
an integrating center, how can the connections between
various levels of the central nervous system be realized?

ANATOMICAL AND PHYSIOLOGICAL PROBLEMS

It is somewhat strange how reluctantly several facts
of spinal integration gathered by neuromorphology or by
various branches of neurophysiology are incorporated into
the current ideas of our own subspecialty. To enumerate

just a few of them:

1) The intermediolateral nucleus has been described by anatomists to be a typical "noyaux ferme" ("closed" nucleus) receiving its input almost exclusively via its lateral side, i.e. from the lateral funiculus, any neurone system (and those neurones only) projecting into the lateral funiculus may therefore have access to this nucleus (Réthelyi, 1972).

2) No monosynaptic connections between spinal primary sensory (or medullospinal descending) fibers and the sympathetic preganglionic neurones have been proven. A group of spinal interneurons (processing mostly information of cutaneous origin) have been shown to be localized in the deeper laminae of the dorsal horn and another one in even deeper parts of the central gray, i.e. in the basal portions of the intermediate region. In the latter there is a heavy convergence of cutaneous, muscular and visceral afferents (Réthelyi & Szentágothai, 1973). Both regions send fibers into the lateral funiculus.

3) With respect to its macroscopic buildup, neuronal and neuropil architecture, cell density and connections, the intermediate region of the spinal gray is analogous to the brain stem reticular formation. Its role in somatomotor integration is well established; this is the part of the spinal segmental apparatus which has been likened (Réthelyi & Szentágothai, 1973) to a "general central 'computer' with built in functional programs (or subroutines) in the different segmental groups (like the brachial segments for the fore-limb movements)...", etc.; it is hard to believe that the spinal autonomic neurones are inaccessible to this system.

4) The role of presynaptic inhibition in the regulation of the impulse flow in sensory channels has been known for decades (Schmidt, 1971). Spinal connections and descending tracts bringing about primary afferent hyperpolarization or depolarization in the spinal terminals of cutaneous, muscular and visceral afferents and leading thereby to facilitation or inhibition of segmental pathways, are familiar to all of us. We have experienced the announcement of the original form of the gate control theory (Melzack & Wall, 1965), we have followed the lively discussions triggered by this - we may, perhaps, use the expression - revolutionary idea, we have met its modifications, extensions, etc. (Knyihár-Csillik & Csillik, 1981; Wall, 1980), and finally we have classified

it into the domain of sensory physiology. Its almost certain role also in autonomic nervous function has not been elaborated upon.

5) The vestibular nerves contain - from our present point of view at least - afferents like the spinal ones: their stimulation (or natural activation) leads to a variety of autonomic reflexes, including activation and inhibition of the electrical activity of sympathetic nerves. The most important papers of the field have been reviewed previously (Erdélyi, 1982; Erdélyi, Mitsányi & Tóth, 1981). Although the vestibulo-cerebellar connections were recognized rather early, the possiblity of cerebello-autonomic interactions were definitely denied by Karplus in 1937. The first paper on the modification of vasomotor reflexes due to paleocerebellar stimulation came out a year later (Moruzzi, 1938). The present state of our knowledge has been summarized by Martner (1975). In his words: "The results... indicate that the cerebellum is involved in the regulation of a variety of autonomic functions, perhaps according to principles, similar to those valid for cerebellar somatomotor control. The cerebellar influence is not only confined to... autonomic responses...associated with e.g. particular somatomotor adjustments ... but appears to affect virtually all types of autonomic mechanisms, including reflexes engaged in bulbospinal, 'homeostatic' mechanisms and resulting in cardiovascular, gastrointestinal or urinary bladder adjustments. Probably the cerebellar influence takes the form of a modulating and fine-adjusting influence which is exerted mainly at spinal and bulbar levels but it appears likely that cerebellar autonomic interactions may occur also at higher levels by means of e.g. fastigial projections on hypothalamic and limbic structures." Haines et al. (1984) have recently added some new data to the last mentioned possibility. Nevertheless the fact that cerebellar stimulation in decerebrate animals can influence the activity of spinal autonomic neurones proves that the spinal cord and the lower brain stem together comprise a very powerful integrating system even without the contribution of higher autonomic centers. The very close connections between the cerebellum and essentially all the afferents of spinal, bulbar (including vestibular) and even higher origin, and the observation that stimulation of neighboring and distant afferent channels are able to bring about presynaptic inhibition or facilitation on

almost any given input system (Schmidt, 1971) lend support to the idea that these mechanisms may play very important roles also in autonomic integration.

METHODS AND RESULTS

For technical details and detailed results we refer to our previous papers (Erdélyi & Mitsányi, 1977; Erdélyi et al., 1977; Erdélyi et al., 1979; Erdélyi et al., 1977). For this presentation figure 1 is intended to illustrate our (very simple) experimental approach and a few of the results. In the case shown, high intensity stimulation was applied to a cutaneous and to a muscle nerve, both with cervicothoracic segmental inputs. In row 1, the animal was under light ether anaesthesia. The pressor reflexes consisted of transient peaks and of consecutive maintained phases. Higher frequencies and stimulation of cutaneous nerves favored the appearance of the transients, whereas real tonic components were more readily evoked by lower frequencies and by excitation of muscle afferents.

After induction of a deep chloralose-urethane anaesthesia, the effectiveness of muscle nerve stimulation decreased slightly, whereas cutaneous nerve stimulation became almost ineffective (2nd row). A moderate dose of picrotoxin brought back the cutaneous reflex, enhanced the inverse frequency dependence of the responses which were present under control conditions, and led to some disturbances in the organization of both types of reflexes (3rd row). After administration of strychnine, muscular afferent stimulation evoked a moderate tonic reflex, whereas cutaneous stimulation was followed by a phasic, high amplitude and low frequency blood pressure oscillation.

In figure 2 we demonstrate several responses which were collected in 3 acutely spinalized, non-anaesthetized cats. Again, intense electrical stimulation was applied to different muscle and skin nerves. Essentially, no distinct responses could be recorded in the control period (1st row). After injection of picrotoxin (first four panels in row 2) or strychnine (last panel in the row), more or less distinct reflexes were evoked in all of the experiments. Having given the second drug to the animals (row 3), a marked increase in the magnitude of the reactions could be seen. Stimulation of cutaneous afferents was more effective than that of the muscular ones and only the first type of intervention led to the appearance of distinct phasic and tonic components in the responses.

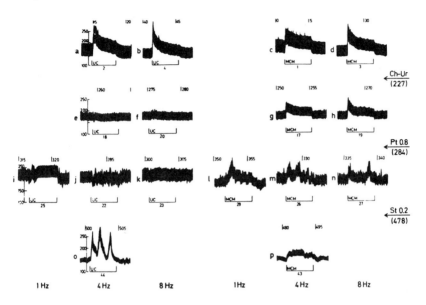

Figure 1. Blood pressure (BP) reflexes in intact cats elicited by electric stimulation of the medial cutaneous nerve of the forelimb (UC) and of the muscular branch of the musculocutaneous nerve(MCM). First row: under light ether anaesthesia (a-d). Second row: after administration of a mixture of chloralose and urethane (Ch-Ur; e-h), 50 and 300 mg/kg, respectively. Third row: after administration of 0.8 mg/kg picrotoxin (Pt; i-n). Last row: after a dose (0.2 mg/kg) of strychnine (St; o-p). Stimulation parameters: 16 V, 0.5 ms, 1-4-8 Hz, as marked at the bottom of the figure, duration 4 min. BP calibration in mm Hg. Numbered bars on the top of each record and in parentheses at the arrows: running time in min. Numbers under stimulation signals: numbering of events.

DISCUSSION

Evaluation of the results of a great number of experiments similar to that shown in figure 1 led to the conclusion that two neural mechanisms must participate in the organization of the reflexes: one of them being responsible for the tonic, the other for the phasic component. Muscular (or, more correctly, locomotor) and also visceral afferents seem to have direct access to the first, while cutaneous ones may project to the second. The two mechanisms must be interconnected and under normal conditions the activity generated in one of them spreads to the other; their interconnction is probably via some interneuronal system, the conduction in which seems to be different in the two directions. Our observations suggest the existence of several different inhibitory mechanisms in the whole system: one of them is picrotoxin sensitive and at least partly presynaptic, being able to modify (in decreasing order) the effective-

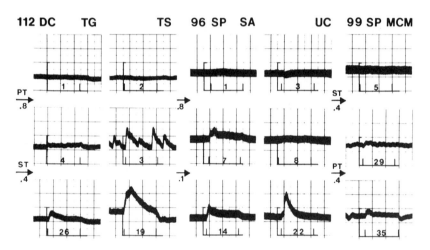

Figure 2. A collection of BP reflexes in unanaesthetized cats under control conditions (1st row), then (2nd row) after administration of either picrotoxin (PT, first four responses) or strychnine (ST, last response) and, lastly (3rd row) after administration of ST (first four responses) or PT (last response). Doses in mg/kg. First two columns: exp. No. 112, decapitated (DC), stimulation of the nerve from the gastrocnemius muscle (TG) and the sural nerve (TS). Third and fourth columns: exp. No. 96, C_1-C_2 spinal cord section (SP), stimulation of the saphenous (SA) and UC (see Fig. 1). Stimulation parameters: 16 V, 0.5 ms, 4 Hz, 4 min. BP calibration (vertical bars on the left side of the panels): 0-100 mm Hg. Time: horizontal bar attached to bottom of BP calibration: 5 min. Stimulus marking: short vertical bars on time calibration.

ness of cutaneous, muscular and visceral afferents; the other is strychnine sensitive (postsynaptic?) braking the activity in the subsystem receiving cutaneous input; there are certainly several more acting on the output of the "tonic" mechanism and perhaps on the interneurones connecting this mechanism with the "phasic" one.

The results of experiments in spinal animals prove that the mechanisms responsible for the phasic and tonic manifestations of the reflexes are complete at the spinal level already. We do not have therefore any reason to suppose that in an intact nervous system descending pathways must bypass these structures and contact the preganglionic sympathetic neurones directly. The almost total irresponsiveness of the spinal cord deprived of descending influences may be due to an enormous increase of the picrotoxin sensitive inhibition; because of the difference in the reflexes produced by stimulation of skin and muscle nerves in spinal animals this inhibition may be presynaptic. It is generated by spinal structures and, in an intact central nervous system, it is under the control of another inhibition driven by activity of supraspinal origin and by segmental high threshold afferents. The above mentioned difference suggests, however, that some change other than the increase of presynaptic inhibition must be brought about by cutting the spinal cord. The relative irresponsiveness of the spinal animal to stimulation of muscle afferents (in contrast to the situation in deeply anaesthetized animals, in which the excitability of this channel is hardly decreased) may be explained by assuming that the activity of the "tonic" system and, moreover, the hypothesized pathway conducting its activity back to the "phasic" mechanism, are also under the control of some inhibition(s), the level of which too, might have been increased as a consequence of cord section.

We have summarized the results of our experiments in figure 3 taking the morphological data and also some of the knowledge accumulated in other fields of physiology into consideration (there are many newer findings which could not be included, e.g. the peptide transmitters or modulators, the sympathetic preganglionic neurones outside of the IML nucleus, etc.). The segmental integrative system shown contains three main subsystems.

One of them, marked "1.", occupies the reticular core of the spinal gray, a neuronal system with a cell density of several times ten thousand per cubic millimeter, containing excitatory and inhibitory interneurones of

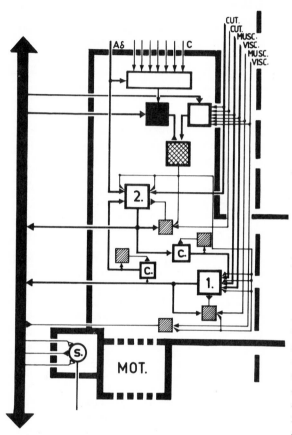

Figure 3. Proposed segmental integrating circuit. Field bordered by thick line: cross-section of one half of the spinal gray (midline on the right). Small "boxes": ventral horn (MOT) and IML nucleus (S). Thick double arrow: propriospinal and long pathways of the lateral funiculus. Empty squares: excitatory systems. Cross-hatched square: presynaptic inhibition, driven by the afferent input via a hypothetical interneurone group and inhibited postsynaptically by another one (unmarked empty and filled squares, resp.). The latter is driven by high threshold afferents (C, A-delta), via neuronal circuits in lam. 1-3 (empty rectangle). Hatched square: strychnine sensitive inhibition. Closely hatched ones: postsynaptic inhibitions with unknown mediation. Square No. 1: neuronal system in the intermediate zone, organizing the "tonic" components of the responses. Square No. 2: neuronal system in the deeper laminae of the dorsal horn, responsible for the "phasic" components. Squares marked by "C": connections between 1 and 2. Cutaneous, muscular and visceral inputs: parallel lines in the right upper corner. Arrowheads on lines: excitatory synapses. Inverted, filled triangles: postsynaptic inhibitory synapses. Obliquely filled triangles: presynaptic inhibitory synapses.

different (mostly unknown) function, intersegmental and more distant connections and an unthinkably great capacity to process (and probably also to store) information, streaming in continuously via tens of thousands of muscular and visceral afferents and receiving a preprocessed selection of the information flow in the cutaneous channels, as well. Adjacent segmental "discs" build up larger functional units in the well known "column of poker chips' fashion and, although the lower levels are certainly subordinated to the higher "centers", nothing speaks in favor of the hypothesis that these higher levels could continuously adjust the organism to the ever changing external and internal requirements without the preprocessed information supplied by the lower levels of the hierarchy.

The second subsystem, marked "2.", is in the deeper layers of the dorsal horn and it is involved in the processing of information arriving via the receptors on the body surface. It is known that the corresponding primary afferents and the postsynaptic neurones are organized into longitudinally oriented lamellae, the units of which are connected to each other via diverging and converging afferents and axon collaterals of the secondary neurones. Apart from its specific role in sensory function this system has something to do with the normal sequence of the sleep-wakefulness cycles, with temperature regulation, with locomotor coordination and probably it participates in many other functions as well. This subsystem feeds into the previous one (and most probably vice versa, too) and the two together must have a decisive influence on the activity leaving the segment(s) via the corresponding efferents.

The third subsystem may by composed of all the local and distant neural elements being able to modify the level of presynaptic inhibition. it has been shown by Polosa and his group some 17 years ago (1969) that about 10-30 times more picrotoxin needs to be given to spinal compared to normal animals to bring about convulsions and to induce a typical oscillatory pattern in blood pressure and in sympathetic activity (i.e. to suppress presynaptic inhibition). We have also supplied some evidence in this regard (Erdélyi et al., 1977). We cannot exclude for the time being the possibility that the main factor of making the isolated spinal cord transiently irresponsive is the loss of descending influences (by disconnecting the pathway between the thick arrow and the filled square in figure 3) restraining under intact conditions the level of this inhibition.

Summing up our ideas, we wish to stress that we do not want to deny the importance of supraspinal structures in the organization of sympathetic activity. We only question the role of supraspinal influences and hesitate to accept the prevalent hypothesis, according to which the highest ranking component in a hierarchy of regulatory systems exerts a direct effect on the output of the lowest level, thereby severely disturbing ongoing programs, sometimes of vital importance. We favor instead the alternative possibility of higher levels acting on the input to the executing member of the hierarchy, assuring in this way smooth changes in the output variables instead of potentially harmful sudden "jumps".

REFERENCES

Erdélyi A (1982). Vestibular Control of Somato-vegetative Integration: a New Interpretation of Orthostatic Compensation. In Lissák K (ed): "Recent developments of neurobiology in Hungary," Vol 9, Budapest: Akademiai Kiado, p 137.

Erdélyi A, Mitsányi A (1977). Interactions of spinal afferents in the integration of vasomotor reflexes elicited by sustained stimulation of somatic nerves. Acta Physiol. Acad. Sci. hung. 50: 135.

Erdélyi A, Mitsányi A, Morava I (1977). Effect of pharmacological disinhibition on vasomotor reactions elicited by electric stimulation of cutaneous and muscular afferents in anaesthetized and in acutely spinalized cats. Acts physiol. Acad. Sci. hung. 50: 245.

Erdélyi A, Mitsányi A, Morava I (1979). Organization of blood pressure reflexes elicited by low intensity stimulation of cutaneous and muscular afferents. Acta Physiol. Acad. Sci. hung. 53: 93.

Erdélyi A, Mitsányi A, Morava I, Pavlik G, Tálasi A (1977). Characteristics of blood pressure and nictitating membrane reflexes elicited by electric stimulation of sciatic nerve in conscious and in anaesthetized cats. Acta Physiol. Acad. Sci. hung. 49: 75.

Erdélyi A, Mitsányi A, Tóth T (1981). Tonic vestibular modulation of cardiovascular function: facts, hypotheses and perspectives. In Kovách AGB, Sándor P, Kollai M (eds): "Adv. Physiol. Sci. Vol 9, Cardiovascular Physiology, Neural Control Mechanisms," Budapest" Pergamon - Akadémiai Kiadó, p 95.

Haines DE, Dietrichs E, Sowa TE (1984). Hypothalamo-- cerebellar and cerebello-hypothalamic pathways: a review and hypothesis concerning cerebellar circuits which may influence autonomic centers and affective behavior. Brain Behav. Evol. 24: 198.

Karplus JP (1937). Die Physiologie der vegetativen Zentren. (Auf Grund experimenteller Erfahrungen.) In Bumke O, Foerster O (Hrsg.): "Handbuch der Neurologie, Band 2. Allgemeine Neurologie II. Experimentelle Physiologie," Berlin: Springer, p 402.

Knyihár-Csillik E, Csillik B (1981). Selective 'labelling' by transsynaptic degeneration of substantia gelatinosal cells: an attempt to decipher intrinsic wiring in the Rolando substance of primates. Neurosci. Lett. 23: 131.

Koizumi K, Brooks CMcC (1984). The spinal Cord and the Autonomic Nervous System. In Davidoff RA (ed): "Handbook of the Spinal Cord. Vols. 1-2," New York: Marcell Dekker, p 779.

Martner J (1975). Cerebellar influences on autonomic mechanisms. An experimental study in the cat with special reference to the fastigial nucleus. Acta Physiol. Scand. Suppl. 425: 1.

Melzack R, Wall PD (1965). Pain mechanisms: a new theory. Science 150: 971.

Moruzzi G (1938). Azione del paleocerebellum sui riflessi vasomotori. Arch. Fisiol. 38: 36.

Polosa C, Rosenberg P, Mannard A, Wolkove N, Wyszogrodski I (1969). Oscillatory behavior of the sympathetic system induced by picrotoxin. Canad. J. Physiol. Pharmacol. 47: 815.

Rethélyi M (1972). Cell and neuropil architecture of the intermediolateral (sympathetic) nucleus of cat spinal cord. Brain Res. 46: 203.

Rethélyi M (1974). Spinal transmission of autonomic processes. J. Neural Transmission, Suppl. XI: 195.

Rethélyi M, Szentágothai J (1973). Distribution and connections of afferent fibres in the spinal cord. In Iggo A (ed): "Somatosensory System; Handbook of Sensory Physiology, Vol II," Berlin: Springer, p 207.

Schmidt RF (1971). Presynaptic inhibition in the verte-
    brate central nervous system. Ergebn. Physiol. 63:
    20.
Wall PD (1980). The role of Substantia Gelatinosa as a
    Gate Control. In Bonica JJ (ed): "Pain," New York:
    Raven Press, p 205.

Organization of the Autonomic Nervous System:
Central and Peripheral Mechanisms, pages 307–314
© 1987 Alan R. Liss, Inc.

A DIENCEPHALIC CONTROL OF THE BARORECEPTOR REFLEX AT THE
LEVEL OF THE NUCLEUS OF THE TRACTUS SOLITARIUS

K. Michael Spyer, Steven W. Mifflin and
Deborah J. Withington-Wray

Department of Physiology, Royal Free Hospital
School of Medicine, Rowland Hill Street,
London NW3 2PF, England

INTRODUCTION

It is a general feature of cardiovascular control
exerted by the central nervous system that the performance
of cardiovascular reflexes is often modulated as part of
the patterning of the autonomic outflows (see Spyer, 1981).
Indeed there is a large literature describing the modifications of the cardiac component of the baroreceptor reflex
as a consequence of stimulating either peripheral nerves or
the brainstem and cerebellum. These effects have been
attributed to the non-linear relationship between vagal
activity and heart-rate (Levy and Zieske, 1969) on the one
hand and the influence of changes in central respiratory
activity that accompany such stimulus evoked responses on
the other (Spyer, 1981, 1984). In the latter case it is now
established on the basis of neurophysiological studies that
vagal motoneurones, which exert a negative chronotropic
influence, are under a direct inhibitory control arising
from medullary inspiratory neurones (Gilbey, Jordan, Richter
and Spyer, 1984). Respiratory influences on sympathetic
preganglionic neurones also affect the sensitivity of these
neurones to other inputs, and particularly to baroreceptor
inputs (Seller and Richter, 1971). In one situation,
however, there is evidence that not only the cardiac component but also the vascular component of the baroreceptor
reflex may be suppressed. This is during the defence
reaction that can be evoked during stimulation of hypothalamus, and amygdala, in the cat (Hilton, 1966) and results
from a central inhibition of the inputs from the baroreceptor afferents (Coote, Hilton and Perez-Gonzalez, 1979).

The site of this interaction has been suggested to be the nucleus of the tractus solitarius (NTS) as neurones within this nucleus that are excited on electrical stimulation of the sinus nerve (SN) (McAllen, 1976; Adair and Manning, 1975), or natural activation of the carotid sinus baroreceptors (McAllen, 1976), are also inhibited by stimulating within the hypothalamus. Subsequently, Jordan and Spyer (1979) were able to demonstrate that this inhibition did not result from primary afferent depolarisation of SN afferents, thereby eliminating presynaptic inhibition of baroreceptor afferent terminals as the basis for the defence area inhibition of the NTS neurones.

Since both the extent and synaptic basis of the interaction have yet to be resolved, the current series of investigations were undertaken. These have involved making both extra- and intracellular recordings within the NTS and observing the influence of SN, aortic (AN) and vagal (VN) nerve stimulation on these neurones with, and without, conditioning stimuli delivered to the hypothalamic defence area. Hypothalamic sites were carefully selected to ensure that stimulation elicited a suppression of the cardio-vascular effects of SN stimulation.

METHODS

The studies were undertaken on anaesthetized (40 mg/kg Sagatal given i.p. and supplemented as required) and paralyzed (2-4 mg/kg i.v./hr gallamine) cats which were artificially ventilated and given a bilateral pneumothorax. Ventilation was adjusted to maintain arterial pCO_2, pH and pO_2 within physiological levels and arterial blood samples were routinely analysed and infusions of HCO_3^- were administered as required. Central respiratory activity was monitored by recording phrenic nerve activity.

The hypothalamus was stimulated (1.0 ms, 50-300 μA at 70 Hz through concentric bipolar electrodes) to identify sites from which the cardiovascular components of the defence reaction, including inhibition of the baroreceptor reflex, could be evoked. The effects of stimulating such sites (10-30 ms trains, 500 Hz) on the discharge of NTS neurones was then investigated. These neurones were also tested for their response to electrical stimulation of the

SN, AN and VN. In some cases the response of NTS neurones to inflation of the ipsilateral carotid sinus using a balloon tipped catheter was studied to discriminate specific baroreceptor inputs.

RESULTS

The basic pattern of interaction was determined in a series of extracellular studies. Here many NTS neurones were identified which responded to stimulation of the SN, AN and VN at a range of latencies. In a proportion of those excited by SN stimulation, inflation of the balloon tipped catheter also elicited an excitatory response indicating that the neurones received a baroreceptor input (see Fig. 1a). The excitatory response to SN stimulation in those neurones excited by inflation of the intrasinus balloon was invariably suppressed by a conditioning stimulus applied to the hypothalamus. Hypothalamic stimulation alone exerted an inhibitory influence on those NTS neurones showing ongoing activity, and an inhibition of SN evoked discharge when SN stimulation followed hypothalamic stimulation by periods as great as 250 ms. 67% of NTS neurones excited by SN were inhibited by hypothalamic stimulation. These observations are reminiscent of those reported by McAllen (1976). Convergent excitatory inputs from the AN and VN onto these neurones were affected similarly by hypothalamic stimulation. A smaller number of NTS neurones were inhibited by SN stimulation, and in a proportion of these inflation of the carotid sinus also led to inhibition of ongoing discharge. In approximately one-half of these neurones hypothalamic stimulation evoked an excitatory response.

In several cases following characterization of the various inputs to individual neurones, as described above using extracellular recording, the cell was impaled and a detailed study of the membrane events underlying the various responses was obtained.

E.p.s.p.s in NTS neurones to SN stimulation

In a group of neurones, SN stimulation evoked an e.p.s.p. with an onset latency of 3.5-10.5 ms (see Fig 1b).

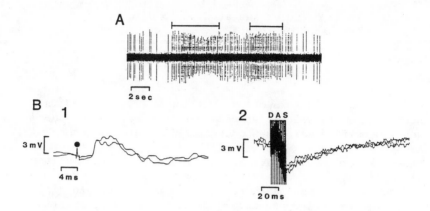

Figure 1. Response of unit with carotid sinus baroreceptor input to defence area stimulation. (A) Extracellularly recorded increase in action potential discharge evoked by stimulation of the carotid sinus baroreceptors. The inflations of the intrasinus balloon are indicated by the bars above the neurogram unit recording. (B) Intra-cellularly recorded responses of the same unit to: 1) electrical stimulation of the carotid sinus nerve (stimulus artifact indicated by filled circle): two sweeps superimposed;   2) electrical stimulation of the hypothalamic defence area. The hypothalamus was stimulated for 20 ms, 500 Hz, 1 msec pulses of 120 µA during the period indicated by the DAS. Three sweeps superimposed.

In a further group such stimulation elicited an e.p.s.p./ i.p.s.p. sequence with an onset latency of 4.3-6.3 ms. The latencies and magnitude of such excitatory and inhibitory changes in membrane potential were unaffected by the timing of the stimulus within the respiratory cycle or in relation to whether the lungs were inflated or deflated (Mifflin, Spyer and Withington-Wray, 1986b). Equally there were no fluctuations in membrane potential in relation to respiration. This would seem to be good evidence that any respiratory "gating" of the baroreceptor reflex as a consequence of respiration is exerted at a later stage in the reflex pathway since many of these neurones were also shown to be affected by specific baroreceptor stimulation.

In the majority of neurones excited by SN stimulation, hypothalamic stimulation produced an i.p.s.p. of long duration (82-195 ms). The amplitude of this hyper- polarization varied from 1.2-7.3 mV (see Fig. 1B) and both the duration and magnitude of this effect could be modified by varying the duration of hypothalamic stimulation (Mifflin, Spyer and Withington-Wray, 1986a). Using the hypothalamic stimulus as a conditioning stimulus, prior to SN stimulation, resulted in a reduction in the magnitude and duration of the SN-evoked e.p.s.p. over condition testing intervals of up to 100 ms. This was not simply a consequence of the membrane hyperpolarization accompanying hypothalamic stimulation as passing negative current through the electrode to hyperpolarize the cell failed to diminish the magnitude of the e.p.s.p., which conversely was enhanced. Hypothalamic stimulation was effective since it elicited an i.p.s.p. and the cell's input resistance was reduced by 15-40%, resulting in the shunting of the evoked e.p.s.p. The i.p.s.p.s recorded were Cl^- dependent since they could be reversed by either the injection of Cl^- into the cell or by the passage of hyperpolarizing currents. Consequently, it appears that the inhibitory synaptic connections are made on the soma and/or proximal dendrites of these NTS neurones.

I.p.s.p.s to SN stimulation

In a smaller population of NTS neurones, stimulation of the SN evoked a hyperpolarization of significant magnitude and short latency (6.4-10.7 ms). It could be reversed to a depolarizing wave by both Cl^- injection or the delivery of hyperpolarizing currents. In approximately 50% of these cases hypothalamic stimulation elicited an excitatory influence and this was seen also in those few NTS neurones which were inhibited by baroreceptor activation.

DISCUSSION

The results of this study provide unequivocal evidence that the suppression of the baroreceptor reflex accompanying defence area activation is in part a consequence of the postsynaptic inhibition of those NTS neurones that integrate baroreceptor inputs. In this respect, these observations expand the suggestions of both

McAllen (1976) and Adair and Manning (1975) which had
indicated that some action of descending inputs from the
hypothalamus might modify the baroreceptor reflex at this
site. They expand these by demonstrating that it is a
postsynaptic action rather than a presynaptic modification
of afferent transmission confirming the results of the
study of Jordan and Spyer (1979). The inhibitory influence
of stimulation within the hypothalamic defence area is not
restricted to those neurones receiving a SN, and
specifically baroreceptor, input within the NTS as it is
now clear that medullary respiratory neurones receive
inhibitory inputs from the same hypothalamic site
(Ballantyne, Jordan, Spyer and Wood, 1986) and there is a
direct inhibition of cardiac vagal motoneurones (Spyer,
1984). However, stimulation at hypothalamic sites beyond
those defined in this report as being within the defence
region fail to evoke consistently an inhibitory control of
those NTS neurones excited by the baroreceptor input.

There is a need to consider the physiological
significance of these observations. The demonstration that
hypothalamic stimulation can exert such a profound
influence on these NTS neurones does not imply that the
activation of the hypothalamic defence area results in an
all or none suppression of the baroreceptor reflex. There
is clearly the facility for spatial and temporal summation
of the action of descending inputs leading to a graded
synaptic response just as the influence of the arterial
baroreceptors can be varied. Equally there is evidence,
first, that at least a portion of the suppression of the
baroreceptor-vagal reflex is due to a direct hypothalamic
inhibitory input to preganglionic vagal motoneurones
(Spyer, 1984) and, secondly, through an enhancement of the
inspiratory related inhibition of these vagal neurones
(Gilbey et al. 1984). Notably we have failed to reveal any
respiratory 'gating' of the effects of SN or baroreceptor
inputs at the level of the NTS.

Interestingly, in the rabbit the activation of the
central nucleus of the amygdala results in an activation of
NTS neurones that are excited on stimulating the AN (Cox,
Jordan, Moruzzi, Schwaber, Spyer and Turner, 1986). The
cardiovascular effects of such stimulation are a depressor
response with a marked vagally mediated bradycardia, that
in the conscious animal is accompanied by a suppression of
motor activity (Kapp, Gallagher, Underwood, McNall and

Whitehorn, 1982).

Together these processes allow a precise and marked modification of baroreceptor control so that at one extreme the effectiveness of the reflex can be totally abbrogated. The modification of reflex action is one of the many means by which rostral brainstem and cortical areas can exert a control of motor performance and it may be important that the same general feature applies to autonomic, and specifically cardiovascular, regulation. This study provides an example of a potential mechanism whereby stress related inputs may exert profound changes in the ability of the arterial baroreceptors to regulate the cardiovascular system. Whether acute and reversible changes of the type described are on repetition converted to maintained and prolonged modifications of cardiovascular regulation remains to be resolved.

Acknowledgements. Steven W. Mifflin is a British-American Heart Association Fellow. The study was supported by an M.R.C. Grant to K. Michael Spyer.

REFERENCES

Adair JR, Manning JW (1975). Hypothalamic modulation of baroreceptor afferent unit activity. Am J Physiol 229: 1357-1364.
Ballantyne D, Jordan D, Spyer KM, Wood LM (1986). Differential changes in the synaptic rhythm of caudal expiratory bulbospinal neurones in response to hypothalamic stimulation in the cat. J Physiol 371: 117P.
Coote JH, Hilton SM, Perez-Gonzalez JF (1979). Inhibition of baroreceptor reflex on stimulation in the brainstem defence centre. J Physiol 288: 549-560.
Cox GE, Jordan D, Moruzzi P, Schwaber JS, Spyer KM, Turner SA (1986). Amygdaloid influences on brainstem neurones in the rabbit. J Physiol in press.
Gilbey MP, Jordan D, Richter DW, Spyer KM (1984). Synaptic mechanisms involved in the inspiratory modulation of vagal cardio-inhibitory neurones in the cat. J Physiol 356: 65-78.
Hilton SM (1966). Hypothalamic regulation of the cardiovascular system. Brit Med Bull 22: 243-248.

Jordan D, Spyer KM (1979). Studies on the excitability of sinus nerve afferent terminals. J Physiol 297: 123-134.

Kapp BS, Gallagher M, Underwood M, McNall C, Whitehorn P (1982). Cardiovascular responses elicited by electrical stimulation of the amygdala central nucleus in the rabbit. Brain Res 234: 251-262.

Levy MN, Zieske H (1969). Autonomic control of cardiac pacemaker activity and atrioventricular transmission. J Appl Physiol 27: 465-470.

McAllen RM (1976). Inhibition of the baroreceptor input to the medulla by stimulation of the hypothalamic defence area. J Physiol 257: 45-46P.

Mifflin SW, Spyer KM, Withington-Wray DJ (1986a). Hypothalamic inhibition of baroreceptor inputs in the nucleus of the tractus solitarius in the cat. J Physiol 373: 58P.

Mifflin SW, Spyer KM, Withington-Wray DJ (1986b). Lack of respiratory modulation of baroreceptor inputs in the nucleus of the tractus solitarius in the cat. J Physiol in press.

Seller H, Richter DW (1971). Some quantitative aspects of the central transmission of the baroreceptor activity. In Kao FF, Koizumi K, Vassalle M (eds): "Research in Physiology", Bologna: Auto Gaggi Publisher, pp 541-545.

Spyer KM (1981). Neural organisation and control of the baroreceptor reflex. Rev Physiol Biochem Pharmacol 88: 12-124.

Spyer KM (1984). Central control of the cardiovascular system. In Baker PF (ed): "Recent Advances in Physiology, 10" Edinburgh: Churchill Livingstone, pp 163-200.

Organization of the Autonomic Nervous System:
Central and Peripheral Mechanisms, pages 315–325
© **1987 Alan R. Liss, Inc.**

DOES THE HYPOTHALAMUS CONTAIN NEURONES INTEGRATING THE
DEFENCE REACTION?

S.M. Hilton and W.S. Redfern

Department of Physiology, The Medical School,
University of Birmingham, Birmingham B15 2TJ

The term, defence reaction, was first used by Hess to
refer to the characteristic behaviour of a cat in response
to a noxious or threatening stimulus (Hess & Brügger, 1943).
This consists of a retaliatory threatening display, culminating in attack or flight, and it is accompanied by visceral
and hormonal changes most of which are best understood as
adaptions which prepare the animal to cope with an emergency
and, if necessary, to perform extremes of muscular exertion
(Cannon, 1929). These changes include hyperventilation and
a cardiovascular pattern consisting of an increased cardiac
output which is directed mainly to skeletal muscle, the
heart and brain at the expense of the splanchnic organs,
kidneys and skin (see Hilton, 1981 for review). These
cardiorespiratory adjustments are fully developed in the
early, alerting stage of the behavioural response and we
have therefore referred to them collectively as the visceral
alerting response (Timms, 1981; Hilton, 1982). The actual
behaviour which then ensues depends to some extent upon the
species, the nature of the threatening or noxious stimulus
and the environment, but the pattern of visceral and hormonal changes which precedes and accompanies it is basically
the same for all mammalian species studied so far, including
man (Hilton, 1982).

The Hypothetical Role of the Hypothalamus

Until very recently, the hypothalamus has generally
been assumed to be the main integrating area for the whole
complex defence reaction. From the earliest, beginning even
with Goltz (1892), attempts to define the regions of the
brain responsible for emotional defensive behaviour showed

that subcortical structures were important for their organisation. It was the work of Bard (1928), however, which
pointed to the hypothalamus as the crucial structure for
full expression of sham rage in the cat. He made decere-
brations at different levels and found, in long-term
experiments, that if transections had been made caudal to
the hypothalamus the response to a variety of stimuli was
attenuated. He concluded that an intact hypothalamus was
essential for the full and organised expression of sham
rage.

In the course of the meticulous mapping work of Hess
who used localized electrical stimulation of the hypothalamus in conscious cats, he identified a strip of tissue
running through the perifornical hypothalamus from which
could be evoked the characteristic feline threat display, or
flight. He stated (1954) that, in regard to the defence
reaction, "... the hypothalamus must mediate the autonomic
mechanisms as well as the somatomotor signs ..." Evidence
was soon obtained in support of this view. In 1960,
Abrahams, Hilton and Zbrożyna reported that electrical
stimulation of sites which in conscious cats had elicited
the behavioural defence reaction, evoked in anaesthetized
cats the whole visceral alerting response including the
characteristic pattern of cardiovascular changes. This
paper was also concerned with the extension of the "defence
area" from the hypothalamus into the periaqueductal grey
matter of the mid-brain and later papers described regions
in the amygdala (Hilton & Zbrożyna, 1963) and hind-brain
(Coote, Hilton & Zbrożyna, 1973) from which the defence
reaction could be elicited by electrical stimulation.

In the course of this series of studies, the possible
roles and functions of these regions had naturally been discussed, and emphasis was placed on the longitudinal arrangement along the length of the neuraxis of the regions which
appeared to act as a reflex centre for the defence reaction
as a whole. But this did little to affect the view, which
was by then well-established, that the hypothalamus was the
key location of neurones organising emotional responses.
One of the most influential papers, in this regard, had been
that of Bard & Macht (1958); for they had reported that,
whereas most elements of the sham rage responses could be
obtained in mesencephalic cats, the stimulus needed to be
stronger and the responses were not as well coordinated as
in cats with an intact hypothalamus — and these results

were obtained in animals that had been maintained for
several months.

Recent Experiments

In more recent times, the rat has been emerging as a
species of choice for neuroanatomical studies and for
investigations of behaviour and central nervous control of
cardiovascular function. This led Yardley and Hilton (1986)
to map the regions of the hypothalamus and mid-brain from
which the behavioural and cardiovascular components of the
defence reaction could be elicited by electrical stimulation. These maps are extremely detailed, and show a continuous region extending from the pre-optic area through the
ventral hypothalamus and into the mid-brain central grey
matter and tegmentum.

A well-aired problem with electrical stimulation is
that it activates axons of passages at least as readily as
neuronal perikarya. For a few years now, micro-injection of
excitatory amino acids has been employed to stimulate
neurones alone (McLennan, 1975), so we explored the newly-
defined hypothalamic defence area of the rat, using a
cannula-electrode for comparing drug injection with
electrical stimulation. Using the anaesthetic alphaxalone-
alphadolone, we were unable to evoke the cardiovascular
components of the defence reaction by micro-injections of
cholinergic agonists, so we tested our method by micro-
injecting D,L-homocysteic acid (DLH), which is more potent
than L-glutamate, in volumes of 0.1 μl. We found that DLH
did not mimic the responses to electrical stimulation at any
site tested within the hypothalamus, whereas its injection
into the dorsal periaqueductal grey matter (shown as area 1
in Fig. 1) reproduced the full pattern of visceral and
somatic responses characteristic of the defence reaction,
viz. hyperpnoea, tachypnoea, hindlimb vasodilatation, renal
vasoconstriction, tachycardia, elevation of arterial blood
pressure, twitching of the vibrissae, palpebral retraction,
mydriasis and raising of the tail (Hilton & Redfern, 1983).
This region has also been shown to yield some of the cardiovascular components of the defence reaction when stimulated
by micro-injections of L-glutamate in rabbits (Tan &
Dampney, 1983) and cats (McDougall et al., 1985).

These results are in keeping with a report by Bandler

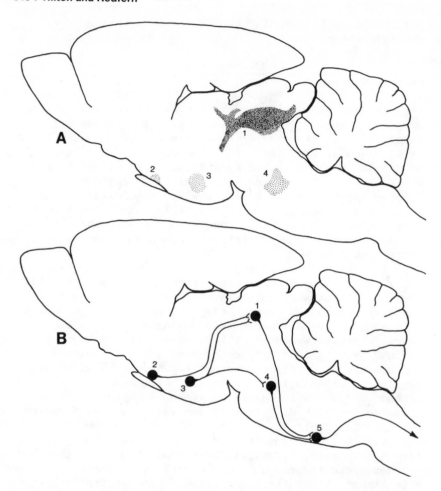

Figure 1. Diagrammatic paramedian sections of rat brain.
A, with stippling indicating mid-brain area (1, heavy
stippling) containing neurones integrating the defence
reaction (behavioural and autonomic), hypothalamic region
(3) and pontine area (4) containing neurones initiating an
'adrenaline-like' response only, and suprachiasmatic area
(2) containing neurones which elicit a cardiovascular
pattern which includes renal vasoconstriction.
B, with schematic neurones illustrating the major
known efferent connections (see text for details) between
areas 1, 2, 3, 4 and nucleus paragigantocellularis
lateralis (5) in ventrolateral medulla which is the
location of presympathetic cardiovascular neurones.

(1982) that micro-injection of L-glutamate did not elicit
the characteristic threat display of the cat when injected
into the hypothalamus in the conscious animal, whereas its
injection into the mid-brain periaqueductal grey matter
readily did so. More recently, Bandler has worked with rats
also and has reported the characteristic defensive flight
behaviour of this species on micro-injection of glutamate,
aspartate or DLH into the mid-brain periaqueductal grey
matter (Bandler et al., 1985).

In our experiments, DLH was not without effect on the
hypothalamus, however. From points in the tuberal region,
scattered between the dorsomedial and ventromedial nuclei,
micro-injection of DLH evoked a small increase in ventilation with tachycardia, a fall of blood pressure and vasodilation in muscle with no vasoconstriction in the kidney
(Hilton & Redfern, 1986). This pattern of response could
have been caused by adrenaline (released from the adrenal
medulla): it was accompanied by the facial signs of alerting. The region from which this 'adrenaline-like' response
was elicited is indicated as area 3 in Fig. 1. A similar
response pattern was elicited from a small region in the
lateral pontine tegmentum, medial to the lateral lemniscus
and ventral to the brachium conjunctivum (area 4 in Fig. 1).
Interestingly, similar responses were also evoked from a
compact rostral region in the anterobasal hypothalamus,
immediately dorsal to the optic chiasma on each side of the
mid-line just medial to the supraoptic nucleus (area 2 in
Fig. 1): there was a difference, however, in that a small
renal vasoconstriction formed part of the pattern evoked
from this area.

Injections of DLH (0.2 μl) in conscious rats evoked
brisk exploratory locomotion when made into this suprachiasmatic region, and a characteristic combination of
darting and freezing, culminating in flight, when made into
the dorsal PAG. Such injections evoked no behavioural signs
of the defence reaction when made into the tuberal hypothalamus, although at sites at which electrical stimulation
readily evoked the full response (Yardley & Hilton, 1986).
The pontine tegmentum was equally 'negative'.

Possible Explanations of the New Findings

In seeking an explanation for the difference between

electrical and chemical stimulation in the tuberal hypothalamus several possibilities must be considered. Firstly,
this region may contain neurones which organize the entire
defence reaction, which for some reason micro-injection of
DLH is unable to excite adequately. It may be that the
neuronal cell bodies are fairly scattered, and electrical
stimulation could be more effective due to a larger
effective stimulation zone, or because it can activate a
widespread terminal field synapsing onto hypothalamic
neurones distal from the stimulus site. Moreover, it is
possible that DLH can activate these neurones but that the
behavioural and vasoconstrictor elements are not expressed
because of some neural gating mechanism, which is somehow
over-ridden by electrical stimulation.

Neither of these suggestions may seem highly plausible,
however, in which case the possibility must be considered
that the tuberal hypothalamus does not contain neurones
which integrate or even initiate the defence reaction, and
that electrical stimulation activates merely fibres of
passage. In this connection a number of older observations
must be recalled. Hunsperger (1956), for example, reported
that bilateral destruction of the perifornical region of the
hypothalamus in the cat did not impair the expression of a
full defence reaction to an attacking dog. Ellison & Flynn
(1968) prepared cats in which the hypothalamus had been dis-
connected from the rest of the brain: such animals were
motionless when not stimulated but displayed a complete and
well-coordinated defence reaction if the skin was pinched.
Adams (1968) reported that he could readily find neurones in
the dorsal PAG of conscious cats which fired when a defence
reaction was evoked, but he found none in the perifornical
hypothalamus. Closer to Bard's work is that of Bignall &
Schramm (1974) who showed that cats which had been subject
to pre-collicular decerebration as kittens displayed normal
behavioural defence reactions. All this leaves us with the
impression that the dorsal PAG of the mid-brain is an
important integrating area for the defence reaction, containing neurones which can initiate the full response and
the inputs through which they can be excited reflexly (cf.
Adams, 1979; Hilton & Redfern, 1986).

For the rat at least, there seems little need to go
beyond this simple conclusion; for it has long been known
that adult rats decerebrated at the rostral mid-brain level
show more coordinated defence behaviour than do cats simil-

arly prepared (Woods, 1964). In the cat, however, the cardiovascular pattern characteristic of alerting is not obtained reflexly in acutely decerebrated preparations in response to noxious stimuli (Abrahams et al., 1960) or to the peripheral chemoreceptor stimulation (Hilton & Marshall, 1982), unless the level of decerebration is sufficiently far rostral as to spare the hypothalamus. Therefore, if there are indeed no neurones in the tuberal hypothalamus which can initiate the defence response, there seem at least to be inputs to the mid-brain (and specifically to the dorsal PAG) which originate in the hypothalamus and which act tonically to lower the threshold of the mid-brain 'defence' centre. The bulk of the so-called hypothalamic defence area as defined by electrical stimulation, however, probably consists of axons of passage.

One possible source of such nerve fibres is the neuronal cell group overlying the optic chiasma (area 2 in Fig. 1). Neurones within this region provide a direct input to the dorsomedial PAG in the rat (Beitz, 1982; Marchand & Hagino, 1983; Marson, 1984). They also provide axons which course through the hypothalamus (Swanson & Cowan, 1975; Conrad & Pfaff, 1976) and may contribute fibres which would respond to electrical stimulation within the classical "hypothalamic defence area". These fibre connections are indicated in the diagram of Fig. 1b. Another possible source of such fibres is the amygdala. Pathways from the amygdala which course through the hypothalamus are known from several neuroanatomical studies (Nauta, 1961; Millhouse, 1973; Palkovits & Zaborszky, 1979), and have been inferred from physiological investigation of the amygdaloid region from which defence reactions can be evoked (Hilton & Zbrożyna, 1963; Timms, 1981). The latter have revealed a pathway which runs into the lateral hypothalamus, passing just dorsal to the optic tract. The amygdala may be an essential link in conditioned defence reactions, particularly their cardiovascular component (for studies in the rabbit, see e.g. Kapp et al., 1979). Moreover, bilateral lesions in the tuberal hypothalamus in baboons can abolish the cardiovascular components of the defence reaction in response to an auditory conditioned stimulus without affecting the response to the unconditioned, noxious stimulus (Smith et al., 1980).

Finally, a third possible source of input to, or through, the hypothalamus may be provided by the neurones in the mid-line thalamic nuclei described at this meeting by Gebber et al. (1987).

The cardiovascular responses which we obtained on micro-injection of DLH into the hypothalamus were evoked from points scattered rather dorsally and laterally in the tuberal region (area 3). We earlier designated these responses as "adrenaline-like"; but they could perhaps be regarded as incomplete visceral alerting responses. It may be significant that a similar pattern of responses was evoked from the small area in the lateral pontine tegmentum (area 4) as this could be an area of relay from the tuberal hypothalamus to the nucleus paragigantocellularis lateralis (PGL) in the ventrolateral medulla, which is the site of synapses essential to the expression of the cardiovascular components of the visceral alerting response in the cat (Hilton et al., 1983; Hilton & Smith, 1984) and rat (Marson, 1984; Brown & Guyenet, 1985).

There are few direct projections from the so-called hypothalamic defence area to PGL in the cat (Lovick, 1985) or rat (Marson, 1984; Li & Lovick, 1985); but the region we have designated as area 3 contains neurones projecting to PAG (Beitz, 1982; Marchand & Hagino, 1983) and the lateral pontine tegmentum (Jackson & Crossman, 1981) both of which provide major projections to PGL (Marson, 1984). These connections are all summarised diagrammatically in Fig. 1b.

In conclusion, whereas there are neurones scattered through the tuberal hypothalamus that can evoke an "adrenaline-like" cardiorespiratory response, possibly through some of the connections described above, the bulk of the region hitherto called the hypothalamic defence area has probably produced defence reactions as a result of elect-rical stimulation of fibres of passage rather than cell bodies; and efforts must now be devoted to identifying with certainty the regions of the forebrain which are the sites of their cells of origin.

REFERENCES

Abrahams VC, Hilton SM, Zbrożyna AW (1960). Active muscle vasodilatation produced by stimulation of the brain stem: its significance in the defence reaction. J Physiol 154: 491.

Adams DB (1968). The activity of single cells in the mid-brain and hypothalamus of the cat during affective defense behaviour. Arch Ital Biol 106:243.

Adams DB (1979). Brain mechanisms for offense, defense and submission. Behav Brain Sci 2:201.

Bandler R (1982). Induction of 'rage' following micro-injections of glutamate into midbrain but not hypothalamus of cats. Neurosci Lett 30:183.

Bandler R, Depaulis A, Vergnes M (1985). Identification of midbrain neurones mediating defensive behaviour in the rat by microinjections of excitatory amino acids. Behav Brain Res 15:107.

Bard P (1928). A diencephalic mechanism for the expression of rage with special reference to the sympathetic nervous system. Am J Physiol 84:290.

Bard P, Macht MB (1958). The behaviour of chronically dec-erebrate cats. In Wolstenholme GEW, O'Connor CM (eds): "Neurological Basis of Behaviour," London: J & A Church-ill, p 55.

Beitz AJ (1982). The organization of afferent projections to the midbrain periaqueductal gray of the rat. Neuro-science 7:133.

Bignall KE, Schramm L (1974). Behaviour of chronically dec-erebrated kittens. Exp Neurol 42:519.

Brown DL, Guyenet PG (1985). Electrophysiological study of cardiovascular neurones in the rostral ventrolateral medulla in rats. Circ Res 56:359.

Cannon WB (1929). Bodily changes in Pain, Hunger, Fear and Rage. 2nd Edition. Appleton, New York.

Conrad LCA, Pfaff DW (1976). Efferents from medial basal forebrain and hypothalamus in the rat. I. An autoradio-graphic study of the medial preoptic area. J Comp Neurol 169:185.

Coote JH, Hilton SM, Zbrożyna AW (1973). The ponto-medullary area integrating the defence reaction in the cat and its influence on muscle blood flow. J Physiol 229:257.

Ellison GD, Flynn JP (1968). Organized aggressive behaviour in cats after surgical isolation of the hypothalamus. Arch Ital Biol 106:1.

Gebber GL, Varner KJ, Barman SM, Huang Z-S (1987). The medial thalamus as a generator of sympathetic tone. This volume.

Goltz F (1892). Der Hund ohne Grosshirn. Pflügers Arch 51:570.

Hess WR (1954). "Diencephalon: Autonomic and Extrapyramidal

Functions." New York: Grune and Stratton.
Hess WR, Brügger M (1943). Das subkorticale Zentrum der affectiven Abwehrreaktion. Helv physiol acta 1:33.
Hilton SM (1981). The physiology of stress. Part 1 - emotion. In Edholm OG, Weiner JS (eds) "Principles and Practice of Human Physiology," London: Academic Press, p 397.
Hilton SM (1982). The defence-arousal system and its relevance for circulatory and respiratory control. J exp Biol 100:159.
Hilton SM, Marshall JM (1982). The pattern of cardiovascular responses to carotid chemoreceptor stimulation in the cat. J Physiol 326:495.
Hilton SM, Marshall JM, Timms RJ (1983). Ventral medullary relay neurones in the pathway from the defence areas of the cat and their effect on blood pressure. J Physiol 345:149.
Hilton SM, Redfern WS (1983). Exploration of the brain stem defence areas with a synaptic excitant in the rat. J Physiol 345:134P.
Hilton SM, Redfern WS (1986). A search for brain stem cell groups integrating the defence reaction in the rat. J Physiol 378 (in press).
Hilton SM, Smith PR (1984). Ventral medullary neurones excited from the hypothalamic and mid-brain defence areas. J Auton Nerv Sys 11:35.
Hilton SM, Zbrożyna AW (1963). Amygdaloid region for defence reactions and its efferent pathway to the brain stem. J Physiol 165:160.
Hunsperger RW (1956). Affektreaktionen auf elektrische Reizung in Hirnstamm der Katze. Helv physiol acta 14:70.
Jackson A, Crossman AR (1981). Basal ganglia and other afferent projections to the peribrachial region in the rat: a study using retrograde and anterograde transport of horseradish peroxidase. Neuroscience 6:1537.
Kapp BS, Frysinger RC, Gallagher M, Haselton JR (1979). Amygdala central nucleus lesions: effect on heart-rate conditioning in the rabbit. Physiol Behav 23:1109.
Li P, Lovick TA (1985). Excitatory projections from hypothalamic and mid-brain defense regions to nucleus paragigantocellularis lateralis in the rat. Exp Neurol 89:543.
Lovick TA (1985). Projections from the diencephalon and mesencephalon to nucleus paragigantocellularis lateralis in the cat. Neuroscience 14:853.
Marchand, JE, Hagino N (1983). Afferents to the periaque-

ductal gray in the rat. A horseradish peroxidase study. Neuroscience 9:95.

Marson L (1984). Neuronal pathways involved in the defence reaction. PhD Thesis, University of Birmingham.

McDougall A, Dampney RAL, Bandler R (1985). Cardiovascular components of the defence reaction evoked by excitation of neuronal cell bodies in the midbrain periaqueductal grey of the cat. Neurosci Lett 60:69.

McLennan H (1975). Excitatory amino acid receptors in the central nervous system. In Iversen LL, Iversen SD, Snyder SH (eds): "Handbook of Psychopharmacology, section 1, vol. 4: Amino Acid Neurotransmitters," New York: Plenum Press, p 211.

Millhouse OE (1973). Certain ventromedial hypothalamic afferents. Brain Res 55:89.

Nauta WJH (1961). Fibre degeneration following lesions of the amygdaloid complex in the monkey. J Anat 95:515.

Palkovits M, Zaborszky L (1979). Neural connections of the hypothalamus. In Morgane PJ, Panksepp J (eds): "Handbook of the Hypothalamus, vol. 1: Anatomy of the Hypothalamus," New York: Marcel Dekker, p 379.

Smith OA, Astley CA, DeVito JL, Stein JM, Walsh KE (1980). Functional analysis of hypothalamic control of the cardiovascular responses accompanying emotional behaviour. Fed Proc 39:2487.

Swanson LW, Cowan WM (1975). The efferent connections of the suprachiasmatic nucleus of the hypothalamus. J Comp Neurol 160:1.

Tan E, Dampney RAL (1983). Cardiovascular effects of stimulation of neurones within the 'defence area' of the hypothalamus and midbrain of the rabbit. Clin Exp pharmacol physiol 10:299.

Timms RJ (1981). A study of the amygdaloid defence reaction showing the value of Althesin anaesthesia in studies of the function of the fore-brain in cats. Pflugers Arch 391:49.

Woods JW (1964). Behaviour of chronic decerebrate rats. J Neurophysiol 27:635.

Yardley CP, Hilton SM (1986). The hypothalamic and brainstem areas from which the cardiovascular and behavioural components of the defence reaction are elicited in the rat. J Auton Nerv Syst 15:227.

Organization of the Autonomic Nervous System:
Central and Peripheral Mechanisms, pages 327–336
© 1987 Alan R. Liss, Inc.

ARGININE VASOPRESSIN: NEW ROLES FOR AN OLD PEPTIDE

Quentin J. Pittman, Colleen L. Riphagen and
Sheilagh M. Martin
Dept. Med. Physiol. & Neuroscience Research
Group, Faculty Medicine, University of Calgary,
Calgary, Alberta, Canada T2N 4N1 (Q.J.P.,
C.L.R.) and Dept. Biology, Mt. St. Vincent
University, Halifax, Nova Scotia, Canada (S.M.M.)

Arginine vasopressin is well known for its peripheral
pressor and cardiovascular actions. Anatomical, electrophysiological and pharmacological studies have now established that magnocellular neurons within the hypothalamic
supraoptic and paraventricular nuclei (PVN) receive
afferent baroreceptor, chemoreceptor and osmoreceptor
information; in response to such stimuli, vasopressinergic, action potentials are generated and travel
down the neurohypophysial axons to the posterior pituitary
where AVP is released into the peripheral circulation
(Renaud et al., 1979). Over the last ten years, numerous
anatomical tracing studies and electrophysiological
reports have revealed that, in addition to its well known
projection to the pituitary, the PVN also contains neurons
which project to many areas of the central nervous system
(Buijs, 1983; Pittman et al., 1981; Swanson and Sawchenko,
1983). Immunohistochemical studies combined with axonal
transport methodology indicate that a substantial number
of these centrally projecting PVN neurons contain arginine
vasopressin; furthermore, immunohistochemical studies at
both the light and electron microscopic level reveal
immunoreactive AVP within axonal processes which make
apparent synaptic contact with neurons throughout the
nervous system (Sofroniew, 1985). It was of particular
interest to us that a number of brain stem and limbic
areas known to be involved in central cardiovascular
control demonstrated not only AVP immunoreactivity, but
also apparent vasopressin receptors (Dorsa et al., 1983).
In light of the known role of the paraventricular nucleus
in central cardiovascular regulation (Ciriello and

Calaresu, 1980) and the presence of AVP in various
autonomic nuclei, we raised the hypothesis that central
vasopressinergic pathways may participate in the neural
control of the cardiovascular system (Pittman et al.,
1982b). To test this hypothesis, we have carried out a
variety of electrophysiological, pharmacological and
physiological studies in rats and rabbits.

Our initial studies, in anaesthetized rats, revealed
that intracerebroventricular (ICV) injection of picomole
quantities of AVP caused dose related increases in blood
pressure and heart rate (Pittman et al., 1982a). We were
subsequently able to obtain similar findings in chronically catheterized, unanaesthetized rabbits (Martin et al.,
1985b) and rats (Fig. 1). As substances administered ICV
can pass quickly via bulk absorption into the circulation,

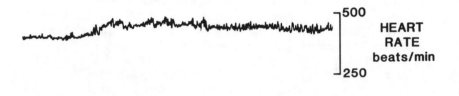

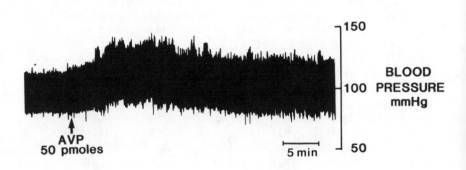

Fig. 1 - Heart rate and blood pressure of a
chronically-cannulated, unanaesthetized,
unrestrained rat given an ICV injection of 50
pmoles of AVP

it was important to eliminate the possibility that these short latency, transient pressor responses were not due to a peripheral action of the AVP due to a direct action on the peripheral vasculature. That this was not likely to be the case was suggested by the fact that pressor responses following centrally administered AVP were accompanied by tachycardia, whereas pressor responses arising from intravenously administered AVP were accompanied by bradycardia. Nonetheless, we monitored urine flow in one group of animals and found that the central administration of AVP caused pressor responses in the absence of any antidiuretic effects. As the kidney responds dramatically to even slight elevations in quantities of circulating AVP, it appeared unlikely that circulating AVP levels were elevated at the time of the blood pressure responses. As it appeared possible that the centrally generated pressor responses resulted from activation of the sympathetic nervous system, pharmacological interference with the autonomic nervous system was expected to antagonize the pressor responses. This indeed proved to be the case as intravenously administered chlorisondamine, a ganglionic blocking agent (Fig. 2) and phenoxybenzamine, an α-adrenergic antagonist, were both effective in abolishing the pressor responses (Martin et al., 1985). Further evidence for involvement of the sympathetic system in these pressor responses comes from studies which have revealed elevated levels of circulating catecholamines in rats (Riphagen & Pittman, 1986) and rabbits (Martin et al., 1985a) following ICV AVP.

Experiments aimed at determining the tissue site which responds to the ICV administered AVP have revealed several possible structures. Microinjection experiments indicate that both the locus coeruleus (Berecek et al., 1984) and the nucleus tractus solitarius (NTS) (Martin et al., 1985b; Matsuguchi, et al., 1982; Vallejo et al., 1984) as possible brain sites for the actions of ICV AVP. In addition, our findings (Pittman et al., 1984) that AVP could be released into the spinal subarachnoid space following PVN stimulation raised the possibility that AVP could also act within the spinal cord to influence cardio-vascular tone. In support of this possibility, we have found that intrathecal administration of only a few picomoles of AVP into the lower thoracic space produced a rapid onset, dose-dependent increase in both blood pres-sure and heart rate. Peripheral administration of an AVP

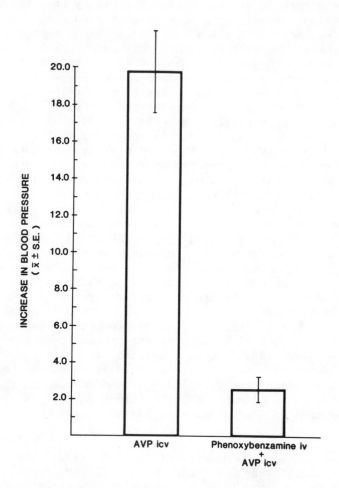

Fig. 2 - Increase in systolic blood pressure following ICV
        injection of 500 pmoles AVP (n=5) compared with
        increase following AVP in 5 other rats which had
        been pretreated with IV phenoxybenzamine (1
        mg/kg)

antagonist did not block these responses, thereby indicating their central origin (Riphagen and Pittman, 1985a).
In this series of experiments, in addition to monitoring

cardiovascular variables, we also measured urine flow and osmolarity. We observed that similar injections of picomolar quantities of AVP, particularly within the lower thoracic areas of the spinal cord caused a reduction in urine output and an increase in urine osmolarity; these mechanisms appeared to be neurally mediated as they were dependent on the presence of an intact innervation to the kidney (Riphagen and Pittman, 1985b). Although the mechanisms by which this antidiuresis is brought about are not yet known, we have recently obtained electrophysiological evidence that renal nerve activity increases following intrathecal administration of AVP.

The actual mechanisms by which AVP acts within the brain are yet unclear. Studies with various structural analogues and antagonists indicate that this effect is mediated by a receptor resembling a V1 receptor (Pittman and Franklin, 1985; Riphagen and Pittman, 1986a; Vallejo et al., 1984). There is evidence from biochemical studies (Tanaka et al., 1977) that some of AVP's central effects may involve the increased turnover of catecholamines. Consequently, we have investigated the possible involve-ment of catecholamines in AVP's central pressor actions by using the neurotoxin, 6-hydroxydopamine, to lesion the central catecholaminergic system. Our results to date indicate that substantial reductions in the amount of norepinephrine and dopamine in the brain of 6-hydroxydopamine treated rats are accompanied by signifi-cant reductions in the magnitude of the pressor responses to AVP. Studies are presently underway to determine if receptor blockade of the catecholaminergic system results in a similar attenuation of the AVP action.

The studies summarized above indicate that applica-tion of exogenous AVP to the central nervous system of rats and rabbits causes activation of the autonomic nervous system resulting in pressor and antidiuretic responses. Although these responses are neurally mediat-ed, they are complementary to the peripheral actions of this hormone on the cardiovascular and renal systems. However, it is required to demonstrate that endogenous AVP can mimic the above actions within the central nervous system. To address this question, we have examined the activity of putative vasopressinergic neurons within the PVN. Electrophysiological studies in which we monitored the activity of PVN neurons projecting to the NTS indicate

that a proportion of such cells respond to peripheral
hypovolemic and osmotic challenges with alterations in
their spontaneous activity (Lawrence and Pittman, 1985a).
In keeping with these observations, Kannan and Yamashita
(1983) found that some PVN neurons which project to the
NTS area receive synaptic input from carotid
baroreceptors. Electrophysiological studies in areas
known to receive projections from the PVN indicate that
PVN stimulation activates sympathetic pre-ganglionic
neurons (Yamashita et al., 1984) as well as neurons in a
variety of other autonomic and limbic areas (Lawrence and
Pittman, 1985b; Rogers and Nelson, 1984; Kannan and
Yamashita, 1985; Disturnal et al., 1985). AVP has been
shown to have post-synaptic actions upon neurons in a
number of these areas (Gilbey et al., 1982; Charpak et
al., 1984) but the relationship between these
post-synaptic effects and those seen following PVN
stimulation are still unclear. Further studies will be
required making use of AVP antagonists to attempt to block
the evoked responses.

If PVN neurons which innervate the brain stem and
spinal cord respond to baroreceptor inputs with changes in
activity, it follows that activation of these neurons
should influence blood pressure. In keeping with this
idea, electrical stimulation of the PVN elevates both
blood pressure and heart rate via neural mechanisms
(Ciriello and Calaresu, 1976; Lawrence et al., 1984). At
least part of these pressor responses results from release
of AVP within brain, as we have been able to show that
microinjection of the AVP antagonist into the NTS
significantly attenuates them (Pittman & Franklin, 1985).

It may be that other centrally mediated pressor
responses also occur via activation of the PVN. For
example, pressor responses due to activation of the
subfornical organ decrease following PVN lesions (Ferguson
and Renaud, 1984). There is also evidence that central
AVP may be released in response to peripheral hypovolemic
or osmotic stimuli (Burnard et al., 1983; Kasting et al.,
1981; Riphagen and Pittman, 1986b). We have attempted to
demonstrate a role of central AVP in maintaining blood
pressure following haemorrhage, but to date have had
little success. Neither the magnitude nor the time course
of the hypotension was altered in rats which received the
AVP antagonist $d(CH_2)_5Tyr(Me)AVP$ given either ICV or

directly into the NTS. It may be that this potent hypovolemic stimulus activates a number of central pathways involved in blood pressure control such that an interference with the AVP system is more than compensated for. Alternately, the AVP neurons activated by such a stimulus may have projections diffuse enough and distant enough from the ventricle that the antagonist was not effective.

The evidence summarized to date convincingly demonstrates that centrally applied AVP can alter blood pressure and kidney function. There is suggestive, but not conclusive evidence that endogenous AVP may participate in cardiovascular and renal control mechanisms. It would appear that certain acute stimuli that are known to be effective in altering circulating AVP levels may also be effective in releasing AVP within the central nervous system. As electrophysiological studies (Zerihun and Harris, 1983; Yamashita et al., 1984; Pittman et al., 1981) indicate the presence of considerable synaptic interaction between neurohypophysial and some caudally projecting PVN neurons, it is possible that AVP may be released simultaneously in the brain and the pituitary to provide a coordinated neural and endocrine response to homeostatic perturbations. The relative importance of the central AVP system within the large number of central and peripheral mechanisms involved in blood pressure control remains to be determined.

ACKNOWLEDGEMENTS

This work was supported by Medical Research Council of Canada, the Canadian Heart Foundation and Mt. St. Vincent University. CLR is an AHFMR Student and QJP is an MRC Scientist and AHFMR Scholar. Thanks to Ms. C. Von Niessen for typing the manuscript.

REFERENCES

Berecek KH, Olpe HR, Jones RSG, Hofbauer KG (1984). Microinjection of vasopressin into the locus coeruleus of conscious rats. Am J Physiol 247:H675-H681.
Buijs RM (1983). Vasopressin and oxytocin - their role in neurotransmission. Pharmacol & Ther 22:127-141.

Burnard DM, Pittman QJ, Veale WL (1983). Increased motor disturbances in response to arginine-vasopressin following hemorrhage or hypertonic saline: evidence for central AVP release in rats. Brain Res 273:59-65.

Charpak S, Armstrong WE, Muhlethaler M, Dreifuss JJ (1984). Stimulatory action of oxytocin on neurones of the dorsal motor nucleus of the vagus nerve. Brain Research 300:83-89.

Ciriello J, Calaresu FR (1980). Role of paraventricular and supraoptic nuclei in central cardiovascular regulation in the cat. Am J Physiol 239:R137-R142.

Disturnal JE, Veale WL, Pittman QJ (1985). Electrophysiological analysis of potential arginine vasopressin projections to the ventral septal area of the rat. Brain Res 342:162-167.

Dorsa DM, Majumdar LA, Petracca FM, Baskin DG, Cornett LE (1983). Characterization and localization of ^{3}H-arginine^8-vasopressin binding to rat kidney and brain tissue. Peptides 4:699-706.

Ferguson AV, Renaud LP (1984). Hypothalamic paraventricular nucleus lesions decrease pressor responses to subfornical organ stimulation. Brain Res 305:361-364.

Gilbey MP, Coote JH, Fleetwood-Walker S, Peterson DF (1982). The influence of the paraventriculo-spinal pathway and oxytocin and vasopressin on sympathetic preganglionic neurones. Brain Res 251:283-290.

Kannan H, Yamashita H (1985). Connections of neurons in the region of the nucleus tractus solitarius with the hypothalamic paraventricular nucleus: their possible involvement in neural control of the cardiovascular system in rats. Brain Res 329:205-212.

Kannan H, Yamashita H (1983). Electrophysiological study of paraventricular nucleus neurons projecting to the dorsomedial medulla and their response to baroreceptor stimulation in rats. Brain Res 279:31-40.

Kasting NW, Veale WL, Cooper KE (1981). Effects of hemorrhage on fever: the putative role of vasopressin. Can J Physiol Pharmacol 59:324-328.

Lawrence D, Ciriello J, Pittman QJ, Lederis K (1984). The effect of the vasopressin antagonist $d(CH_2)_5dTyr$ VAVP on the cardiovascular responses to stimulation of the paraventricular nucleus. Proc West Pharmacol Soc 27:15-17.

Lawrence D, Pittman QJ (1985a). Response of rat paraventricular neurones with central projections to suckling, haemorrhage or osmotic stimuli. Brain Res 341:176-183.

Lawrence D, Pittman QJ (1985b). Interaction between descending paraventricular neurons and vagal motor neurons. Brain Res 332:158-160.

Martin S, Malkinson TJ, Bauce L, Veale WL, Pittman QJ (1985a). Plasma catecholamines after central administration of arginine vasopressin in conscious rabbits. Can J Physiol Pharmacol 63:Axx.

Martin S, Malkinson TJ, Veale WL, Pittman QJ (1985b). Central effect of arginine vasopressin on blood pressure in the rabbit. Brain Res 348:137-145.

Matsuguchi H, Sharabi FM, Gordon FJ, Johnson AK, Schmid PG (1982). Blood pressure and heart rate responses to microinjection of vasopressin into the nucleus tractus solitarius region of the rat. Neuropharmacology 21:687-693.

Olpe H, Baltzer V (1981). Vasopressin activates noradrenergic neurons in the rat locus coeruleus: a microiontophoretic investigation. Eur J Pharmacol 73:377-378.

Pittman QJ, Blume HW, Renaud LP (1981). Connections of the hypothalamic paraventricular nucleus with the neurohypophysis, median eminence, amygdala, lateral septum and midbrain periaqueductal gray: an electrophysiological study in the rat. Brain Res 215:15-28.

Pittman QJ, Franklin LG (1985). Vasopressin antagonist in nucleus tractus solitarius/vagal area reduces pressor and tachycardia responses to paraventricular nucleus stimulation in rats. Neurosci Lett 56:155-160.

Pittman QJ, Lawrence D, McLean L (1982a). Central effects of arginine vasopressin on blood pressure in rats. Endocrinology 110:1058-1060.

Pittman QJ, Riphagen CL, Lederis K (1984). Release of immunoassayable neurohypophyseal peptides from rat spinal cord, in vivo. Brain Res 300:321-326.

Pittman QJ, Veale WL, Lederis K (1982b). Central neurohypophyseal peptide pathways: interactions with endocrine and other autonomic functions. Peptides 5:515-520.

Renaud LP, Pittman QJ, Blume HW (1979). Neurophysiology of hypothalamic peptidergic neurons. In Fuxe K, Hokfelt T, Luft R (eds): "Central Regulation of the Endocrine System", Plenum, pp 119-136.

Riphagen CL, Pittman QJ (1985). Cardiovascular responses to intrathecal administration of arginine vasopressin in rats. Regul Pept 10:293-298.

Riphagen CL, Pittman QJ (1985). Vasopressin influences renal function via a spinal action. Brain Res 336:346-349.

Riphagen CL, Pittman QJ (1986a). Oxytocin and [1-deamino, 8-D-arginine]-vasopressin (dDAVP): intrathecal effects on blood pressure, heart rate and urine output. Brain Res 374:371-374.

Riphagen CL, Pittman QJ (1986b). Arginine vasopressin as a central neurotransmitter. Fed Proc 45:272-276.

Rogers RC, Nelson DO (1984). Neurons of the vagal division of the solitary nucleus activated by the paraventricular nucleus of the hypothalamus. J Autonom Nerv Syst 10:193-197.

Sofroniew MV (1985). Vasopressin, oxytocin and their related neurophysins. In Bjorklund A, Hokfelt T (eds): "Handbook of Chemical Neuroanatomy 6: Neuropeptides", Amsterdam: Elsevier, pp 93-165.

Swanson LW, Sawchenko PE (1983). Hypothalamic integration: organization of the paraventricular and supraoptic nuclei. Ann Rev Neurosci 6:269-324.

Tanaka M, Versteeg DHG, deWied D (1977). Regional effects of vasopressin on rat brain catecholamine metabolism. Neurosci Lett 4:321-325.

Vallejo M, Carter DA, Lightman SL (1984). Haemodynamic effects of arginine-vasopressin microinjections into the nucleus tractus solitarius: a comparative study of vasopressin, a selective vasopressin receptor agonist and antagonist, and oxytocin. Neurosci Lett 52:247-252.

Yamashita H, Inenaga K, Koizumi K (1984). Possible projections from regions of paraventricular and supraoptic nuclei to the spinal cord: electrophysiological studies. Brain Res 296:373-378.

Zerihun L, Harris M (1983). An electrophysiological analysis of caudally-projecting neurones from the hypothalamic paraventricular nucleus in the rat. Brain Res 261:13-20.

Organization of the Autonomic Nervous System:
Central and Peripheral Mechanisms, pages 337–345
© **1987 Alan R. Liss, Inc.**

Carotid Body Chemoreceptors and Forebrain Activation.

M.C.Harris, D.Banks, W.N.Stokes[*] & S.Jamieson.

Depts. of Physiology & [*]Physics, University of
Birmingham, U.K.

Introduction

The time has long passed since the carotid body
chemoreceptor reflex was considered to be an influence
localised within the pontine/medullary region and affecting
only the respiratory and cardiovascular systems. Having said
that, however, there is very little detailed evidence
concerning the influence that the carotid bodies do have on
areas of the brain rostral to the pons.

Most studies suggesting an influence of chemoreceptors
on the forebrain have revolved around its influence on
arousal and the defence reaction. Thus it is clear that
under the right conditions, chemoreceptor stimulation can
give rise to all the cardiovascular components of the
defence reaction in both cats and rats (Marshall,1981;
Hilton & Marshall,1982). In addition, an
electrophysiological study of our own (Harris,Ferguson &
Banks,1984) showed that vasopressin-secreting neurones
within the hypothalamic supraoptic nuclei of the rat were
activated by stimulation of carotid body chemoreceptors.
Moreover, this activation was via a pathway descending
through the medial hypothalamus having first passed more
rostrally by a presumably more lateral route.

These findings suggested that this reflex input might
have a widespread influence throughout the forebrain. We
therefore set out to examine this problem. The experiments
to be described involved the use of ^{14}C-2-deoxyglucose
autoradiography as a scanning procedure for effects of
carotid body chemoreceptor stimulation on the forebrain in
general, and electrophysiology to look in detail at the
influence of that stimulus on individual parts of the
hypothalamus.

Methods

All experiments were performed on male Sprague Dawley rats anaesthetised with a Urethane/Sagatal mixture (1.2-1.4g Kg^{-1} ; 20mg Kg^{-1} I.P.). The procedure for stimulation of the carotid body chemoreceptors was identical in all experiments. A catheter was inserted in one external carotid artery with the tip at the carotid bifurcation. The internal and common carotid arteries were patent. Chemoreceptor stimulation was obtained by the injection down this catheter of 20-50µl 0.15M saline saturated with CO_2 (Band, Cameron & Semple,1970) into the carotid blood flow so that it was carried back up to the carotid body. With this procedure the stimulus could be isolated to one side only. Arterial blood pressure, heart rate and ventilation were monitored continuously throughout the experiment.

Deoxyglucose Autoradiography

The deoxyglucose (2DG) experiments were based on the procedure described by Sokoloff, Reivich, Kennedy, Des Rosiers, Patlak, Pettigrew, Sakurada & Shinohara(1977). ^{14}C-2-deoxyglucose (16.7µCi/100g b.w. sp.A. 56mCi/mmol, Amersham U.K.) was injected intravenously in 0.5ml 0.15M saline at time zero of the experiment. The carotid body was then stimulated at 1min intervals from time zero for 45min. Blood samples were taken at -1min, at rapid intervals over the first 5min, and then at more extended intervals until the end of 45min. At the end of the experiment the animal was killed, the brain removed and rapidly frozen to $-76^{0}C$. The brain was later sectioned (20µ) in a cryostat and the sections exposed to film (Kodak AR5) for 7-10days in the presence of ^{14}C tissue standards (Amersham U.K.). The autoradiograms were subjected to image analysis, and the optical densities converted to glucose utilisation by the formula of Sokoloff et al (1977) utilising the ^{14}C and glucose contents of the blood samples which were measured by scintillation counting and colorimetry respectively.

Two forms of control were used. In the first, the catheterisations were performed, and the 2DG injected, but no stimulus was given. In the second, to control for an effect of CO_2 itself, the CO2 stimulus was given as in the intact animal, but the sinus nerve on the stimulated side only was sectioned, thereby abolishing the reflex. Abolition of the reflex was confirmed as lack of hyperventilation following CO_2 injection and before injection of 2DG.

Lastly, to test for the possible involvement of the ventrolateral medulla in the metabolic changes in the

forebrain following chemoreceptor stimulation, the
experiment was repeated one week after producing a thermal
lesion just rostral to nucleus ambiguus on the stimulated
side only.

Electrophysiology

The ventral surfaces of both the hypothalamus and the
medulla were exposed, and the activity of neurones within
the medial basal hypothalamus was recorded extracellularly
with glass micropipettes (8-10M impedance). Each neurone
located was tested for possible projection to either the
median eminence or the ipsilateral dorsal medulla. The
former was achieved by antidromic invasion following
electrical stimulation of the pituitary stalk/median
eminence junction (SMJ) with a bipolar stimulating electrode
(120-300K impedance), and the latter by stimulation of the
region of the tractus solitarius with a similar electrode.
Stimulation and recording sites were verified
histologically.

Results

2-Deoxyglucose

The effect of carotid body chemoreceptor stimulation on
forebrain metabolic activity was complex and widespread.
There was a powerful and obvious activation within areas
such as the thalamus, the hippocampus and the cortex,
particularly on the stimulated side, but litte obvious
effect on the hypothalamus. As Fig 1 shows, however, closer
examination of the hypothalamus revealed that the arcuate
(ARC) and the supraoptic (SON) nuclei showed much greater
metabolic activity following stimulation than any other part
of the hypothalamus including the paraventricular nuclei
(PVN). Indeed the activity of ARC and SON was more than
double that of any other hypothalamic region. The activity
within ARC and SON was reduced to about the same level by
sectioning the sinus nerve, or by lesioning in the
ventrolateral medulla (VLM). However, the activity in those
nuclei was still greater than in the rest of the
hypothalamus, and was only reduced to that level in those
animals that were not given the CO_2 injections, suggesting
that the CO_2 itself must have been generally increasing
metabolic activity.

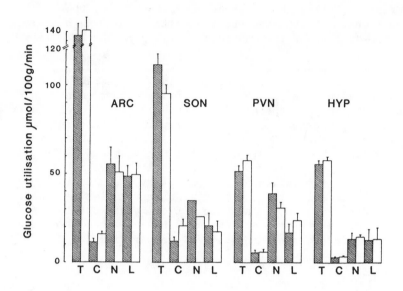

Fig 1. Block diagrams of glucose utilisation (means ± S.E.) in the hypothalamus of anaesthetised rats following stimulation of the carotid body chemoreceptors of one side and ^{14}C deoxyglucose autoradiography. ▨=Stimulated side, ☐=Unstimulated side. T=intact stimulated, C=control unstimulated, N=stimulated with sinus nerve on stimulated side cut, L=stimulated with a lesion in the ventrolateral medulla of the stimulated side. ARC-arcuate nucleus, SON-supraoptic nucleus, PVN-paraventricular nucleus, Hyp-general hypothalamus.

Electrophysiology

It was already known that stimulation of the carotid body chemoreceptors activated vasopressin-secreting neurones in SON (Harris,1979). Since PVN contains apparently identical neurones, however, the lack of increased metabolic activity in that nucleus and the clear increase in ARC was unexpected. Consequently an electrophysiological investigation was performed to see if the 2DG had given a true reflection of neuronal responses.

Recordings were taken from 272 medial hypothalamic neurones, each of which was tested first for projection to either SMJ or the medulla, and secondly for its response to stimulation of the ipsilateral carotid body. From that total, 18 neurones were found to be activated by chemoreceptor stimulation. All but two of those were in the arcuate nucleus and the remaining two were in the ventral thalamus, an area also showing increased metabolic activity with 2DG. Not one PVN neurone showed any activation, even the vasopressin-secreting neurones remaining unaffected.

Within the group of activated ARC neurones, 3 were antidromically invaded from the medulla, 6 from the SMJ, and 7 were unaffected from either site. The response of the neurones to chemoreceptor stimulation varied. Most showed a brief 3-5 spike burst of activity, but others, all projecting to the median eminence, responded with activation lasting many minutes. Moreover, correlation analysis showed that the discharge of those neurones was linked with respiration and occasionally with heart rate as well.

Discussion

That the influence of carotid body chemoreceptors must extend as far rostral as the hypothalamus has been known, at least by implication, for many years. For example, Bizzi, Libretti, Malliani & Zanchetti (1961) reported that hypoxia will cause sham rage in high decerebrate cats providing the hypothalamus is intact, and Cross & Silver (1963) recorded increases in extracellular activity of hypothalamic neurones during hypoxia. More precisely, Hilton & Joels (1965) showed that stimulation of carotid body chemoreceptors would evoke sham rage and muscle vasodilatation in the high decerebrate cat, whilst Marshall (1981) and Hilton & Marshall(1982) demonstrated that using the correct anaesthetic conditions, all the cardiovascular components of the defence reaction could be elicited by carotid body chemoreceptor stimulation in rats and cats.

With this in mind, it is surprising to find that virtually nothing is known of the detailed effects on the fore-brain of carotid body chemoreceptor stimulation. The results presented here form part of a much larger study of this phenomenon.

In performing this investigation we have used two different, but complementary, techniques. That is, ^{14}C-deoxyglucose autoradiography as a means of scanning the entire CNS for increased metabolic activity, and electrophysiological recording from single neurones to further explore the avenues opened by the deoxyglucose.

Although the 2DG showed widespread forebrain activation following chemoreceptor stimulation, for reasons of space we have concentrated in this paper on the hypothalamic effects. Within that region it is clear, by both procedures, that the effects of the chemoreceptor stimulus are confined to the supraoptic and arcuate nuclei. The influence on SON has already been documented (Harris,1979; Harris et al,1984), but the effect on ARC is, so far as we are aware, a new discovery.

The chemoreceptor activation in ARC is complicated by the fact that as shown by the electrophysiology, at least two broad groups of neurones are involved. Those projecting to the median eminence, and those projecting to the hind brain. So far as the former are concerned, the implication must be that they have a neuroendocrine function. Since, however, ARC contains cells secreting many transmitters and peptides many of which have neuroendocrine functions, speculation as to a particular role for this response would not be particularly fruitful without further investigation.

Much the same situation applies to the caudally-projecting neurones. They have been identified more recently (Horst,Luiten & Kuipers,1984; Schwanzel-Fukuda, Morrell & Pfaff,1984) than the tuberoinfundibular neurones and their potential functions are still unclear. They may, however, form part of the pathway described by Lopez, Cipola-Neto & Rocha e Silva (1977) who showed that in barbiturate anaesthetised rats, knife cuts in the medial-basal hypothalamus reduced the pressor response to bilateral carotid occlusion. Further support for this is provided by finding a correlation between neuronal activity and both ventilation and heart rate.

There is almost no information concerning the route taken by the chemoreceptor input to the forebrain. Harris, Ferguson & Banks (1984) reported that activation within SON was abolished by lesions within medial preoptic area rostral to SON. This implied that the pathway ascended by a lateral path and then descended again by the more medial route. It seems not unlikely that it is this path that leads to ARC.

Moreover, the finding that, at least in the hypothalamus, the metabolic activity was reduced to the same extent by a lesion within the ventrolateral medulla supports the finding by Banks & Harris (1984) that thermal and 6-hydroxydopamine lesions in the same region abolished the chemoreceptor activation within SON.The present finding that the metabolic activity was reduced by section of the sinus nerve shows that the majority of the activation was neuronally mediated. But the fact that animals not given any CO_2 injections showed even lower glucose utilisation suggests strongly that the CO_2 itself was in some way increasing metabolic activity in the CNS. This may of course be an artifact of giving the injections at one minute intervals over 45min, or it may not be an electrical event at all; it is probably worthy of further study, however.

In this investigation, the negative results are almost as interesting as the positive ones. In particular the lack of effect, as seen both by deoxyglucose and electrophysiology, of the stimulus on PVN and the major part of the hypothalamus raises some interesting points. The fact that vasopressin-secreting neurones in SON are powerfully activated by chemoreceptor stimulation (Harris,1979), and that PVN contains vasopressin-secreting neurones with apparently identical discharge patterns (Poulain, Wakerley & Dyball,1977) had led us to assume that neurones within PVN would respond in the same manner to the chemoreceptor stimulus as those in SON. This belief was reinforced, moreover, by the finding that PVN neurones were depressed by baroreceptor inputs as are those in SON (Kannan & Yamashita,1983). Consequently, the finding that PVN is apparently totally unaffected by the chemoreceptor stimulus came as a surprise, and raises the possibility of functional differences between the magnocellular neurones of PVN and SON.

The implications of this spread wider than the neurohypophysis, however, because it has long been thought that PVN and surrounding hypothalamic regions were involved in cardiovascular control (Ciriello & Calaresu,1980) and the responses of the defence reaction (Abrahams, Hilton & Zbrozyna,1960). For the latter at least, this would appear not to be the case. Some caution must be exercised in this interpretation because the anaesthetic used in these experiments was Urethane, and it has not been possible to elicit the defence reaction, even with electrical stimulation, using this anaesthetic (Timms, 1981). On the other hand, preliminary experiments in our laboratory, using deoxyglucose to look at chemoreceptor stimulation in Althesin anaesthetised rats, indicate that the pattern of metabolic influence in the hypothalamus is the same as in Urethane anaesthetised animals. This suggests, therefore, that defence responses obtained by electrical stimulation within the hypothalamus come not from groups of cell bodies, but from fibre bundles passing through to more caudal regions.

References
Abrahams VC, Hilton SM, Zbrozyna, AW (1960). Active muscle vasodilatation produced by stimulation in the brain stem. Its significance in the defence reaction. J Physiol

(Lond) 154: 491.

Band DM, Cameron IR, Semple SJG (1970). The effects on respiration of abrupt changes in carotid artery pH and Pco_2 in the cat. J Physiol (Lond) 211: 479.

Banks D, Harris MC (1984). Lesions of the locus coeruleus abolish baroreceptor-induced depression of supraoptic neurones in the rat. J Physiol 355: 383.

Bizzi E, Libretti A, Malliani A, Zanchetti A (1961). Reflex chemoreceptive excitation of diencephalic rage behaviour. Am J Physiol 200: 923.

Ciriello J, Calaresu FR (1980). Role of paraventricular and supraoptic nuclei in central cardiovascular regulation in the cat. Am J Physiol 239: R137.

Cross BA, Silver IA (1963). Unit activity in the hypothalamus and the sympathetic response to hypoxia and hypercapnia. Expl Neurol 7: 375.

Harris MC (1979). Effects of chemoreceptor and baroreceptor stimulation on the discharge of hypothalamic supraoptic neurones in rats. J Endocrinol 82: 115.

Harris MC, Ferguson AV, Banks D (1984). The afferent pathway for carotid body chemoreceptor input to the hypothalamic supraoptic nucleus in the rat. Pflugers Archiv 400: 80.

Hilton SM, Joels N (1965). Facilitation of chemoreceptor reflexes during the defence reaction J Physiol (Lond) 176: 20P

Hilton SM, Marshall JM (1982). The pattern of cardiovascular response to carotid chemorceptor stimulation in the cat. J Physiol (Lond) 326: 495.

Horst GJ, Luiten PGM, Kuipers F (1984). Descending pathways from hypothalamus to dorsal motor vagus and ambiguus nuclei in the rat. J Aut n Syst 11: 59-75

Kannan H, Yamashita H (1983). Electrophysiological studies of paraventricular nucleus neurons projecting to the dorsal medulla and their response to baroreceptor stimulation in rats. Brain Research 279: 31.

Lopez O, Cipola-Neto J, Rocha e Silva M Jr (1977). Hypothalamic component in pressor response to carotid occlusion in the rat. Am J Physiol 233: 240.

Marshall JM (1981). Interaction between the responss to stimulation of peripheral chemoreceptors and baroreceptors: the importance of chemoreceptor activation of defence areas. J Auton Nerv System 3: 389.

Poulain DA, Wakerley JB, Dyball REJ (1977). Electrophysiological differentiation of oxytocin- and vasopressin-secreting neurones. Proc R Soc B 196: 367.

Schwanzel-Fukuda M, Morrell JI, Pfaff DW (1984). Localisation of forebrain neurones which project directly to the medulla and spinal cord of the rat by retrograde tracing with wheatgerm agglutinin. J Comp Neurol 226: 1-20.

Sokoloff L, Reivich M, Kennedy C, Des Rosiers MH, Patlak CS, Pettigrew KD, Sakurada O, Shinohara M (1977). The [^{14}C] deoxyglucose method for the measurement of local cerebral glucose utilisation: theory, procedure and normal values in the conscious and anesthetised albino rat. J Nuerochem 28: 897.

Timms RJ (1981). A study of the amygdaloid defence reaction showing the value of Althesin anaesthesia in studies of the function of the fore-brain in cats. Pflugers Archiv 391: 49.

Aknowledgments

The authors wish to thank the SmithKline Foundation and the Nuffield Foundation for their support. We are grateful to Mrs.J.Dean for her technical assistance.

Organization of the Autonomic Nervous System:
Central and Peripheral Mechanisms, pages 347-361
© **1987 Alan R. Liss, Inc.**

Role Played by Amygdala Complex and Common Brainstem System in Integration of Somatomotor and Autonomic Components of Behaviour

P. Langhorst, M. Lambertz, G. Schulz* and
G. Stock* Institute of Physiology, The Free
University of Berlin, Arnimallee 22, D-1000
Berlin 33, F.R.G.; *Schering AG, Müllerstrasse
170-178, D-1000 Berlin 65, F.R.G.

INTRODUCTION

Everyday life requires a permanent adaptation of the organism to environmental circumstances and internal needs (Hess, 1925). During the development of complex behaviour patterns an adequate adjustment of somatomotor, cardio-vascular and respiratory activity is necessary. In general this is complemented by emotional feelings developing out of the situation, and then the behaviour patterns can be determined by their emotional component (Brady, 1960). The neuronal systems responsible for these coordinations are located in different levels of the neuraxis. More complex and differentiated patterns are represented in higher levels beginning with the brainstem. The reticular formation of the lower brainstem contains a multi-functional system in which basic activity for somatomotor, cardiovascular and respiratory regulation is generated (Langhorst and Werz, 1974; Langhorst et al., 1983; Schulz et al., 1983; Schulz et al., 1985b; Langhorst et al., 1980). Thus the common brainstem system (CBS) has basically a homeostatic function including the function of the so-called ARAS (ascending reticular activating system) necessary for the maintenance of consciousness (Moruzzi, 1972). The hypothalamus is the prominent neuronal structure of the next level. According to the investi-gations of W.R. Hess ergotropic and trophotropic behaviour patterns can be elicited by hypothalamic stimulations (Hess, 1948). The ergotropic behaviour includes the well elaborated concepts of the defence reaction and the emergency state (Hilton, 1974; Cannon, 1928). The high flexibility observed in everyday life is bound to higher sub-cortical brain areas and their interaction with frontal, parietal and temporal structures. One nodal point is the amygdala complex, a sub-cortical group of nuclei deep within the temporal lobe belonging to the limbic system (MacLean, 1949). The nodal function of the amygdala complex is supported by several lines of evidence. The neurones of the amygdala complex receive information already pre-processed by higher cortical areas. Moreover it receives afferents from the hypothalamus and from the CBS (Nauta and Domesick, 1982). The efferent connections of the amygdala complex are partly reciprocal to those mentioned above. Thus, there are connections with the frontal brain, the motor cortex, the hypothalamus and, bypassing the hypothalamus, with the mesencephalon, the CBS, the dorsal vagal nucleus and the nucleus of the solitary tract (Nauta, 1960); Hopkins and Holstege, 1978; Krettek and Price, 1978; Schwaber et al., 1982). The role of the amygdala complex for tuning the somatomotor, the visceral motor and the emotional components of behaviour patterns is elucidated by the symptoms of temporal lobe epilepsy in man. These so-called psychomotor seizures often have their origin in the amygdala. Such seizures start with a vegetative aura, e.g. gastric sensations, changes in heart rate and blood pressure. These vegetative phenomena precede the typical somatomotor automatisms and the EEG manifestations. During the seizure, there is an impairment of consciousness, although the patients are able to perform complex motor acts. The seizures are accompanied by emotions like anxiety, fear, joy, hallucinations (Penfield and Jasper, 1954). The same temporal sequences of at first vegetative and then somatomotor reactions during seizures could be observed in the kindling model of temporal lobe epilepsy (Stock et al., 1979). From the anatomical as well as the physiological point of view it can be assumed that there is a continuum of the amygdala complex via the hypothalamus, the midbrain and the reticular formation responsible for the coordination of vegetative and somatomotor reactions. To get further information on the reciprocal relations between amygdala complex and CBS, single cell recordings were done in two models: on the one hand, in anaesthetized dogs, to investigate the principles of functional organization and the functional properties of the neurones of the CBS, and on the other hand, in the amygdala of conscious freely moving cats, to investigate the reaction patterns of neurones to complex stimuli and their consequence for amygdala influence on cortex, blood pressure, heart rate and somatomotor activity.

METHODS

The methods used in the experiments on anaesthetized dogs and awake cats were described in detail in previous publications (Langhorst et al., 1983; Schulz et al., 1986a). In short: a) Action potentials of single cells, from as many as three simultaneously recorded with one electrode, were obtained from the reticular formation of the lower brainstem of chloralose-urethane-anaesthetized dogs together with blood pressure, respiration, renal sympathetic nerve activity and cortical EEGs. b) Single cell discharges were recorded from the central subnucleus of the amygdala complex in conscious, freely moving cats chronically instrumented for blood pressure, EEG and EMG recordings. In both types of experiments, the responses of the neurones to sensory stimuli were tested. Data recorded on tape were analyzed off-line; the analyses included computations of auto- and crosscovariance histograms and power spectra.

RESULTS

Part A

To investigate the physiological properties of the neurones of the CBS it was necessary to record from several neurones with one electrode under identical conditions. The extracellularly recorded action potentials could be separated and analyzed (Langhorst et al., 1983). All CBS neurones were spontaneously active. Afferents from visceral systems (pressoreceptors, chemo-receptors, lung stretch receptors (see Figs. 4,7,8 in Langhorst et al., 1983) and from somato-sensory systems (skin-, muscle- and joint-receptors, nociceptors) converge on one and the same neurone. A detailed evaluation of pairs of neurons - 2 to 5 neurones were recorded simultan-eously under identical conditions - revealed that visceral afferents influenced nearly all neurones of the CBS in the same way, either increasing or decreasing the activity. Somatosensory afferents had more differentiated effects on these neurones. Only neurones situated closely together received similar combinations of these afferents, whereas in neurones separated by larger distances the combinations were clearly different (see e.g. Figs. 5 and 6 in Schulz et al., 1983). These findings lead to the conclusion that groups of neighbouring neurones can be organized in sub-populations discharging under the influence of somatosensory afferents. In such phases the discharges of neurones of the sub-populations are characterized by similar discharge frequencies between 8 and 16 impulses/s and strong nonrhythmical discharge couplings with latencies of a few milliseconds (see Figs. 5 and 7 in Schulz et al., 1985b).

Under conditions in which the neuronal activity is determined by inputs from the other neurones of the network, the CBS is organized into a functional unit. In this state of functional organization the tendency of the CBS neurones to discharge rhythmically is enhanced.

In the spontaneous activity of the neurones rhythms of different frequency ranges in various combinations can be observed. The different rhythms induce a coupling of the discharges of CBS neurones which is different from the functional coupling into sub-populations by somato-sensory afferents. These rhythmical types of couplings can be observed not only between neighbouring neurones but also between neurones located in a larger area. In periods in which the neuronal network CBS is organized into a functional unit, the oscillations in the activity of CBS neurones are dominated by a typical reticular rhythm in the frequency range of about 0.2 to about 0.07 Hz. This reticular rhythm is not identical with the respiratory rhythm, but both rhythms can influence each other in the sense of relative coordination according to E. von Holst (1939). In this type of functional organiz-ation both rhythms occur in the simultaneously recorded heart frequency, arterial blood pressure, respiration and in the degree of synchronization of the EEG, as shown in Fig. 1. The analysis of different rhythms in the same frequency range is possible only by applying covariance- and spectral analysis.

Part B

The results described here are based on the evalu-ation of the discharge sequences of 20 single neurones from the nucleus amygdala centralis recorded for up to 180 minutes over several sleep and waking periods. In 18

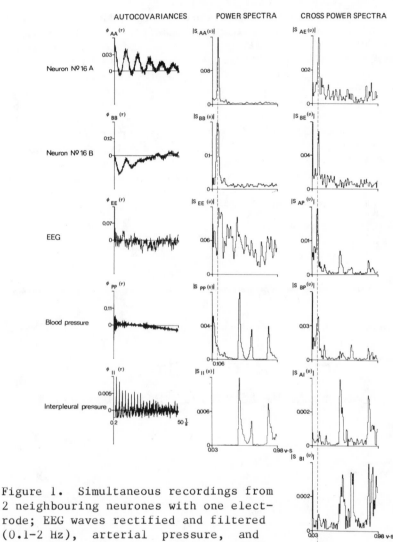

Figure 1. Simultaneous recordings from 2 neighbouring neurones with one electrode; EEG waves rectified and filtered (0.1-2 Hz), arterial pressure, and inspiration (determined by recording intrapleural pressure). Power spectra of both neurones have a common peak of 0.106 Hz (period duration 9.4 s). The same rhythmic component occurs in the power spectra of EEG waves and of arterial pressure and is also indicated by the respective cross power spectra. Spectral analysis reveals that the respiratory rhythm is common to all signals.

neurones the reaction to natural, tactile, acoustic, optic and olfactory stimuli could be tested. Stimuli were applied during states of quiet wakefulness. One example is given in Fig. 2. Eleven neurones reacted to several of these stimuli with an increase or a decrease in frequency, 7 neurones reacted only to one kind of stimulus. In comparing the responses to simple or complex stimuli - e.g. a pure tone or barking dogs, singing of birds; light flashes or presenting a living mouse - complex stimuli elicited much more distinct changes in frequency. It was observed that stimuli of the same modality could lead to different responses; for instance a simple acoustic stimulus could lead to a decrease in frequency, and a complex acoustic stimulus to an increase in frequency in the same neurone and vice versa. That means that it is

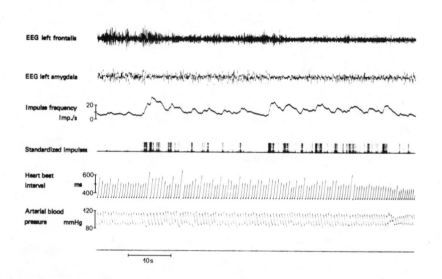

AMYGDALA CENTRALIS K 141

Figure 2. Response to miaowing of another cat (indicated by bars) in the EEGs of left frontal cortex and left amygdala, in single neuronal activity of the right amygdala centralis (shown as an integrated frequency curve and standardized impulses), in heart beat interval and arterial pressure. The impulse frequency increases during the acoustic stimulus; note the simultaneous desynchronization of the amygdala EEG and the arrhythmia.

not the modality which is crucial but the content of the signal. The reactions of the neurones were followed regularly by an arousal reaction indicated by a desynchronization of the cortical EEG. In those cases in which the stimulus evoked a motor reaction, typical sequences were observed in the time course of alterations of physiological variables as shown in Fig. 3. The neurone discharged spontaneously with a mean frequency of 6 impulses/s. The arrow marks the presentation of a complex acoustic stimulus. In response

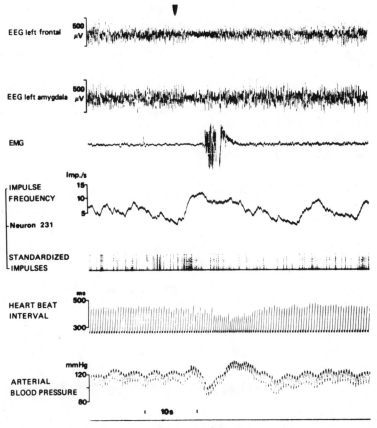

Figure 3. Response to barking of dogs (arrow) in the EEGs of the left frontal cortex, left amygdala, EMG, single neuronal activity of the right amygdala centralis, heart beat interval and arterial blood pressure. For further explanation see text.

to this, the discharge frequency of the neurone increased. Note that the desynchronization of the contralateral amygdala EEG took place at the same time. The autonomic responses shown (a brief increase followed by a decrease and an increase again of blood pressure and tachycardia together with the desynchronization of the frontal suprasylvian EEG) started nearly 1 s after the activation of the neurone. The first signs of somatomotor activity – the cat lifted its head, indicated by EMG activity of the neck muscles – occurred about 2.5 s after the increase of neuronal discharges. The blood pressure fluctuations lasted approximately 15 s. After the response the discharge rate of the neurone fell typically below control values. The spontaneous discharge rates before and after the response were slightly rhythmically modulated. Such modulations were observed in 17 of the 20 neurones. An example is given in Fig. 4. The frequency of such modulations was around 0.1 Hz varying between 0.16 Hz and 0.07 Hz and could be observed in all phases of sleep and wakefulness. Sometimes faster and slower

AMYGDALA CENTRALIS NEURON K 233

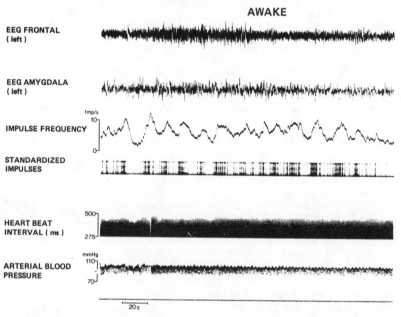

Figure 4. Spontaneous rhythmic activity of a single amygdala neurone with period durations between 10 and 14 s.

modulations were superimposed on these rhythmic discharge patterns. Their frequency was variable and alternated with tonic phases.

In view of the increase in neuronal discharge rates, of the subsequent blood pressure oscillations in response to complex sensory stimuli and the spontaneous rhythmic activity of the neurones, the relation between these rhythmic activities and blood pressure oscillations were investigated by the computations of crosscovariances between neuronal discharges in blood pressure. An example of the results of such computations with 4 different neurones is shown in Fig. 5. In relation to neuronal activity the blood pressure shows increases and decreases with period durations between 8 and 13 s. This means that the influence of amygdala neurones on blood pressure can

Crosscovariances

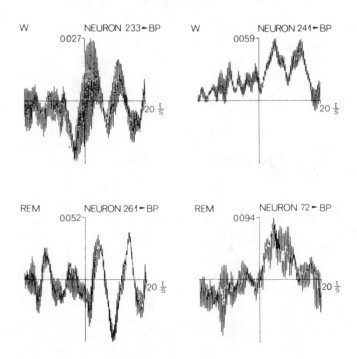

Figure 5. Four crosscovariance histograms between the discharge sequences of 4 different neurones of the right amygdala centralis and arterial blood pressure. For further explanation see text.

be detected by analysis of the rhythmic properties also in the absence of motor activity. This was found in 12 out of 16 neurones investigated in the state of quiet wakefulness, and in 16 out of 18 neurones tested in the state of REM.

DISCUSSION

The distinct convergence of multimodal and multifocal afferents onto the neurones of the CBS may be interpreted in two ways. On the one hand, via the energizer function of the CBS they are the source of basic activity of the entire central nervous system. The contribution to regulatory processes can be seen in their adjusting and maintaining the background activity necessary for different behaviour patterns (Moruzzi, 1969). On the other hand, somatic afferents organize the neurones of the CBS into sub-populations. Experimentally such organization could be induced particularly well by passive movements of the extremities (Schulz et al., 1983). The plasticity of such forms of local organization can be considered as the basis of differentiated patterns of innervation of vegetative and somatomotor systems influenced by the CBS. As shown here, neurones of the nucleus amygdala centralis also receive afferents from different modalities. This is in agreement with reports from other groups (cf. Le Gal la Salle and Ben Ari, 1981). Sawa and Delgado reported that the neurones react in particular to complex stimuli like singing of birds (1963). In contrast to the reticular formation, amygdala neurones react to complex, pre-processed information. The function of the amygdala as postulated by Gloor (1960) is to organize sensory percepts into vegetative and motor programs appropriate to the situations; this view is supported by the results. The same sequence of vegetative and somatomotor patterns was observed also after electrical stimuli in the amygdala centralis (Stock et al., 1978).

From all the experimental evidence we would like to propose a novel hypothesis. Afferents on the one hand lead to arousal via the reticular formation, on the other hand they induce changes in sub-populations which can be used by the patterns initiated by the amygdala complex. This hypothesis is supported by the results presented here. Besides the ability of the reticular formation to organize itself, it is also able to produce

rhythms. As described in our previous papers, the
neurones discharge in respiratory rhythm as well as in a
rhythm resembling that of respiration with a period
duration around 10 s (Langhorst et al., 1984; Langhorst
et al., 1986). These rhythms interacting with each
other are reflected in peripheral patterns of activity,
like peripheral sympathetic activity, blood pressure and
heart rate. They are also reflected in the degree of
synchronization of the EEG. It could also be demonstrated
that amygdala neurones are able to modulate their
discharge frequency rhythmically (Schulz et al., 1985).
The dependence of blood pressure on such rhythms permits
the conclusion that amygdala neurones utilize the rhythmic
properties of the reticular formation. Rhythmic blood
pressure waves with relations to amygdala activity were
reported by Ben Ari et al. (1973) in anaesthetized cats.
Such rhythmic influences of the amygdala complex are found
to be exerted also on cortical activity. After an
increase of the amygdala neuronal activity a desynchronization of the cortical EEG with a fixed temporal relation
is induced lasting 8 to 12 s (Schulz et al., 1985a, Schulz
et al., 1986b, in press). When the amygdala complex is
stimulated electrically, blood pressure increases and a
tachycardia develops (Heinemann et al., 1973; Stock et
al., 1978). In this phase, the effect of baroreceptor
activity is reduced. When baroreceptors are stimulated at
that time, reflex bradycardia is blocked (Schlor et al.,
1984). This blockade can be achieved, as shown before,
by a direct influence of the amygdala neurones on the
processing of baroreceptor information at their first
relay station in the nucleus of the tractus solitarius
(NTS). This is supported by the demonstration of direct
anatomical connections between the amygdala and the NTS
(Hopkins and Holstege, 1978). With ongoing stimulation
of the amygdala the effectiveness of baroreceptors
becomes re-established gradually after approximately 10
s (Schlör et al., 1984). Thus, while the amygdala on
the one hand exerts an influence on the processing of
pressoreceptor afferents, it is in turn controlled by
pressoreceptors, as shown by the detection of a direct
anatomical connection between the NTS and the amygdala,
and by the electrophysiological findings of the
pulse-rhythmically occurring deactivation of amygdala
neurones (Schwaber et al., 1982; Schulz et al., 1986).
These findings support the concept that the functional

relations between the amygdala complex and the CBS are realized by various feedback loops.

REFERENCES

Ben Ari Y, Le Gal la Salle G, Champagnat J (1973). Amygdala unit activity changes related to a spontaneous blood pressure increase. Brain Res 52: 394-398.

Brady JV (1960). Emotional behavior. In Field J, Magoun HW, Hall VE (eds): "Handbook of Physiology", Sect 1 Neurophysiology, Vol III, Washington, DC: Amer Physiol Soc, pp 1529-1552.

Cannon WB (1928). Die Notfallsfunktion des sympathicoadrenalen Systems. Erg Physiol 27: 380-406.

Gloor P (1960). Amygdala. In Field J, Magoun HW, Hall VE (eds): "Handbook of Physiology", Sect 1 Neurophysiology Vol II, Washington, DC: Amer Physiol Soc, pp 1395-1420.

Heinemann H, Stock G, Schaefer H (1973). Temporal correlation of responses in blood pressure and motor reaction under electrical stimulation of limbic structures in unanaesthetized, unrestrained cats. Pflügers Arch ges Physiol 343: 27-40.

Hess WR (1925). Über die Wechselbeziehungen zwischen psychischen und vegetativen Funktionen. Schweiz Arch Neurol 16: 285-306.

Hess WR (1948). Die funktionelle Organisation des vegetativen Nervensystems. Basel: Benno Schwabe & Co.

Hilton SM (1974). The role of the hypothalamus in the organization of patterns of cardiovascular response. In Lederis K, Cooper KE (eds): "Recent Studies of Hypothalamus Function", Basel, Munchen, Paris, London, New York, Sydney: S. Karger, pp 306-314.

Holst EV (1939). Die relative Koordination als Phänomen und als Methode zentralnervöser Functionsanalysen. Erg Physiol 42: 228-306.

Hopkins DA, Holstege G (1978). Amygdaloid projections to the mesencephalon, pons and medulla oblongata in the cat. Exp Brain Res 32: 529-547.

Krettek JE, Price JL (1978). Amygdaloid projections to sub-cortical structures within the basal forebrain and brain stem in the rat and cat. J Comp Neurol 178: 225-253.

Langhorst P, Werz M (1974). Concept of functional organization of the brain stem 'cardiovascular center'. In Umbach W, Koepchen HP (eds): "Central Rhythmic and Regulation", Stuttgart: Hippokrates, p 238.

Langhorst P, Schulz B, Lambertz M, Schulz G, Camerer H (1980). Dynamic characteristics of the 'unspecific brain stem system'. In Koepchen HP, Hilton SM, Trzebski A (eds): "Central Interaction between Respiratory and Cardiovascular Control Systems", Berlin, Heidelberg, New York: Springer-Verlag, pp 30-39.

Langhorst P, Schulz B, Schulz G, Lambertz M (1983). Reticular formation of the lower brain stem. A common system for cardio-respiratory and somatomotor functions: discharge patterns of neighboring neurons influenced by cardiovascular and respiratory afferents. J Auton Nerv Syst 9: 411-432.

Langhorst P, Schulz G, Lambertz M (1984). Oscillating neuronal network of the 'common brain stem system'. In Miyakawa K, Koepchen HP, Polosa C (eds): "Mechanisms of Blood Pressure Waves", Tokyo/Berlin: Japan Sci Soc Press/Springer-Verlag, pp 257-275.

Langhorst P, Lambertz M, Schulz G (1986, in press). Assessment of rhythmicity in the visceral nervous system. In Lown, Malliani, Prosdocimi (eds): "Proceedings of International Symposium on Neural Mechanisms and Cardiovascular Disease", Padua: Fidia Research Series, Liviana Press.

Le Gal la Salle G, Ben Ari Y (1981). Unit activity in the amygdaloid complex. A review. In Ben Ari Y (ed): "The Amygdaloid Complex", INSERM Symposium N 20. Amsterdam: Elsevier, pp 227-238.

MacLean PD (1949). Psychosomatic disease and the 'visceral brain'. Psychosom Med 11: 338-358.

Moruzzi G (1969). Sleep and intrinsic behavior. Arch ital Biol 107: 175-216.

Moruzzi G (1972). The sleep-waking cycle. In Adrian RH et al (eds): "Reviews of Physiology, Biochemistry and Experimental Pharmacology", Vol 64, Berlin: Springer-Verlag, pp 1-65.

Nauta WJH (1960). Limbic system and hypothalamus: anatomical aspects. Physiol Rev 40 (Suppl 4): 102-104.

Nauta WJH, Domesick VB (1982). Neural associations of the limbic system. In "The Neural Basis of Behaviour", Spectrum Publ, pp 175–206.

Penfield W, Jasper H (1954). "Epilepsy and the Functional Anatomy of the Human Brain". Boston: Little, Brown & Co.

Sawa M, Delgado JMR (1963). Amygdala unit activity in the unrestrained cat. EEG Clin Neurophysiol 15: 637–650.

Schlör KH, Stumpf H, Stock G (1984). Baroreceptor reflex during arousal induced by electrical stimulation of the amygdala or by natural stimuli. J Auton Nerv Syst 10: 157–165.

Schulz B, Lambertz M, Schulz G, Langhorst P (1983). Reticular formation of the lower brain stem. A common system for cardio-respiratory and somatomotor functions: discharge patterns of neighboring neurons influenced by somatosensory afferents. J Auton Nerv Syst 9: 433–449.

Schulz G, Lambertz M, Langhorst P (1985). Slow rhythmic rate fluctuations of amygdala neurons and their influence on arterial blood pressure in sleep and quiet waking of unanaesthetized cats. Neurosci Lett 22 (Suppl): 397.

Schulz G, Lambertz M, Stock G, Langhorst P (1985a). Influence of amygdala neurons on cortical activity. Pflugers Arch Eur J Physiol 405: R50.

Schulz G, Lambertz M, Schulz B, Langhorst P, Krienke B (1985b). Reticular formation of the lower brainstem. A common system for cardiorespiratory and somatomotor functions: cross-correlation analysis of discharge patterns of neighboring neurons. J Auton Nerv Syst 12: 35–62.

Schulz G, Stock G, Lambertz M, Langhorst P (1986). Influence of baroreceptor activity on spontaneous discharge sequences of amygdala neurons recorded in the awake cat. Pflugers Arch Eur J Physiol 406: R23.

Schulz G, Lambertz M, Stock G. Langhorst P (1986a, in press). Neuronal activity in the amygdala related to somatomotor and vegetative components of behaviour in cats. J Auton Nerv Syst.

Schulz G, Schulz B, Stock G, Langhorst P, Kazner E (1986b, in press). Single cell recordings of the nucleus amygdalae in conscious cats. A contribution to research of focal epilepsy. Adv Neurosurg.

Schwaber JS, Kapp BS, Higgins GA, Rapp PR (1982). Amygdaloid and basal forebrain direct connections with the nucleus of the solitary tract and the dorsal motor nucleus. J Neurosci 2: 1424-1438.

Stock G, Schlör KH, Heidt H, Buss J (1978). Psychomotor behaviour and cardiovascular patterns during stimulation of the amygdala. Pflügers Arch ges Physiol 376: 177-184

Stock G, Sturm V, Klimpel L, Schlör KH (1979). Cardiovascular change in the course of amygdaloid kindling in cats. Exp Neurol 63: 647-651.

Organization of the Autonomic Nervous System:
Central and Peripheral Mechanisms, pages 363–374
© **1987 Alan R. Liss, Inc.**

Cardiovascular Afferent Inputs to Limbic Neurons

Franco Calaresu

Department of Physiology, University of
Western Ontario, London, Ontario N6A 5C1

INTRODUCTION

Although humoral and metabolic factors appear of
paramount importance in the genesis of human degenerative
cardiovascular diseases (myocardial infarction and
arterial hypertension) emotional factors, probably
mediated by autonomic centres in the central nervous
system, have been implicated in the genesis of these
diseases (Dembroski, Schmidt & Blumchen, 1983). This
suggestion is supported by the demonstration that
emotional stress in humans has a definite influence
on cardiovascular variables (Hickman, Cargill and Golden,
1948). Since 1937, when Papez first suggested that the
limbic brain was involved in emotional behavior, it has
been demonstrated that the limbic system receives
information from the internal and external environments,
and transforms these inputs into modulatory influences on
the hypothalamus and brain stem to elicit behavioral,
humoral and autonomic responses characteristic of the
particular emotion (Mogenson, 1984). Two limbic
structures in particular, the amygdala and the septum,
which have been the subject of two recent monographs
(Ben-Ari, 1981; De France, 1976), appear to be likely
sites for the integration of emotional and autonomic
responses, in particular cardiovascular responses, as
indicated by stimulation studies (Brickman, Calaresu &
Mogenson, 1979; Calaresu, Ciriello & Mogenson, 1976;
Calaresu & Mogenson, 1972; Kaada, 1972; Mogenson, 1976).

The essential components of the central neural control system of the circulation are integrating circuits which receive information from receptors sensing changes in the internal and external environments and issue signals to cardiovascular effector organs to produce changes in the regulated variables according to physiological needs and environmental demands. The early studies of circuits involved in the central control of the circulation consisted of investigating reflex arcs affecting the circulation in animal preparations transected at different levels of the neuraxis (decorticate, decerebrate, encéphale isolé, spinal). Subsequently, through the efforts of several laboratories (e.g. Hilton, 1982; Korner, 1979; Zanchetti, Baccelli & Mancia, 1970), the role of the intact central nervous system on the central control of the circulation was investigated. A picture has emerged of a very complex network of systems interconnected in parallel at multiple levels of the central nervous system and not at all organized in series in a hierarchical segmental fashion, as previously thought.

The objectives of our recent experiments have been to establish functional specificity of connections between cardiovascular receptors and limbic structures involved in emotional behavior. Recording and stimulation techniques were used in selected central "cardiovascular" networks to establish functional properties of the systems studied.

STUDIES ON THE AMYGDALA

This limbic structure is composed of several nuclei reciprocally connected with the cerebral cortex, the hippocampus, the thalamus and the hypothalamus. Experimental evidence obtained using stimulation and ablation techniques, has shown that the amygdala can control somatic, autonomic, endocrine and behavioral responses (Kaada, 1972). Although the different components of these responses are controlled by other structures in the central nervous system, the amygdala plays the essential coordinating role (Ben Ari, 1981). For example, it has been shown in the awake cat that electrical stimulation of the amygdala elicits the "defence reaction" ("fear-flight" or "anger-attack"), a complex set of behavioral responses interpreted as an expression of fear and associated with autonomic reactions, including a well-defined pattern of cardiovascular changes characterized by an increase in arterial pressure, heart rate and skeletal muscle blood flow, and a decrease in mesenteric and skin flows (Zbrożyna, 1972).

We have recently done experiments to investigate whether the amygdala was involved in the integration of signals originating in the cardiovascular system, i.e. whether activation of baro- and chemoreceptors could alter the firing frequency of single units in the amygdala, and to investigate the central pathways of these inputs to the amygdala. Detailed results have been presented fully elsewhere (Cechetto and Calaresu, 1983a, 1983b, 1984, 1985).

In an extensive investigation of spontaneously firing units in the amygdala of the cat under chloralose it was shown that units responding to electrical stimulation of the aortic depressor and carotid sinus nerves were found primarily in the central nucleus of the amygdala (Cechetto and Calaresu, 1983a). In addition, units responding to selective activation of baroreceptors were found primarily in the ventrolateral amygdala, whereas most of the units responding to activation of chemoreceptors were found in the dorsomedial amygdala (Fig. 1): these two regions have been identified by electrical stimulation to be inhibitory and excitatory, respectively, of the defence and arousal responses (e.g. Kaada, 1972). Further experiments aimed at the identification of the central pathways of baro- and chemoreceptors to the amygdala showed unequivocally that these receptors project to and receive information from the parabrachial nuclei, whereas a projection through the paraventricular nucleus could not be demonstrated conclusively (Cechetto and Calaresu 1983b, 1985). These studies have provided new information about cardiovascular afferent inputs to the amygdala and their possible functional significance in the organization of central circuits involved in the defence reaction (Fig. 2).

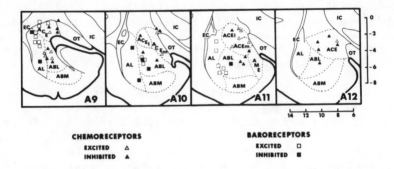

Fig. 1. Diagrams of 4 transverse sections of the amygdala of the cat (9-12 mm anterior to interaural line) showing sites of single units responding to activation of arterial baro- and chemoreceptors. Calibration scales in mm. (Modified after Am. J. Physiol. 246: R832, 1984).

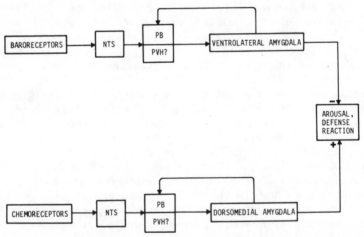

Fig. 2. Schematic diagram of pathways and functional connections to the amygdala from baro- and chemoreceptors. NTS, N. of the solitary tract; PB, parabrachial NN.; PVH, paraventricular N. of the hypothalamus.

STUDIES ON THE SEPTUM

This limbic structure is composed of nuclei and

fiber tracts located ventral to the corpus callosum and medial to the anterior horns of the lateral ventricles. The septum contains cells and bundles of fibers from the hippocampus and amygdala passing through on their way to the hypothalamus and brain stem. The lateral septal nucleus receives its major input from the hippocampus and projects to the medial septum and diagonal band which project back to the hippocampal nuclei. Both medial and lateral septal nuclei have reciprocal connections through the medial forebrain bundle with hypothalamic nuclei (preoptic, anterior, lateral, mammillary). The functional role of the septum appears to be inhibitory of aggressive behavior as suggested by the vicious behavior displayed by rats immediately after septal lesions (Brady & Nauta, 1953). However, it has also been shown that placidity can be induced in rats by lesions of the medial septum (Clody & Carlton, 1969).

The role of the septum in central cardiovascular control is controversial. Although electrical stimulation of the septum in anesthetized animals has been shown to elicit changes in arterial pressure (AP) and heart rate (HR), there are conflicting reports concerning the direction of the responses, i.e. both an increase (Andy & Koshino, 1967; Covian & Timo-Iaria, 1966; Calaresu & Mogenson, 1972; Calaresu, Ciriello & Mogenson, 1976) and a decrease (Calaresu & Mogenson, 1972; Calaresu, Ciriello & Mogenson, 1976; Ranson, Kabat & Magoun, 1935; Korotsu, Sakai, Megawa & Ban, 1958; Manning, Charbon & Cotten, 1963) in AP and HR have been described. More detailed experiments have shown that changes in arterial pressure in the medial (MS) and lateral septum (LS) are in opposite directions and, in addition, opposite responses from both areas could be obtained if different anesthetics were used (Calaresu & Mogenson, 1972). These results could be interpreted to indicate that the opposite changes in arterial pressure elicited by electrical stimulation in animals under different anesthetics were probably due to simultaneous activation of cell bodies and fibers within the septum (Raisman, 1966; Swanson & Cowan, 1979; Watson, Seigel & Seigel, 1985) and to the differential effects of anesthetics on bodies and fibers. We therefore decided to study the effect of selective stimulation of septal cell bodies on the cardiovascular system. A preliminary report of these experiments has been published (Gelsema & Calaresu, 1986). The excitatory aminoacid dl-homocysteic acid, which is known to influence selectively the activity of cell bodies (Goodchild, Dampney & Bandler, 1982), was microinjected (maximum volume = 50 nl) into the septum of rats anesthetized with urethane or α-chloralose. Arterial pressure was consistently decreased after the injection but the changes in heart rate were inconsistent. The responses were similar in the MS and LS and in the two groups of animals under two different anesthetics.

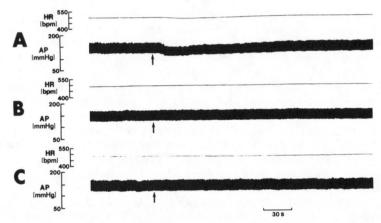

Fig. 3. Characteristic responses of AP (arterial pressure) and HR (heart rate) to microinjections (< 50 nl) of (A) dl-homocysteic acid; (B) isotonic saline; (C) hypertonic (0.45 M) saline into the septum of the rat under urethane.

The demonstration of a reproducible decrease in arterial pressure elicited by activation of cell bodies in the septum prompted us to investigate the possibility that the septum, like the amygdala, also receives an input from cardiovascular receptors. The septum in the urethane-anesthetized rat was therefore explored for spontaneously firing single units responding to activation of baroreceptors (by electrical stimulation of the aortic depressor nerve, which is a purely baroreceptor nerve in the rat; Sapru, Gonzalez and Krieger, 1981) and

chemoreceptors (systemic injection of sodium cyanide).
Approximately 300 spontaneously firing units were
studied. Of the approximately 100 units that responsed
to activation of baroreceptors two-thirds responded with
excitation and one-third with inhibition. The percentages of units with excitatory and inhibitory responses
were similar for the LS and MS. Most responsive units
were found throughout the MS and in the dorsal LS. Of
the 30 units in the MS and LS responding to activation
of chemoreceptors the majority were excited. Characteristic responses of septal units to activation of
baro- and chemoreceptors are shown in Fig. 4. A
preliminary report of these experiments has been
published (Miyazawa, Gelsema & Calaresu, 1986).

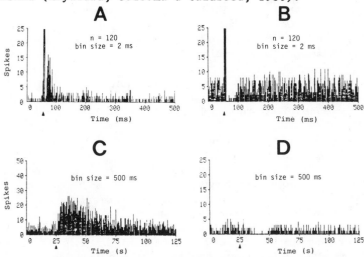

Fig. 4. A, B: peristimulus time histograms of two
septal units responding with excitation (A) and
inhibition (B) to activation of baroreceptors. C, D:
continuous frequency histograms of two units responding
with excitation (C) and inhibition (D) to activation of
chemoreceptors; arrow indicates time of stimulation.

FUNCTIONAL IMPLICATIONS

A novel finding of our studies is the demonstration
that activation of cardiovascular receptors influences
the activity of neurons in the amygdala and septum.
Although this may not be surprising in view of the

multiplicity of anatomical connections of these two limbic structures and of the demonstration of units in the amygdala (Le Gal, La Salle & Ben Ari, 1981) and in the septum (Hayat & Feldman, 1974) responding to many sensory inputs the significance of our observations is clear. We would like to propose that in the execution of complex physiological and behavioral activities, often essential for survival, these two limbic structures must receive and analyze sensory inputs from receptors monitoring the level of arterial pressure and blood gases. These long-loop reflexes provide the neuro-physiological substrate for the regulatory mechanisms involved in complex physiological adjustments. With regard to the septal units responding to activation of baroreceptors it is interesting to note that it has been reported recently that units in the medial septum and the diagonal band of Broca of the rat, antidromically identified by stimulation of the supraoptic nucleus, are excited by increases in arterial pressure (Jhamandas & Renaud, 1986); this evidence suggests that the septal region is a component of a reflex pathway for the control of release of neurohypophyseal hormones.

Two additional conclusions can be drawn from the experiments on the amygdala. The first is that most of the chemoreceptor information was found to project to the dorsomedial amygdala whereas most of the baro-receptor information projected ventrolaterally. As these two areas have an excitatory and an inhibitory influence, respectively, on the alertness of the animal (e.g. Kaada, 1972) the physiological significance of this complex reflex arc is based on the observation that activation of chemoreceptors by hypoxia increases alertness in dogs and has obvious survival value (Bowes et al., 1981). The second significant finding of these studies is the existence of reciprocal connections between the amygdala and the parabrachial nuclei (PB). These connections could operate as a negative feedback mechanism, from amygdaloid neurons receiving sensory cardiovascular information back to the lower-order sensory station in the PB. This arrangement could provide stability to neuronal circuits.

With regard to the chemical stimulation experiments on the septum our observations are at variance with

our previous results obtained by electrical stimulation. In our earlier experiments arterial pressure
changes induced by electrical stimulation in the MS
and LS were in opposite directions as well as being
affected differentially by the two anesthetics used,
α -chloralose and urethane. We must conclude that our
past results were probably due to simultaneous activation
of cell bodies and of fibers of passage and to the
differential effects of anesthetics on bodies and
fibers. This interpretation raises the general issue of
the validity of results obtained by electrical
stimulation. It would appear that selective activation
of cell bodies by the use of discrete pressure injection
of excitatory chemical substances is a much more
selective technique of stimulation of sites in the
central nervous system.

CONCLUSIONS

The role of limbic structures in the central control
of the circulation has not been studied as extensively as
the role of hypothalamus and brain stem. Recent
neuroanatomical and neurophysiological evidence has
demonstrated that limbic structures receive and integrate
a variety of sensory information. We have reported
evidence for the existence of projections from arterial
baro- and chemoreceptors to the amygdala and septum.
These findings combined with the demonstration that
activation of neurons in these two limbic structures can
influence cardiovascular variables provide evidence for
the existence of long-loop reflexes controlling the
cardiovascular system during complex behavioral and
physiological responses.

ACKNOWLEDGEMENTS

I thank the Medical Research Council of Canada for
research support. I thank Drs. G. J. Mogenson and
L. C. Weaver for critical comments on the manuscript.
Rebecca Woodside and Kim Clarke have provided excellent technical and secretarial assistance.

REFERENCES

Andy OJ, Koshino K (1967). Duration and frequency patterns of the afterdischarge from septum and amygdala. Electroenceph clin Neurophysiol 22: 167.

Ben-Ari Y (1981). (ed) "The Amygdaloid Complex. Amsterdam Elsevier, p V.

Brickman AL, Calaresu FR, Mogenson GJ (1979). Bradycardia during stimulation of the septum and somatic afferents in the rabbit. Am J Physiol 235: R225.

Bowes G, Townsend ER, Kozar LF, Bromley SM, Phillipson EA (1981). Effect of carotid body denervation on arousal response to hypoxia in sleeping dogs. J Appl Physiol 51 (1): 40.

Brady JV, Nauta WJH (1953). Subcortical mechanisms in emotional behavior: affective changes following septal forebrain lesions in the albino rat. J Comp Physiol Psychol 46: 339.

Calaresu FR, Mogenson GJ (1972). Cardiovascular responses to electrical stimulation of the septum in the rat. Am J Physiol 223 (4): 777.

Calaresu FR, Ciriello J, Mogenson GJ (1976). Identification of pathways mediating cardiovascular responses elicited by stimulation of the septum in the rat. J Physiol 260: 515.

Cechetto DF, Calaresu FR (1983a). Response of single units in the amygdala to stimulation of buffer nerves in cat. Am J Physiol 244: R646.

Cechetto DF, Calaresu FR (1983b). Parabrachial units responding to stimulation of buffer nerves and forebrain in the cat. Am J Physiol 245: R811.

Cechetto DF, Calaresu FR (1984). Units in the amygdala responding to activation of carotid baro- and chemoreceptors. Am J Physiol 246: R832.

Cechetto D, Calaresu FR (1985). Central pathways relaying cardiovascular afferent information to amygdala. Am J Physiol 248: R38.

Clody DE, Carlton PL (1968). Behavioral effects of lesions of the medial septum in rats. J Comp Physiol Psychol 67: 344.

Covian MR, Timo-Iaria C (1966). Decreased blood pressure due to septal stimulation: parameters of stimulation, bradycardia, baroreceptor reflex. Physiol Behav 1: 37.

De France JF(1976). "The Septal Nuclei." New York: Plenum Press.

Dembroski TM, Schmidt TH, Blumchen G (1983). "Biobehavioral Bases of Coronary Heart Disease." Basel: S. Karger.

Gelsema AJ, Calaresu FR (1985). Microinjection of homocysteic acid into the septum elicits arterial depressor responses in the rat. Proc Can Fed Biol Soc 29: 79.

Goodchild AK, Dempney RAL, Bandler R (1982). A method for evoking physiological responses by stimulation of cell bodies, but not axons of passage, within localized regions of the central nervous system. J Neurosci Meth 5: 351.

Hayat A, Feldman S (1974). Effects of sensory stimuli on single cell activity in the septum of the cat. Exp Neurol 43: 298.

Hickman JB, Cargill HH, Golden A (1948). Cardiovascular reactions to emotional stimuli. Effect on the cardiac output, arteriovenous oxygen difference, arterial pressure, and peripheral resistance. J Clin Invest 27: 290.

Hilton SM (1982). The defence-arousal system and its relevance for circulatory and respiratory control. J Exp Biol 100: 159.

Jhamandas JH, Renaud LP (1986). Diagonal band neurons may mediate arterial baroreceptor input to hypothalamic vasopressin-secreting neurons. Neurosci Let 65: 214.

Kaada BR (1972). Stimulation and regional ablation of the amygdaloid complex with reference to functional representations. In Eleftheriou BE (ed): "The Neurobiology Of The Amygdala," New York: Plenum Press, p. 205.

Korner PI (1979). Circulatory homeostasis - Role of reflex interactions. Proc Austr Physiol Pharmacol Soc 10: 102.

Korotsu T, Sakai A, Megawa A, Ban T (1958). The changes in blood pressure and gastric motility induced by electrical stimulation in the preoptic and septal areas. Med J Osaka Univ 9: 201.

Le Gal La Salle G, Ben-Ari Y (1981). Unit activity in the amygdaloid complex: a review. In Ben-Ari Y (ed): "The Amygdaloid Complex," Amsterdam: Elsevier/North Holland, P. 227.

Manning JW, Charbon GA, Cotten M de V (1963). Inhibition of tonic cardiac sympathetic activity by stimulation of the brain septal region Am J Physiol 205: 1221.

Miyazawa T, Gelsema AJ, Calaresu FR (1986). Baro-receptors project to a depressor area in the septum of the rat. Soc Neurosci Abs 12: 579.

Mogenson GJ (1976). Septal-hypothalamic relationships. In De France JF (ed): "The Septal Nuclei," New York: Plenum Press. p. 149.

Mogenson GJ (1984). Limbic-motor integration - with emphasis on initiation of exploratory and goal-directed locomotion. In Bandler R (ed): "Modulation of Sensory Motor Activity During Alterations in Behavioral States," New York: Alan R Liss Inc, p. 121.

Papez JW (1937). A proposed mechanism of emotion. Arch Neurol Psychiatry 38: 725.

Raisman G (1966). The connexions of the septum. Brain 89: 317.

Ranson SW, Kabat H, Magoun HW (1935). Autonomic responses to electrical stimulation of hypothalamus, preoptic region and septum. Arch Neurol Psychiatry 33: 457.

Sapru HN, Gonzalez E, Krieger AJ (1981). Aortic nerve stimulation in the rat: cardiovascular and respiratory responses. Brain Res Bull 6: 393.

Swanson LW, Cowan WM (1979). The connections of the septal region in the rat. J Comp Neurol 186: 621.

Watson RE, Jr, Siegel HE, Siegel A (1985). A [^{14}C] 2-deoxyglucose analysis of the functional neural pathways of the limbic forebrain in the rat. V. The septal area. Brain Res 346: 89.

Zanchetti A, Baccelli A, Mancia G (1970). Cardiovascular effects of emotional behavior. In Bartorelli C, Zanchetti A (eds): "Cardiovascular Regulation in Health and Diseases," Milano: Elli and Pagani.

Zbrozyna AW (1972). The organization of the defence reaction elicited from the amygdala and its connections. In Eleftheriou BE (ed): "The Neuro-biology of the Amygdala," New York: Plenum Press, p. 597.

SECTION VI: Cellular Mechanisms for Hypothalamic Regulation: The Magnocellular Neurosecretory Neuron

The hypothalamus has a key role in central regulation of the autonomic nervous system. Many of the homeostatic functions attributed to the hypothalamus (e.g. temperature regulation) require the existence of intricate connections with neurons located at other levels of the neural axis (e.g. intermediolateral cell column) in order to "effect" the response, i.e. vasodilation or vasoconstriction. One other "effector" mechanism resides within the hypothalamus itself, i.e. the hypothalamo-neurohypophysial complex. In the mammalian brain, this complex is composed of the magnocellular oxytocin- and vasopressin-secreting neurons in the supraoptic and parventricular nuclei as well as scattered accessory magnocellular cell groups. Representing the classical neurosecretory neurons, these cells are capable of integrating data pertinent to the status of plasma osmolality, blood volume, arterial pressure and visceral afferents and effecting a response by releasing oxytocin or vasopressin into the systemic circulation of the neurohypophysis. Quite clearly, these events are only a fraction of the integrative capabilities of the hypothalamus. Nonetheless, these magnocellular neurosecretory cells (MNGs) presently represent one of the most intensely studied outflow projections of the central autonomic axis. Hence, there is justification for including in this volume a series of chapters that reflect recent advances in our understanding of their electrophysiological and integrative properties.

Organization of the Autonomic Nervous System:
Central and Peripheral Mechanisms, pages 377–386
© 1987 Alan R. Liss, Inc.

INTRINSIC AND SYNAPTIC FACTORS CONTROLLING NEURONAL AFTER-
DISCHARGES IN THE SUPRAOPTIC NUCLEUS

F. Edward Dudek and Valentin K. Gribkoff,
Department of Physiology, Tulane University
School of Medicine, New Orleans, Louisiana, USA.

INTRODUCTION

The magnocellular neuroendocrine cells (MNC's) of the supraoptic nucleus are known to fire burst discharges during periods of maximal secretion of oxytocin and vasopressin (Poulain and Wakerley, 1982). A wide range of studies have suggested that oscillations of intrinsic membrane conductances could be responsible for or contribute to the burst discharges of oxytocinergic and vasopressinergic neurons. However, synaptic inputs from nearby hypothalamic areas and other regions of the brain are also important for regulation of burst discharges in neurons of the supraoptic nucleus (SON). A characteristic of bursting neurons, particularly intrinsic bursters, is that they tend to fire a long-lasting train of action potentials that persist after brief electrical stimuli. These spike afterdischarges would presumably augment hormone secretion from neuroendocrine cells. The studies summarized below were aimed at understanding both intrinsic and synaptic mechanisms that promote afterdischarges and burst firing in SON neurons.

In vivo electrophysiological studies provided the first evidence that MNC's might possess intrinsic mechanisms for burst firing. Antidromic stimulation, suprathreshold to the recorded cell, evoked afterdischarges in phasically firing SON neurons (Dreifuss et al., 1976). Intracellular electrophysiological experiments using hypothalamic slices have provided new evidence for intrinsic burst generation (Andrew and Dudek, 1983, 1984). This chapter will briefly review some of the data supporting the hypothesis for endogenous bursting in MNC's, with particular emphasis on afterdischarges.

Specific physiologic stimuli trigger release of neuro-hypophyseal peptides (e.g., suckling for oxytocin secretion and hemorrhage for vasopressin secretion); therefore, synaptic inputs must play an important role in burst regulation. An interaction of intrinsic mechanisms and synaptic inputs presumably controls burst firing. Hatton et al. (1983) recently found that extracellular stimulation dorsolateral to the SON could trigger afterdischarges in phasically firing MNC's; electrical stimulation in this area would be expected to activate a population of local neurons, including putative cholinergic cells. We have recently extended these findings and observed a synaptically activated slow depolarization that initiates and contributes to afterdischarges in SON neurons (Gribkoff and Dudek, 1985). Data supporting the hypothesis that this slow depolarization can occur independent of intrinsic mechanisms, such as summation of depolarizing afterpotentials, will also be reviewed briefly below.

METHODS

Coronal slices (300-600 µm) of rat hypothalamus (Fig. 1) were prepared and maintained with standard procedures described previously (Hatton et al., 1980; Andrew and Dudek, 1984; Dudek and Gribkoff, submitted). Most intracellular recordings were obtained with 3 M K-acetate micro-

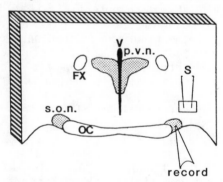

Figure 1. Schematic diagram of hypothalamic slice preparation.

pipettes and an M-707 electrometer (WP Instr.), which had a bridge circuit for intracellular currrent injection. Bipolar, 90 % platinum-10 % iridium wires (76 µm diameter) were used for extracellular stimulation of the area dorsolateral to SON.

RESULTS

Several criteria have been established for identification of intrinsic burst generation versus network-mediated bursting (e.g., Johnston and Brown, 1984). Electrophysiologic data fulfilling the criteria for intrinsic bursting have been obtained with intracellular recordings from in vitro systems. Intracellular injection of steady currents could modify burst duration and frequency (Andrew and Dudek, 1983, 1984), suggesting that in these neurons intrinsic voltage-dependent conductances regulated these burst characteristics. A brief, suprathreshold current pulse injected intracellularly into a single SON neuron could evoke an afterdischarge lasting tens of seconds (Fig. 2A). The afterdischarge appeared to arise from summation

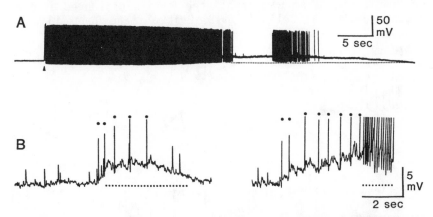

Figure 2. Intrinsic afterdischarges and depolarizing afterpotentials. A. Spike burst triggered by brief depolarizing pulse of intracellular current (arrow). B. Summation of depolarizing afterpotentials during interburst interval (left) and at onset of spontaneous spike burst (right). Closed circles indicate action potentials, which have been truncated by the chart recorder. Reproduced from Andrew and Dudek, 1984, with permission.

of depolarizing afterpotentials. During the interburst interval or at the onset of a spontaneous burst (Fig. 2B) in a phasically firing SON neuron, a depolarizing afterpotential frequently followed individual spikes. Summation of depolarizing afterpotentials, when interspike intervals are brief, represents a regenerative mechanism for burst firing and afterdischarges. Some MNC's possess this intrinsic mechanism, which does not require synaptic inputs.

Electrophysiologic and anatomic data have suggested that electrical stimulation of a region dorsolateral to the SON, which included a population of cholinergic neurons, could evoke afterdischarges and phasic firing in MNC's (Hatton et al., 1983; Mason et al., 1983). These initial physiologic studies did not consider intrinsic mechanisms (see above), and we have undertaken additional studies to evaluate the contribution of intrinsic versus synaptic mechanisms to these extracellularly evoked afterdischarges (Gribkoff and Dudek, 1985). Single electrical stimuli to the dorsolateral area (Fig. 1) synaptically evoked a brief afterdischarge, and repetitive stimulation caused a slow depolarization that was associated with a prolonged afterdischarge in many cells (Fig. 3, Gribkoff and Dudek, 1985).

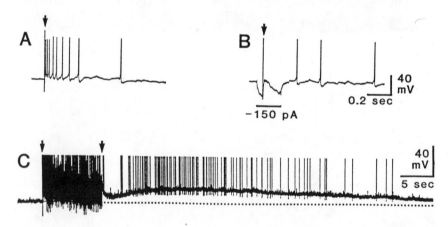

Figure 3. Synaptic activation of afterdischarge and slow depolarization. A. Brief afterdischarge to single stimulus (arrow). B. EPSP revealed with hyperpolarizing current pulse. C. Prolonged afterdischarge and slow depolarization resulting from repetitive stimulation (between arrows).

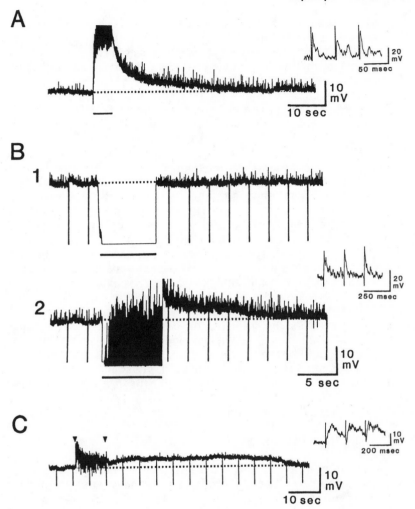

Figure 4. Evidence that slow depolarization from dorso-lateral stimulation is not due to an intrinsic mechanism. A. Repetitive stimulation (bar) at an intensity sub-threshold for the impaled SON neuron. B. Action potentials prevented with injection of hyperpolarizing current (bar). Upper trace (1) shows hyperpolarizing current alone; lower trace shows slow depolarization when current was injected during stimulation. C. Action potentials blocked with intracellular QX 314. Downward deflections in B and C show truncated current pulses, and insets show EPSP's evoked during train.

Several independent experiments were used to evaluate whether the slow depolarization could be a long-lasting EPSP, independent of intrinsic mechanisms (i.e., depolarizing afterpotentials). First, the slow depolarization could be observed after stimulation at intensities that did not cause action potentials in the impaled neuron (Fig. 4A). Second, hyperpolarizing current was used to block action potentials in the recorded cell during repetitive stimulation of the dorsolateral area. A slow depolarization could still be obtained after dorsolateral stimulation, even though membrane potential was kept below resting levels throughout the duration of the stimulus train (Fig. 4B). Finally, recordings were obtained with electrodes containing QX 314, which blocked sodium-dependent action potentials (Connors and Prince, 1982). Since calcium-dependent action potentials have a higher threshold, it was possible to stimulate the dorsolateral area repetitively without evoking action potentials in the impaled neuron. In some cells recorded with an electrode containing QX 314, a slow depolarization could still be observed (Fig. 4C). Low-$[Ca^{2+}]$, high-$[Mg^{2+}]$ solutions, which blocked chemical synaptic transmission, reduced or eliminated the slow depolarization. Therefore, although endogenous mechanisms may contribute to afterdischarge of SON neurons evoked with dorsolateral stimulation, at least a substantial component of the slow depolarization is not intrinsic to the recorded cell.

DISCUSSION AND CONCLUSION

A wide range of in vivo electrophysiologic studies have indicated that both oxytocinergic and vasopressinergic MNC's fire bursts of action potentials during periods of maximal hormone release (e.g., Brimble and Dyball, 1977; Poulain et al., 1977; see also Poulain and Wakerley, 1982 for review). In particular, considerable attention has focused on the mechanisms of phasic firing in vasopressinergic MNC's, neurons that showed afterdischarges to neurohypophyseal stimulation in vivo (Dreifuss et al., 1976). Several in vitro studies have been aimed at elucidating the membrane mechanisms of phasic firing (Andrew and Dudek, 1983, 1984; Bourque et al., 1986; Legendre et al., 1982). Recent studies with combined intracellular staining and immunocytochemistry have shown that most phasically bursting neurons in vitro are vasopressinergic (Cobbett et al., 1986; Theodosis et al., 1983; Yamashita et al., 1983), a finding that should allow for more detailed studies of the membrane mechanisms responsible for this firing pattern.

It has been impossible in this brief chapter to review all of the data supporting the hypothesis that some MNC's possess intrinsic mechanisms for afterdischarges and burst generation. Hatton (1982) found that some paraventricular neurons in vitro could still fire phasic bursts after chemical synapses were blocked with low-$[Ca^{2+}]$, high-$[Mg^{2+}]$ solutions. Andrew and Dudek (1982, 1984) showed that brief trains of action potentials in MNC's evoked with intracellular current pulses could trigger afterdischarges (Fig. 2), which is a criterion for intrinsic burst generation. In some MNC's, a depolarizing afterpotential followed each action potential; these events could sum during repetitive firing and lead to bursts. The ionic conductance mechanisms responsible for depolarizing afterpotentials may generate the slow oscillations in membrane potential occasionally seen in phasic bursters. Other intrinsic mechanisms may also contribute to phasic firing (Bourque et al., 1986). Large plateau potentials, which may be analogous to the summed depolarizing afterpotentials observed in hypothalamic slices, have been observed in cultured MNC's (Legendre et al. 1982; Theodosis et al., 1983). Biophysical studies on identified MNC's are now needed to specify the actual conductance mechanisms for afterdischarges and phasic firing.

Several mechanisms involving conventional chemical synapses may also contribute to phasic firing and afterdischarges in MNC's. Spontaneously occurring phasic PSP's have been observed in hypothalamic cultures (Gahwiler and Dreifuss, 1979) and slices (Andrew and Dudek, 1984). This result suggests that the bursts of some MNC's derive from phasic synaptic inputs by another bursting neuron.

Although conventional chemical synapses causing fast changes in membrane conductance probably regulate burst discharges, slow synaptic mechanisms could have important modulatory actions. A slow depolarization, resulting from repetitive orthodromic stimulation (Fig. 4), was observed most frequently in phasic neurons; this event was associated with afterdischarges (Gribkoff and Dudek, 1985). At least three types of experiments indicated that postsynaptic action potentials were unnecessary for the occurrence of this synaptically activated slow depolarization (Fig. 4). Afterdischarges and slow depolarizations could result from activation of cholinergic inputs alone (Hatton et al., 1983; Mason et al., 1983), possibly involving a synaptic feedback loop from SON to the dorsolateral area of the hypothalamus (Leng, 1982; Mason et al., 1984). Activation of non-cholinergic fibers of passage near the area of stimulation could also be responsible for the responses. The slow depolarization may be a long-lasting EPSP or due to an increase in extracellular $[K^+]$ from repetitive firing of many MNC's. Additional experiments are required to resolve these issues.

Therefore, both intrinsic and synaptic mechanisms are involved in afterdischarges and burst firing of supraoptic MNC's. During membrane depolarization, the afterdischarge to an extracellular stimulus train could far outlast the underlying slow depolarization, thus suggesting that intrinsic mechanisms involving depolarizing afterpotentials augment and prolong the effects of synaptic activation. Future studies should now be directed toward understanding the biophysical mechanisms of these events, the nature of their interactions and the physiological role of these processes in the intact animal.

ACKNOWLEDGMENTS

Supported by NS07625, NS16877, and BNS-00162 from NIH and NSF.

REFERENCES

Andrew RD, Dudek FE (1983). Burst discharge in mammalian neuroendocrine cells involves an intrinsic regenerative mechanism. Science 221:1050-1052.
Andrew RD, Dudek FE (1984). Analysis of intracellularly recorded phasic bursting by mammalian neuroendocrine cells. J Neurophysiol 51:552-565.
Bourque CW, Randle JCR, Renaud LP (1986). Non-synaptic depolarizing potentials in rat supraoptic neurones recorded in vitro. J Physiol. 376:493-506.
Brimble MJ, Dyball REJ (1977). Characterization of the response of oxytocin and vasopressin secreting neurones

in the supraoptic nucleus to osmotic stimulation. J Physiol 271:253-271.

Cobbett P, Smithson KG, Hatton GI (1986). Immunoreactivity to vasopressin- but not oxytocin-associated neurophysin antiserum in phasic neurons of rat hypothalamic paraventricular nucleus. Brain Res 362:7-16.

Connors BW, Prince DA (1982). Effects of local anesthetic QX-314 on the membrane properties of hippocampal pyramidal neurons. J Pharmacol Exptl Ther 220:476-481.

Dreifuss JJ, Tribollet E, Baertschi AJ, Lincoln DW (1976). Mammalian endocrine neurones: control of phasic activity by antidromic activation potentials. Neurosci Lett 3:281-286.

Dudek FE, Gribkoff VK (submitted). Synaptic activation of slow depolarization in rat supraoptic nucleus neurones in vitro.

Gahwiler BH, Dreifuss JJ (1979). Phasically firing neurons in long-term cultures of the rat hypothalamic supraoptic area: pacemaker and follower cells. Brain Res 177:95-103.

Gribkoff VK, Dudek FE (1985). Afterdischarge in rat supraoptic neurons following repetitive orthodromic stimulation: role of synaptic and intrinsic factors. Soc Neurosci Abstr 11.:1236.

Hatton GI (1982). Phasic bursting activity of rat paraventricular neurones in the absence of synaptic transmission. J Physiol 327:273-284.

Hatton GI, Doran AD, Salm AK, Tweedle CD (1980). Brain slice preparation: hypothalamus. Brain Res Bull 5:405-414.

Hatton GI, Ho YW, Mason WT (1983). Synaptic activation of phasic bursting in rat supraoptic nucleus neurones recorded in hypothalamic slices. J Physiol 345:297-317.

Johnston D, Brown TH (1984). Mechanisms of neuronal burst generation. In Schwartzkroin PA, Wheal HV (eds): "Electrophysiology of Epilepsy," New York: Academic, pp 277-301.

Legendre P, Cooke IM, Vincent JD (1982). Regenerative responses of long duration recorded intracellularly from dispersed cell cultures of fetal mouse hypothalamus. J Neurophysiol 48:1121-1141.

Leng G (1982). Lateral hypothalamic neurones: osmosensitivity and the influence of activating magnocellular neurosecretory neurones. J Physiol 326: 35-48.

Mason WT, Ho YW, Eckenstein F, Hatton GI (1983). Mapping of cholinergic neurons associated with rat supraoptic nucleus: combined immunocytochemical and histochemical identification. Brain Res Bull 11:617-626.

Mason WT, Ho YW, Hatton GI (1984). Axon collaterals of supraoptic neurones: anatomical and electrophysiological evidence for their existence in the lateral hypothalamus. Neuroscience 11:169-182.

Poulain DA, Wakerley JB (1982). Electrophysiology of hypothalamic magnocellular neurones secreting oxytocin and vasopressin. Neuroscience 7:773-808.

Poulain DA, Wakerley JB, Dyball REJ (1977). Electrophysiological differentiation of oxytocin- and vasopressin-secreting neurones. Proc R Soc Lond B 196:367-384.

Theodosis DT, Legendre P, Vincent JD, Cooke IM (1983). Immunocytochemically identified vasopressin neurons in culture show slow, calcium-dependent electrical responses. Science 221:1052-1054.

Yamashita H, Inenaga K, Kawata M, Sano Y (1983). Phasically firing neurons in the supraoptic nucleus of the rat hypothalamus: immunocytochemical and electrophysiological studies. Neurosci Lett 37:87-92.

Organization of the Autonomic Nervous System:
Central and Peripheral Mechanisms, pages 387–396
© 1987 Alan R. Liss, Inc.

INTRINSIC FEATURES AND CONTROL OF PHASIC BURST ONSET IN
MAGNOCELLULAR NEUROSECRETORY CELLS

Charles W. Bourque

M.R.C. Neuropharmacology Research Group,
Department of Pharmacology,
The School of Pharmacy, University of London,
29/39 Brunswick Square, London WC1N 1AX, U.K.

INTRODUCTION

When the physiological demand for oxytocin or vasopressin is at a premium, magnocellular neurosecretory cells
(MNCs) in the rat adopt distinct bursting patterns of electrical activity (cf. Poulain and Wakerley,1982). This response is significant because the amount of hormone released
by each action potential is potentiated during burst firing
(Dutton and Dyball, 1979; Bicknell and Leng, 1981; Cazalis
et al., 1985). Recent intracellular recordings obtained in-
vitro have revealed much of the mechanism involved in the
generation of phasic bursting by putative vasopressin-secreting cells (Mason, 1983; Andrew and Dudek, 1983; 1984; Bourque, 1984; 1986; Bourque et al., 1986; Bourque and Renaud,
1985a). Part of this mechanism is reviewed below, with attention to the features which may be modulated to change the
rate and pattern of firing in MNCs.

BASIC MEMBRANE PROPERTIES OF MNCs

Intracellular recordings of MNCs in hypothalamic slices
(Dudek et al.,1980; MacVicar et al.,1982; Mason, 1980; 1983;
Abe and Ogata, 1982; Andrew and Dudek, 1983; 1984) or perfused explants (Bourque, 1984; 1986; Bourque et al.,1985;1986;
Bourque and Renaud, 1985a; 1985b) have revealed resting membrane potentials ranging from -75 to -55 mV and a spike
threshold near -60 mV. The action potential of these cells
is carried by a low threshold Na^+, and a high threshold Ca^{++}
current (Bourque and Renaud, 1985b). A selective enhancement

of the Ca^{++} component has also been shown to accompany the
activity-dependent broadening of their action potential
(Bourque and Renaud, 1985a). In current-clamp (Mason, 1983;
Andrew and Dudek, 1984; Bourque and Renaud, 1985b) and in
voltage-clamp (Bourque, 1986) MNCs display a high input resistance (80-360 MΩ), which does not vary between -85 and
-60 mV. At more depolarized levels however, their steady-
state current-voltage (I-V) relation shows a strong outward
rectification (Fig. 1), a component of which may be Ca^{++}-
dependent (Bourque and Renaud, 1985b). During prolonged hyperpolarizing current pulses (0.5-2 seconds) a small depolarizing sag becomes apparent at potentials below ca. -75 mV.
Under voltage-clamp conditions, this is reflected as a slow
inward relaxation of the membrane current which imparts a
slight inward rectification to the I-V relation below -85 mV
(Fig. 1).

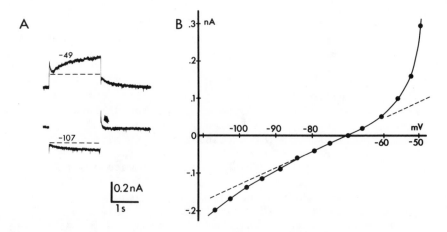

Figure 1. Membrane current responses of an MNC voltage-clamped in the presence of 0.3 μM tetrodotoxin. A, two traces
show the currents flowing during 2 second clamp commands
from -70 mV, to the potentials indicated. Depolarization
evokes a transient (arrow) and a late, persistent outward
current. Hyperpolarization induces a slow inward relaxation
and on repolarization, a transient outward current (arrow).
In B, the steady-state I-V relation of this cell was obtained by measuring the amplitude of the current flowing at the
end of the 2 second steps, and plotting it as a function of
the command voltage. The broken line extrapolates the linear
portion of the I-V relation. Note the outward rectification
above -60 mV. From Bourque, 1986.

GENERAL FEATURES OF PHASIC BURST ONSET

Several salient features of phasic bursting have been
revealed by the recent observations of Andrew and Dudek
(1983;1984). Individual action potentials in MNCs are followed by a transient after-hyperpolarizing potential (AHP) and
a late 1-4 mV depolarizing after-potential (DAP). Summation
of DAPs appears to establish a small (<10 mV) depolarizing
plateau which initiates and sustains firing during each
burst (Fig. 2). The strong steady-state outward rectification present above -60 mV (Fig. 1) combines with spike-acti-
vated outward currents (eg. the AHP) to prevent excessive
depolarization during this process, which would otherwise
lead to spike inactivation. Interestingly, termination of a
burst does not result from a progressive hyperpolarization
during the active phase (Fig. 2). Rather, it appears that
the generation of DAPs and their capacity to sum and maintain a plateau decreases as the burst progresses (Andrew and
Dudek, 1984). Because this refractoriness recovers slowly
after firing has stopped, a new burst can only be initiated
following a silent interval (Fig. 3).

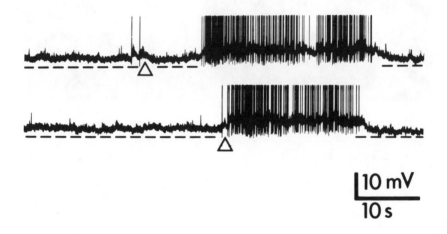

$$\left\lfloor \frac{10\,mV}{10\,s} \right.$$

Figure 2. Intracellular recording of two consecutive bursts
in a phasically active MNC. Individual action potentials are
followed by a late DAP (Δ). At the onset of a burst, DAPs
sum to establish a plateau which sustains firing. Note that
the bursts are not preceded by a slow depolarizing wave, or
accompanied by a progressive decrease of plateau amplitude.
The spike amplitude was 94 mV. The broken line is at -75 mV.

In most phasically active MNCs individual bursts are not preceded by a slow depolarizing wave (SDW) (Fig. 2). This finding agrees with the lack of a region of negative resistance in their steady-state I-V relation (Fig 1.). The origin of the SDW observed in some phasic MNCs (eg. Fig. 5) is therefore unclear. While the steady-state I-V relation of MNCs fails to show a region of negative resistance, persistent and opposing currents may nevertheless be active in the steady-state. Time-dependent, or even synaptically-mediated changes in such standing currents could effectively lead to a SDW. This possibility and its implications for the generation of phasic bursting requires further study.

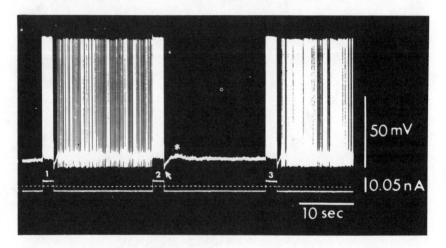

Figure 3. Voltage responses (upper traces) of this MNC to current injection (lower traces) illustrate the refractory properties of the plateau-forming mechanism. At the beginning of the trace the cell was silent and the depolarizing stimulus (1) triggered an after-discharge because DAP summation during the pulse established a plateau sufficiently large to exceed threshold. Application of an identical pulse (2) during the after-discharge interrupted firing because of the brief AHP (arrow) and firing did not resume because the amplitude of the subsequent plateau (*) failed to reach the spike threshold. Later, another identical current pulse (3) could re-initiate firing because the refractoriness of the plateau-forming mechanism was removed during the silent interval. This MNC continued to display alternating responses to the periodic application of identical depolarizing stimuli. From Bourque, 1984.

ROLE OF DEPOLARIZING TRANSIENTS IN PHASIC BURST ONSET

Whether or not they are preceded by a SDW, the onset
of phasic bursts is largely dependent on the presence of depolarizing transients to trigger the initial spikes whose
DAPs sum to establish a plateau (Andrew and Dudek, 1984).
In MNCs, this role is fulfilled by two populations of depolarizing transients. On one hand, conventional excitatory
post-synaptic potentials (EPSPs) are reported to trigger
spikes during intracellular recordings in hypothalamic slices
(Dudek et al., 1980; Mason, 1980; 1983; Andrew and Dudek,
1983; 1984). In a more recent study however, a population of
non-synaptic depolarizing potentials (NSDPs) has also been
found to occur in MNCs (Bourque et al., 1986). These transients differ from EPSPs in their shape, duration, voltage-
sensitivity and resistance to the presence of tetrodotoxin
or elevated concentrations of Mg^{++} (Fig. 4). Because they
appear at potentials within 5-10 mV of the spike threshold
(ie., above -70 mV), NSDPs are an effective and intrinsic
source of prepotentials capable of triggering spikes. Their
presence can therefore explain the occurrence of spontaneous
activity in MNCs, including phasic firing, during synaptic
blockade (Hatton, 1982; Bourque and Renaud, 1983).

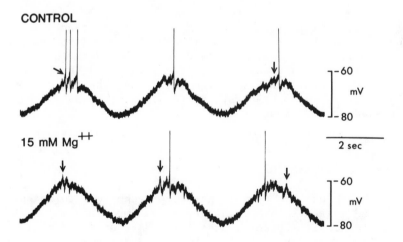

Figure 4. Membrane voltage responses of an MNC to the application of a sinusoidal current wave. Non-synaptic depolarizing potentials (arrows) appear only when the membrane potential rises above ca. -70 mV. Note that they are not blocked
by adding 15 mM Mg^{++} to the perfusate. From Bourque, 1984.

In a cell whose phasic bursts are preceded by a SDW,
NSDPs will appear when the membrane potential rises above
-70 mV and facilitate burst onset by triggering spikes in
rapid succession (Fig. 5). However, because the plateau-
forming mechanism becomes refractory with time during a burst,
neither NSDPs or EPSPs need to occur in a patterned way to
yield phasic bursting. As long as spikes are occasionnally
triggered by either of these depolarizing transients, bursts
of activity will recur periodically.

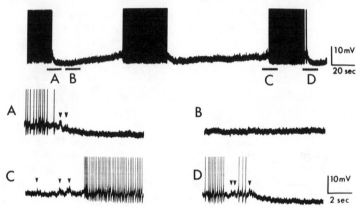

Figure 5. Phasic firing in an MNC. A-D are expanded segments of the top trace. The spike amplitude was 96 mV. In
this cell, bursts were preceded by a SDW. Note the appearance of NSDPs (arrows) immediately before (C) and near the
end (A,D), but not between each burst (B). The peak potential during the inter-burst hyperpolarization was -75 mV.
Modified from Bourque et al., 1986.

VOLTAGE-DEPENDENCE OF THE PLATEAU-FORMING MECHANISM

The recent use of voltage-clamp techniques to measure
membrane currents in MNCs has revealed important information
about the ionic mechanism underlying DAPs and plateau formation (Bourque, 1986). Application of a voltage-clamp after
1-5 current-evoked spikes reveals an early outward, and a
late inward current (Fig. 6). Because they underlie the AHP
and DAP recorded in current-clamp, these after-currents are
respectively termed AHC and DAC. The DAC is at least one
order of magnitude more prolonged than the AHC and decays

exponentially with a time constant of ca. 2 seconds. From a
threshold near -85 mv, the amplitude of the DAC increases as
the post-spike voltage is clamped to more positive potentials
(Fig. 6). Furthermore, beginning at -65 mv, activation of the
DAC effectively imparts a region of negative resistance to
the I-V relation of MNCs (Fig. 6 C). Because this region
crosses the spike threshold, activation of the DAC from potentials near -65 mV will depolarize the cell, and bring the
membrane potential within the region of negative resistance.
This will cause the cell to depolarize regeneratively and
induce a spike. Thus, while the DAC can depolarize the cell
(ie., induce a DAP) at all potentials from which it can be
activated, its effect will be maximized and sustain firing

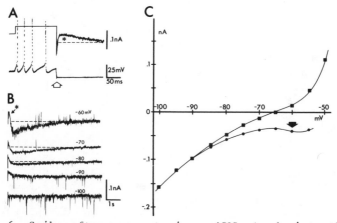

Figure 6. Spike after-currents in an MNC. A, depicts the
procedure employed to reveal the after-currents. A depolarizing current pulse (upper trace) was applied to the cell and
4 spikes were triggered (lower trace). Immediately after the
pulse (arrow) the cell was voltage-clamped to -80 mV, revea-
ling the early outward (*) current which normally underlies
the AHP of MNCs (Bourque et al., 1985). B, shows on a slower
time scale, the after-currents revealed by this procedure
when the cell was clamped to the various potentials indicated. Note that the early outward (*) current is followed by
the slower decaying inward DAC. In C, the filled squares
illustrate the steady-state I-V relation of this cell. The
curve drawn through the filled circles shows the net current
flowing 500 ms after the onset of the clamp (peak DAC). Note
that activation of the DAC induces a region of negative resistance between -65 and -60 mV. The arrow indicates the
spike threshold in this cell. From Bourque, 1986.

when triggered from potentials near -65 mV. Termination of firing at the end of a burst probably results from a use-dependent decrease of DAC amplitude and loss of the negative resistance characteristics.

DISCUSSION

The advent of in-vitro preparations of mammalian hypo-thalamic tissue has permitted the application of current- and voltage-clamp techniques to analyze the electrical beha-viour of MNCs. The information obtained should complement extracellular studies in-vivo, by describing functionally identified ionic mechanisms which are potentially available as targets for the action of neurotransmitters. An important feature of MNCs is their ability to change not only their rate, but also their pattern of firing, to adjust the release of neurohypophyseal peptides to the prevailing physiological requirements. The role of afferent inputs must therefore be examined in terms of their ability to modify the pattern, as well as the rate (or usually the excitability) of firing in MNCs.

Although it is far from complete, the description of the mechanism of phasic bursting described above already indicates how synaptic afferents may mediate such changes. First, the marked voltage-dependence of the plateau-forming mechanism (and NSDPs) implies that slow and discrete changes in membrane potential will strongly influence the intensity of firing within, as well as the duration of phasic bursts. Second, a direct modulation of the activation and inactiva-tion characteristics of the DAC, or currents with which it interacts, can be expected to produce changes in the pattern of firing.

The voltage-clamp experiments described above were sup-ported by a programme grant to professor D.A. Brown from the M.R.C. of the U.K. The author is a Post-Doctoral Fellow of the M.R.C. of Canada.

REFERENCES

Abe H, Ogata N (1982). Ionic mechanism for the osmotically induced depolarization in neurons of the guinea-pig supra-optic nucleus in-vitro. J Physiol 327: 157-171.

Andrew RD, Dudek FE (1983). Burst discharge in mammalian neuroendocrine cells involves an intrinsic regenerative mechanism. Science 221: 1050-1052.

Andrew RD, Dudek FE (1984). Analysis of intracellularly recorded phasic bursting by mammalian neuroendocrine cells. J Neurophysiol 51: 552-566.

Bicknell RJ, Leng G (1981). Relative efficiency of neural firing patterns for vasopressin release in-vitro. Neuroendocrinol 33: 295-299.

Bourque CW (1984). Membrane properties of supraoptic nucleus neurons in-vitro. PhD Thesis, McGill University, Montreal 325 pp.

Bourque CW (1986). Calcium-dependent spike after-current induces burst firing in magnocellular neurosecretory cells. Neurosci Lett (in press).

Bourque CW, Randle JCR, Renaud LP (1985). Calcium-dependent potassium conductance in rat supraoptic nucleus neurosecretory neurons. J Neurophysiol 54: 1375-1382.

Bourque CW, Randle JCR, Renaud LP (1986). Non-synaptic depolarizing potentials in rat supraoptic neurones recorded in-vitro. J Physiol 376:493-505.

Bourque CW, Renaud LP (1983). Activity patterns and osmosensitivity of rat supraoptic neurones in perfused hypothalamic explants. J Physiol 349: 631-642.

Bourque CW, Renaud LP (1985a). Activity-dependence of action potential duration in rat supraoptic neurosecretory neurones recorded in-vitro. J Physiol 363: 429-439.

Bourque CW, Renaud LP (1985b). Calcium-dependent action potentials in rat supraoptic neurosecretory neurones recorded in-vitro. J Physiol 363: 419-428.

Cazalis M, Dayanithi G, Nordmann JJ (1985). The role of patterned burst and interburst interval on the excitation-coupling mechanism in the isolated rat neural lobe. J Physiol 369: 45-60.

Dudek FE, Hatton GI, MacVicar BA (1980). Intracellular recordings from the paraventricular nucleus in slices of rat hypothalamus. J Physiol 301: 101-114.

Dutton A, Dyball REJ (1979). Phasic firing enhances vasopressin release from the rat neurohypophysis. J Physiol 290: 433-440.

Hatton GI (1982). Phasic bursting activity of rat paraventricular neurones in the absence of synaptic transmission. J Physiol 327: 273-284.

Macvicar BA, Andrew RD, Dudek FE, Hatton GI (1982). Synaptic inputs and action potentials of magnocellular neuropeptidergic cells: Intracellular recording and staining in slices of rat hypothalamus. Brain Res Bull 8: 87-93.

Mason WT (1980). Supraoptic neurones of rat hypothalamus are osmosensitive. Nature 287: 154-157.

Mason WT (1983). Electrical properties of neurons recorded from the rat supraoptic nucleus in vitro. Proc R Soc Lond 217: 141-161.

Poulain DA, Wakerley JB (1982). Electrophysiology of hypothalamic magnocellular neurosecretory neurones secreting oxytocin and vasopressin. Neuroscience 7: 773-808.

Organization of the Autonomic Nervous System:
Central and Peripheral Mechanisms, pages 397–405
© 1987 Alan R. Liss, Inc.

GABAergic INHIBITION IN SUPRAOPTIC NUCLEUS NEUROSECRETORY
NEURONS - POSSIBLE ROLE IN A CENTRAL BAROREFLEX PATHWAY.

Leo P. Renaud, Jack H. Jhamandas and John
C.R. Randle

Neurosciences Unit, Montreal General Hospital
and McGill University, Montreal, Quebec,
Canada.

INTRODUCTION

Intracellular recordings obtained from in-vitro
hypothalamic slices and explants (see chapters by
Bourque, also Dudek and Gribkoff) reveal that the
vasopressin (VP) and oxytocin (OXY)-synthesizing
magnocellular neurosecretory neurons of the supraoptic
(SON) and paraventricular (PVN) nuclei are endowed with a
variety of intrinsic conductances that can determine
firing patterns and discharge frequencies. It is also
clear from extracellular recordings obtained in-vivo in
anesthetized preparations that these cells do not
function in isolation but rather that their neuronal
excitability can be modulated by a variety of extrinsic
stimuli. For example, cells increase their activity in
hyperosmolar (Brimble and Dyball, 1977) and hypovolemic
(Poulain et al., 1977) states, and in response to
activation of carotid chemoreceptors (Harris, 1979) or to
suckling (Lincoln and Wakerley, 1974). Alternatively, a
reduction in their excitability can be detected following
electrical stimulation in specific brain areas notably
the amygdala and septum (eg. Cirino and Renaud, 1985),
nucleus accumbens (Shibuki, 1984), subfornical organ (see
chapter by Ferguson) and diagonal band (Jhamandas and
Renaud, 1986b). The latter stimulus is unique in that
the depressant response preferentially affects putative
VP-secreting neurons, i.e. cells that fire in a phasic
manner (Poulain et al., 1977) and whose activity is
arrested transiently by a brief increase in mean
arterial pressure sufficient to activate peripheral

baroreceptors (Kannan and Yagi, 1978; Harris, 1979).

Given that afferent pathways to neurosecretory neurons are influential in regulating their excitability, and hence the release of VP and OXY into the systemic circulation, efforts have been made to identify both the neurotransmitter(s) involved in such pathways and their physiological role. With respect to the depressant response of a brief hypertension on VP-secreting cell activity referred to above, initial attention was focused on the rich catecholamine innervation of SON and PVN, and, in particular, on noradrenaline. An inhibitory action for this transmitter was originally proposed based on its beta-mediated depressant effects on SON and PVN neurons when applied by iontophoresis (Barker et al., 1971; Moss et al., 1972), and ability to suppress vasopressin secretion from organ-cultured hypothalamic explants (Armstrong et al., 1982). However, as reviewed elsewhere (see chapter by Day), the physiological role for noradrenaline in this system is most likely excitatory to promote an alpha 1 receptor mediated membrane depolarization (Randle et al., 1986b) and VP release (Randle et al., 1986c; Armstrong et al., 1986).

More recently, the search for an inhibitory transmitter to neurosecretory cells has focused on γ-aminobutyric acid, or GABA. Iontophoretic studies reveal that GABA has a potent, bicuculline sensitive, depressant action on SON neurosecretory neurons (Nicoll and Barker, 1971). Moreover, there is now clear ultrastructural evidence for GABAergic synapses on SON neurons (Van den Pol, 1985; Theodosis et al., 1986). The following section reports on the electrophysiology of a potent inhibitory input to SON neurosecretory neurons whose action mimics exogenously applied GABA, and whose role involves final mediation of a baroreceptor-activated depressant input to VP-secreting neurons.

DIAGONAL BAND-EVOKED IPSPs IN SON NEURONS

In perfused hypothalamic explants, intracellular recordings obtained with potassium acetate-filled micropipettes reveal the presence of spontaneous 1-20 mV inhibitory postsynaptic potentials (IPSPs) in SON neurons (Randle, Bourque & Renaud, 1986a). These IPSPs rise to peak in 3-5 msec and decay exponentially with a mean time constant of 20.2 msec i.e. 1.5 fold greater than the membrane time constant of 13.8 msec (n=9 cells). In most SON neurons electrical stimulation applied to the ventral surface of the diagonal band also evokes a prominent compound IPSP after a mean latency of 6.8 msec, rising to peak in 3-10 msec and decaying exponentially over 60-100 msec (Fig. 1 A,C). In 16 cells, the mean evoked IPSP time constant of decay was 37.0 msec, approximately 2.5 times their mean cell time constant.

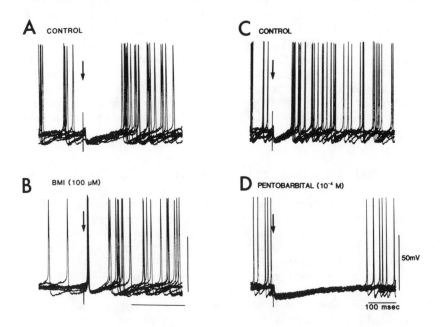

Figure 1: Superimposed oscilloscope traces of intracell-ular in-vitro recordings from an SON neuron in a perfused hypothalamic explant illustrate features of the IPSP evoked by an electrical stimulus (arrow) applied to the ventral surface of the diagonal band. Control sweeps (A,C) demonstrate a clear membrane hyperpolarization and a reduction in excitability during the IPSP. In the presence of bicuculline (B), the IPSP is lost and an underlying EPSP that evokes an action potential becomes apparent. In contrast, pentobarbitol (D) produces a marked prolongation in the duration of the IPSP and associated reduction in cell excitability.

As illustrated in Fig. 1 A,C, the membrane hyper-polarization during evoked IPSPs is accompanied by a reduction in cell excitability reflecting a marked increase in membrane conductance. Estimates of this conductance change vary widely between 0.17 and 3.0 nS for spontaneous IPSPs and between 0.8 and 22.0 nS for evoked IPSPs. These conductances represent an increase in membrane permeability to chloride ions. In control media, IPSP reversal potentials approximate -80 mV (Fig. 2C,D) but this can be shifted to more depolarized levels by intracellular injection of chloride ions or by changing the extracellular chloride ion concentration. Evoked IPSPs are further characterized by their sensitivity to bicuculline, which may unmask an underlying excitatory input (Fig. 1B), and by an almost 5-fold prolongation in their duration in the presence of barbiturates (Fig. 1D). Since these features collectively suggest a GABA-mediated inhibition, SON cells were examined for their sensitivity to this amino acid.

GABA-EVOKED INHIBITION IN SON NEURONS

Applications of GABA (30-50 uM) to the media perfusing hypothalamic explants consistently depress spontaneous activity of all SON neurons. In all cells this effect is associated with a prominent reduction in their membrane resistance (Fig. 2A,B). These changes in input resistance correspond to conductances of 10-50 nS. At these lower GABA concentrations, 60% of neurons display a transient membrane hyperpolarization (Fig. 2A) which has a similar reversal potential to that of evoked IPSPs (Fig. 2D). Muscimol, a GABA-A agonist, produces a similar change in membrane potential and conductance but with a 20 fold increase in potency (Fig. 2B). The slope of log-log plots of ligand induced currents as a function of ligand concentration is approximately 1.7 for both GABA and muscimol suggesting that two molecules combine to activate the ionophore, which in this situation is specific for chloride ions. The latter conclusion is based on arguments outlined previously for IPSPs and includes the sensitivity of GABA and muscimol-induced conductance and potential changes to alterations in intracellular and extracellular chloride ion concentrations and selective blockade by bicuculline (Fig. 2c; also Randle and Renaud, 1987).

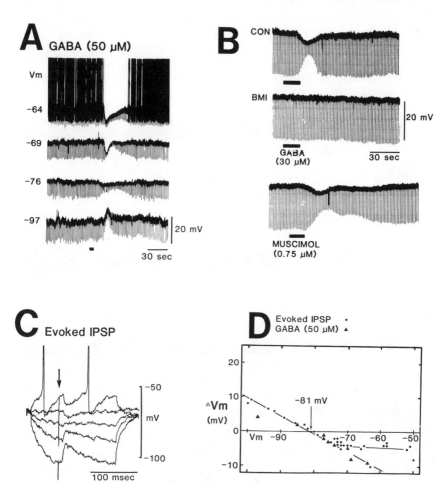

Figure 2: Relationship between the hyperpolarizing response to GABA and the IPSP evoked by diagonal band stimulation. In (A), GABA was administered to the bath while the membrane potential was adjusted by steady intracellular current injection and the sign and amplitude of the membrane voltage responses (Δ Vm) were plotted in (D) as a function of the membrane potential (Vm). Similarly in (C), the sign and amplitude of the IPSP was monitored as the membrane potential was adjusted by intracellular current pulses and Δ Vm plotted in (D) as a function of membrane potential. Note the virtually identical reversal potentials. The panels in (B) illustrate that the membrane response to GABA (30 uM) is blocked by bicuculline (100 uM) and mimicked by the GABA-A receptor agonist muscimol (0.75 uM).

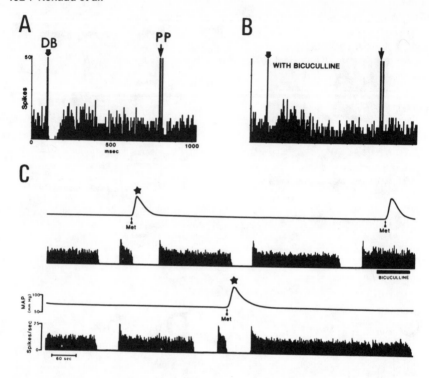

Figure 3: A: Poststimulus histogram (200 sweeps, 4 msec per bin) of data obtained from a VP-secreting SON neuron reveals a prominent reduction in excitability following a single stimulus in the diagonal band (DB; stimulus current 150 uA). For control, the histogram also contains the antidromic response to a posterior pituitary (PP) stimulus. B: In the presence of bicuculline (100 uM) applied by pressure from an adjacent pipette, the depressant response is lost and actually replaced in this instance by a longer latency increase in excitability. C: Two continuous ratemeter records from another SON VP-secreting neuron reveal several spontaneous phasic bursts. Above each ratemeter are simultaneous mean arterial pressure (MAP) tracings. Note that a brief increase in MAP induced by an intravenous injection of metaraminol (Met) prematurely arrests ongoing phasic firing in control conditions (*). This depressant action is transiently lost in the presence of bicuculline (100 uM) applied locally by pressure injection from an adjacent pipette.

IN-VIVO CORRELATES: GABA MEDIATES A CENTRAL BAROREFLEX
INHIBITION

Although in-vivo recordings from SON neurosecretory
neurons are necessarily extracellular, they do have the
distinct advantage in permitting a distinction to be made
between data from VP and OXY-secreting neurons, based on
their firing patterns and selective depressant influence
of peripheral baroreceptor activation on the excitability
of VP-secreting neurons (Harris, 1979). Electrical
stimulation in the diagonal band of Broca evokes a
selective depression in the excitability of VP-secreting
neurons and this depression can be reversibly blocked by
locally applied bicuculline in concentrations similar to
those that block both the in-vitro evoked IPSPs and the
actions of exogenously applied GABA (Fig. 3A,B).
Furthermore, we have observed that bicuculline, a GABA-A
receptor antagonist, but not other receptor antagonists
(eg. timolol, prazosin and strychnine) can also reversibly block the depressant influence of peripheral baroreceptor activation on VP-secreting neurons (Fig. 3C).
There are two reasons to infer an involvement of diagonal
band neurons in a central baroreflex pathway. First,
electrical stimulation in this site evokes a bicuculline-
sensitive inhibition that is selective for VP-secreting
neurons (Fig. 3A,B; also Jhamandas and Renaud, 1986b).
Second, a population of diagonal band neurons that
project to the SON area increase their firing rate in a
reciprocal manner to SON VP-secreting neurons when mean
arterial pressure is increased (Jhamandas and Renaud,
1986a). Collectively, these observations support the
notion of an endogenous GABAergic projection from the
diagonal band of Broca that may mediate the baroreflex
input selectively to vasopressinergic neurons of the SON.
At present, available morphological and immunocytochemical data do not allow for a precise localization of
the GABA interneuron to either the diagonal band or the
perinuclear zone of the SON.

Supported by the M.R.C. of Canada. JHJ and JCRR are
recipients of MRC Fellowships.

REFERENCES

Armstrong WE, Gallagher MJ, Sladek CD (1986) Noradrenergic stimulation of supraoptic neuronal activity and
vasopressin release in vitro: mediation by an α_1-
receptor. Brain Res 365:192-197.

Armstrong WE, Sladek CD, Sladek JR Jr. (1982) Characterization of of noradrenergic control of vasopressin
release by the organ-cultured rat hypothalamoneurohypo-
physeal system. Endocrinology 111:273-279.

Barker JL, Crayton JW, Nicoll RA (1971) Noradrenaline
and acetylcholine responses of supraoptic neurosecretory cells. J Physiol 218:19-32.

Brimble MJ Dyball REJ (1977) Characterization of the
responses of oxytocin- and vasopressin-secreting
neurones in the supraoptic nucleus to osmotic stimulation. J Physiol 271:253-271.

Cirino M, Renaud LP (1985) Influence of lateral septum
and amygdala stimulation on the excitability of
hypothalamic supraoptic neurons. An electrophysiological study in the rat. Brain Res 326:357-361.

Harris MC, (1979) Effects of chemoreceptor and baroreceptor stimulation on the discharge of hypothalamic
supraoptic neurones in rats. J Endocrinol 82:115-125.

Jhamandas JH, Renaud LP (1986a) Diagonal band neurons
may mediate arterial baroreceptor input to hypothalamic
vasopressin-secreting neurons. Neurosci Lett 65:214-
218.

Jhamandas JH, Renaud LP (1986b) A gamma aminobutyric
acid- mediated baroreceptor input to supraoptic vasopressin neurones in the rat. J Physiol (in press).

Kannan H, Yagi K (1978) Supraoptic neurosecretory
neurones: evidence for the existence of converging
inputs from carotid baroreceptors and osmoreceptors.
Brain Res 145:385-390.

Lincoln DW, Wakerley JB (1974) Electrophysiological
evidence for the activation of supraoptic neurones
during the release of oxytocin. J Physiol 242:533-554.

Moss RL, Urban I, Cross BA (1972) Microiontophoresis of
cholinergic and aminergic drugs on paraventricular
neurons. Am J Physiol 233:310-318.

Nicoll RA, Barker JL (1971) The pharmacology of
recurrent inhibition in the supraoptic neurosecretory
system. Brain Res 15:501-511.

Poulain DA, Wakerley JB, Dyball REJ (1977) Electro-physiological differentiation of oxytocin- and vasopressin-secreting neurones. Proc R Soc Lond B 196:367-384.

Randle JCR, Bourque CW, Renaud LP (1986a) Characterization of spontaneous and evoked inhibitory postsynaptic potentials in rat supraoptic neurosecre-tory neurons in vitro. J Neurophysiol (in press).

Randle JCR, Day TA, Jhamandas JH, Bourque CW, Renaud LP (1986b) Neuropharmacology of supraoptic nucleus neurons: noradrenergic and GABAergic receptors. Fed Proc 45:2312-2317.

Randle MCR, Mazurek M, Kneifel D, Dufresne J, Renaud LP (1986c) α1-adrenergic receptor activation releases vasopressin and oxytocin from perfused rat hypothalamic explants. Neurosci Lett 65:219-223.

Randle JCR, Renaud LP (1987) Actions of gamma-aminobutyric acid in rat supraoptic nucleus neurosecretory neurones in vitro. J Physiol (in press).

Shibuki K (1984) Supraoptic neurosecretory cells: synap-tic inputs from the nucleus accumbens in the rat. Exp Brain Res 53:341-348.

Theodosis DT, Paul L, Tappaz ML (1986) Immunocyto-chemical analysis of the GABAergic innervation of oxytocin- and vasopressin-secreting neurons in the rat supraoptic nucleus. Neurosci 19:207-222.

Van Den Pol A (1985) Dual ultrastructural localization of two neurotransmitter-related antigens: colloidal gold-labeled neurophysin-immunoreactive supraoptic neurons receive peroxidase-labeled glutamate decarboxy-lase- or gold-labeled GABA-immunoreactive synapses. J Neurosci 5:2940-2954.

Organization of the Autonomic Nervous System:
Central and Peripheral Mechanisms, pages 407–416
© **1987 Alan R. Liss, Inc.**

THE EFFECTS OF GAMMA-AMINOBUTYRIC ACID ON ELECTRICAL
ACTIVITY OF NEURONS IN THE GUINEA-PIG SUPRAOPTIC NUCLEUS IN
VITRO

Nobukuni Ogata

Department of Pharmacology, Faculty of Medicine,
Kyushu University, Fukuoka 812, Japan

INTRODUCTION

The supraoptic nucleus contains high levels of γ-aminobutyric acid (GABA) and the enzyme responsible for its biosynthesis, glutamic acid decarboxylase (GAD), (Tappaz et al., 1977). The magnocellular neurons in the supraoptic nucleus are surrounded by GAD-positive puncta (Vincent et al., 1982). Although these neurochemical findings strongly implicate a major role for GABA in the hypothalamo-neurohypophysial regulation, the functional significance of GABA in this neuroendocrine regulation is poorly understood.

The inhibitory postsynaptic potential (IPSP) occurs in supraoptic neurons after pituitary stalk stimulation (Nicoll et al., 1970; Yamashita et al., 1970). However, the transmitter involved in such recurrent inhibition remains to be identified. GABA consistently depressed the activity of supraoptic neurons (Arnauld et al., 1983) and influenced the release of posterior pituitary hormones (Feldberg and Silva, 1978), suggesting that GABA may be a transmitter of the recurrent inhibition in the supraoptic nucleus.

We investigated the mode of action of GABA in the supraoptic nucleus using the brain slice preparation, where intracellular activity can be recorded for extended periods and drugs can be applied under modified ionic environments. The findings obtained in the supraoptic nucleus were compared with observations in the hippocampus and the anterior hypothalamus, in order to characterize the significance of GABA-mediated action in the supraoptic nucleus.

METHODS

Adult guinea-pigs of either sex were decapitated, and coronal slices of the hypothalamus (400–600 μm thick) were prepared using a vibratome. Slices prepared from the hippocampus (Inoue et al., 1985a) or the anterior hypothalamus (Ogata and Abe, 1982) were also used. Procedures for incubation and recording were as described (Inoue et al., 1985a).

Intracellular recordings were made from the posterior half of the supraoptic nucleus through conventional glass micro-electrodes filled with 2M potassium acetate. Electrical signals were led through a high input resistance DC amplifier and recorded on a pen-recorder. To facilitate illustration of the spike component, a pen-recorder with a relatively broader high-frequency band width but with a non-linear amplification was used for some of the illustrations.

A single electrical pulse of 50 μsec duration was applied to an area adjacent to the tip of the recording electrode (about 0.5–1 mm distance) through twisted tungsten needles (diameter, 50 μm) insulated except for the tips. Membrane input resistance was measured routinely by passing hyperpolarizing current pulses (0.4 Hz, 0.5 sec duration) of known intensity through the recording electrode. Drugs were applied to the bathing solution in fixed concentrations.

RESULTS

GABA consistently depolarized the membrane, decreased the input resistance, and suppressed the spontaneous firings throughout the concentrations used (10^{-7}-10^{-3}M)(see Fig. 1). Spike generations were consistently suppressed. The action of GABA was completely antagonized by bicuculline (10^{-6} – 10^{-5}M) which did not affect, per se, electrical activity.

Fig. 1 shows the response of the supraoptic cell to GABA at various membrane potentials produced by polarizing DC current injections. The firing pattern at periods indicated by broken lines is shown at the bottom of respective traces. The reversal potential for the depolarization induced by GABA was about 26mV positive to the resting membrane potential.

To examine the specificity of the GABA-response in the

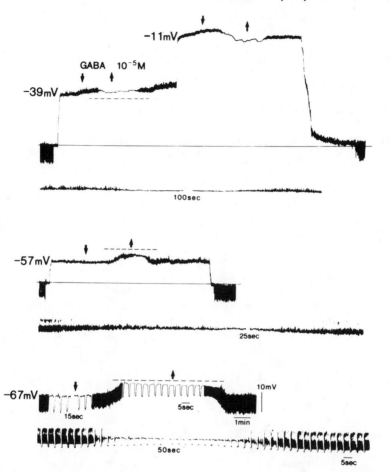

Fig. 1. Voltage dependence of the GABA-induced depolarization in the supraoptic nucleus. In this and subsequent
Figures: downward and upward arrows represent the duration
of superfusion of test solution; repetitive negative
deflections reflect the electrotonic potentials to inward
current injections of constant intensity; the recorder speed
was intermittently accelerated to display voltage transients
produced by current injection; time shown under gaps in the
trace indicates an omitted period; spikes were almost
entirely eliminated from the traces due to the limited
frequency band width of the pen-recorder; upward deflection
represents positive polarity; and inset traces were recorded
by a pen-recorder having a broader high-frequency band
width.

supraoptic nucleus, the action of GABA was examined in several brain regions. The action of GABA in the hippocampus was multiphasic comprising depolarizing and hyperpolarizing components (Fig. 2).

HIPPOCAMPUS

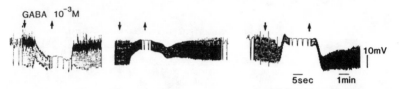

Fig. 2. Effects of GABA on the electrical activity of hippocampal CA3 pyramidal cells. Traces were recorded from different neurones.

GABA (10^{-6} - 10^{-5} M) consistently induced a hyperpolarization in the anterior hypothalamus. Fig. 3 shows the voltage-dependence of the GABA-induced hyperpolarization. The reversal point was about 13 mV negative the resting membrane potential ($n=3$). The hyperpolarization induced by GABA (10^{-5} M) was reversed to depolarization when the concentration of Cl^- in the medium was reduced to 10.2 mM.

Baclofen (β-chlorophenyl-GABA), a derivative of GABA and an agonist for bicuculline-resistant Cl^--independent $GABA_B$ receptors, had no detectable effect on the electrical activity in the supraoptic nucleus in concentrations up to 10^{-4} M, whereas this drug (10^{-7}-10^{-5} M) induced potent hyperpolarizations in the hippocampus and the anterior hypothalamus (Fig. 4).

Depolarizing potentials, either spontaneous (Fig. 5A) or evoked by electrical stimulation of an area adjacent to the recording electrode (Fig. 5B-E), were observed in the supraoptic nucleus. These potentials seemed to be spontaneous or evoked synaptic potentials (PSPs), since they often had a spike superimposed, disappeared in Ca^{2+}-free medium and had reversal level at about 30mV positive to the resting membrane potential (see Fig. 5A).

Fig. 5B summarizes the effects of d-tubocurarine on the evoked (upper traces) and spontaneous (lower traces) PSPs.

ANTERIOR HYPOTHALAMUS

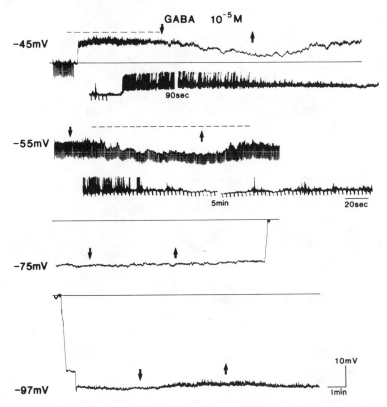

Fig. 3. Voltage dependence of the GABA-induced hyperpolarization in the anterior hypothalamus.

These PSPs were reversibly blocked by d-tubocurarine. Atropine exerted a minimal effect on the EPSP (Fig. 5C, upper traces), whereas the spike on the EPSP was blocked. Atropine also depressed the spontaneous firings (Fig. 5C, lower trace). Our systematic study of the evoked response in which the stimulating electrode was moved arbitrarily around the recording electrode revealed that almost all the PSPs were sensitive to d-tubocurarine, although this does of course not exclude a possible involvement of different types

of synaptic potentials. In no case, we found any hyperpolarizing response which could be discriminated from the
spike afterhyperpolarization.

Since GABA consistently depolarized the cell in the
supraoptic nucleus, it may be that the PSPs were mediated by
endogenously released GABA. However, as shown in Fig. 5D,
when the stimulus intensity was successively augmented, the
synaptic potential enlarged inducing a spike generation,
thereby indicating an excitatory nature. Furthermore, a
high concentration of bicuculline exerted no detectable
action on the synaptic potential (Fig. 5E).

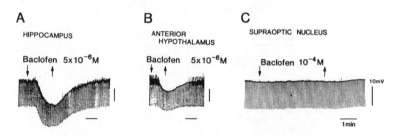

Fig. 4. Effects of baclofen on electrical activities in the
hippocampal (A), anterior hypothalamic (B) and supraoptic
(C) neurones.

Fig. 6 confirms that the GABA-mediated recurrent
inhibitory mechanism does operate in the hippocampus. The
mossy fiber stimulation evoked an IPSP (A, left). When
bicuculline (10^{-5}M) was added to the medium, the IPSP
disappeared and epileptiform discharges were generated (A,
right). Substitution of NaCl in the medium with an equimolar
amount of Na-isothionate resulted in an explosive excitation
of neurons, as revealed by a repetitive generation of burst
discharges (see inset in Fig. 6B). The replacement of total
external NaCl with an equimolar amount of Na-isothionate
shifted a DC potential level. However, this shift was
mostly due to a change in liquid junction potentials (Inoue
et al., 1985b). These observations are in remarkable
contrast with the finding in the supraoptic nucleus. Neither
the low Cl$^-$ medium nor bicuculline by themselves had
effect on either the input resistance or cellular firing
pattern.

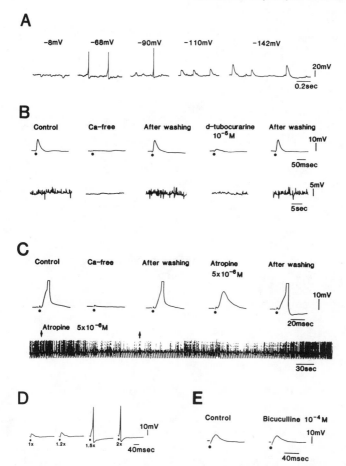

Fig. 5. Effects of drugs on the evoked potentials recorded intracellularly in the supraoptic nucleus. A, spontaneous EPSPs recorded at different membrane potential levels produced by inward and outward DC current injections. B and C: upper traces, responses to the local electrical stimulation delivered to an area about 0.5–1 mm dorsal to the recording electrode; lower traces, spontaneous activity. In D, the stimulus intensity was augmented successively to 1.2, 1.5 and 2 times the control. Traces in A were recorded on X-ray film. Traces in B–E were recorded on a storage oscilloscope and written on an X-Y recorder, except for lower traces of B and C which were recorded with a pen-recorder having a broader high-frequency band width. Dots in B–E represent the local electrical stimulation.

Hippocampus

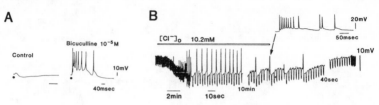

Fig. 6. Effects of bicuculline (A) and low external Cl⁻ on the hippocampal CA3 neurons. A, responses to a single electrical pulse of 50 sec duration applied to the mossy fibers (dots) recorded on an X-ray photograph. B, At the period indicated by a bar, NaCl in the medium was totally replaced by equimolar amounts of Na-iscthionate. The change in external Cl⁻ concentration caused artifactual DC shift (see text). The inset illustrates the epileptiform burst recorded on an X-ray photograph and which is reflected on the pen-recording as a sharp positive deflection.

DISCUSSION

The action of GABA in the supraoptic nucleus was consistently depolarizing throughout a wide range of concentration, and its reversal potential was positive to the resting membrane potential. I have reported that the depolarization induced by GABA was sensitive to a change in the external Cl⁻ concentration and readily blocked by a low concentration of bicuculline (Ogata, 1986). Thus, the action of GABA in the supraoptic nucleus may be mediated by classical GABA$_A$ receptors linked to Cl⁻ channels.

The biphasic pattern of the GABA response in the hippocampus has been explained by a rapid redistribution of Cl⁻ subsequent to activation of a single class of Cl⁻ channels. However, I have shown that the biphasic GABA response in the hippocampus is mediated by at least two receptor-ionophore complexes: one, low-affinity receptors linked to the picrotoxin-sensitive Cl⁻ channel and responsible for the depolarizing action; the other, high-affinity receptors linked to the K⁺ channel and responsible for the hyperpolarizing action (Inoue et al., 1985b).

GABA exerts a variety of membrane effects on vertebrate neurons (for review see Iversen, 1978). It is tempting therefore to speculate that the diversity of the GABA response noted in various central neurons may arise from the multiplicity of GABA receptors rather than from the different electrochemical gradient for Cl^- ions. In this respect, supraoptic neurons would possess only one type of receptor, i.e., those linked to Cl^- channels. This speculation would be strengthened by the finding that baclofen, which appears to share the hyperpolarizing action with GABA possibly through activation of the postsynaptic $GABA_B$ receptors linked to K^+ channels (Inoue et al., 1985a), had no effect on the supraoptic neurons whereas this drug in much lower concentrations causes prominent hyperpolarizations in hippocampal and anterior hypothalamic neurons which were in fact hyperpolarized by GABA.

The mechanism underlying inhibition of cellular firings subsequent to antidromic activation of magnocellular neuroendocrine cells remains controversial. In our intracellular recordings from supraoptic neurons, the action of GABA was consistently a depolarization and we failed to demonstrate an IPSP. Thus, GABA may not be a transmitter responsible for the hyperpolarizing IPSP at least in the guinea pig supraoptic nucleus. In this respect, it was recently shown that a Ca^{2+}-activated K^+ conductance, rather than recurrent synaptic inhibition, apparently causes hyperpolarization following spikes and is at least partly responsible for the pause in firings after spikes in magnocellular neurons (Andrew and Dudek, 1984).

The depolarizing IPSPs mediated by GABA have been demonstrated in several brain regions (e.g.,Brown and Scholfield, 1975). It is unlikely, however, that GABA in the supraoptic nucleus plays such a role, since neither an application of bicuculline nor a reduction of external Cl^-, which would lead to a drastic increase in cellular excitability, had any detectable effect in this tissue. This finding might alternatively implicate that the GABAergic terminals impinging onto the supraoptic neurons originate from cells outside the supraoptic nucleus.

REFERENCES

Andrew RD, Dudek FE (1984). Intrinsic inhibition in magnocellular neuroendocrine cells of rat hypothalamus. J Physiol 353: 171–185.

Arnauld E, Cirino M, Layton BS, Renaud LP (1983). Contrasting actions of amino acids, acetylcholine, noradrenaline and leucine enkephalin on the excitability of supraoptic vasopressin-secreting neurons. Neuroendocrinology 36: 187–196.

Brown DA, Scholfield CN (1979). Depolarization of neurones in the isolated olfactory cortex of the guinea-pig by γ-aminobutyric acid. Brit J Pharmacol 65: 339–345.

Feldberg W, Rocha E Silva JR M (1978). Vasopressin release produced in anaesthetized cats by antagonists of γ-aminobutyric acid and glycine. Brit J Pharmacol 62: 99–106.

Inoue M, Matsuo T, Ogata N (1985a). Baclofen activates voltage-dependent and 4-aminopyridine sensitive K^+ conductance in guinea-pig hippocampal pyramidal cells maintained in vitro. Brit J Pharmacol 84: 833–841.

Inoue M, Matsuo T, Ogata N (1985b). Characterization of pre- and postsynaptic actions of (–)-baclofen in the guinea-pig hippocampus in vitro. Brit J Pharmacol 86: 515–524.

Iversen LL (1978). Biochemical psychopharmacology of GABA. In Psychopharmacology: A Generation of Progress, ed. Lipton MA, Dimascio A, Killam RF pp. 25–38. New York: Raven.

Nicoll RA, Crayton JW, Barker JL (1970). Antidromic and orthodromic responses in supraoptic neurosecretory cells. Physiologist 13: 272.

Ogata N (1986). Gamma-aminobutyric acid causes consistent depolarization of neurons in the guinea-pig supraoptic nucleus due to an absence of $GABA_B$ recognition sites. Brain Res (in press).

Ogata N, Abe H (1982). Neuropharmacology in the brain slice: effects of substance P on neurons in the guinea-pig hypothalamus. Comp Biochem Physiol 72 C: 171178.

Tappaz ML, Brownstein MJ, Kopin JJ (1977). Glutamate decarboxylase (GAD) and γ-aminobutyric acid (GABA) in discrete nuclei of hypothalamus and substantia nigra. Brain Res 125: 109–121.

Vincent SR, Hökfelt T, Wu JY (1982). GABA neuron systems in hypothalamus and the pituitary gland. Neuroendocrinology 34: 117–125.

Yamashita H, Koizumi K, Brooks C McC (1970). Electrophysiological studies of neurosecretory cells in the cat hypothalamus. Brain Res 20: 462–466.

Organization of the Autonomic Nervous System:
Central and Peripheral Mechanisms, pages 417–423
© 1987 Alan R. Liss, Inc.

THE EFFECTS OF NORADRENALINE ON SUPRAOPTIC AND
PARAVENTRICULAR CELLS OF MICE *IN VITRO*

Hiroshi Yamashita, Richard E.J. Dyball[*], Kiyotoshi
Inenaga and Hiroshi Kannan

Department of Physiology, University of
Occupational and Environmental Health, [*]School of
Medicine, Kitakyushu 807 Japan: permanent
address, Department of Anatomy, University of
Cambridge, Cambridge CB2 3DY, UK

INTRODUCTION

Many hypothalamic nuclei receive a profuse ascending
input from the noradrenergic system of the brainstem. The
cells in the A1 region project, among other regions, to the
magnocellular nuclei and also to the periventricular region
of the paraventricular nucleus but the periventricular
region appears more complex since it also receives input
from the A2 and A6 areas (Swanson and Sawchenko, 1981).
Despite earlier reports that iontophoretically applied
noradrenaline (NA) inhibited cells in the magnocellular
nuclei (Barker et al. 1971; Moss et al. 1972) it was found
that stimulation of the A1 region excited these cells (Day
et al. 1984; Day and Renaud, 1984; Kannan et al. 1984). The
present experiments were undertaken in an attempt to resolve
this apparent inconsistency and to investigate the receptor
subtype involved in the noradrenergic control of the
magnocellular nuclei.

METHODS

Conventional brain slices 350-500 μ thick were cut
either coronally or sagittally from mouse brains and
incubated in a modified Yamamoto's medium (with NaCl 124 mM
and $CaCl_2$ 2.1 mM) at 35-36°C and bubbled continuously with
O_2 (95%) and CO_2 (5%). Recordings were made with
extracellular glass micropipettes filled with 0.5 M sodium
acetate and 2% Pontamine-sky blue.

The fluorescent catecholaminergic fibres were stained using the glyoxylic acid method and subsequently counterstained with cresyl violet to determine the outlines of the different hypothalamic nuclei.

RESULTS

The fluorescent micrograph (Figure 1) shows that the hypothalamus receives a profuse catecholaminergic input which is particularly profuse in the ventral part of the supraoptic nucleus (SON).

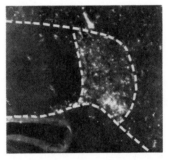

Figure 1. Fluorescent catecholaminergic fibres in the hypothalamus induced by the glyoxylic acid method. The triangular outline of the supraoptic nucleus can be discerned and the intensity of fluorescence seems to be more intense ventrally.

Stimulation at different sites round the supraoptic nucleus in the slice showed that cells in the nucleus can respond to afferent stimulation by both excitation and by inhibition.

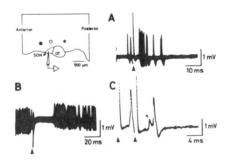

Figure 2. The diagram (upper left) shows, in a parasagittal

slice, the approximate positions of the stimulation sites which (with pulses of 0.3 ms duration and 0.5 mA) gave excitation ($\bullet$, A) inhibition (O,B) or antidromic activation (*, C) of supraoptic cells; arrowheads indicate the time of application of stimulus pulses and, in C the small arrowhead, fractionation of the antidromic spike.

Application of noradrenaline to the slices excited 41 of 43 cells tested in the supraoptic nucleus and the only 2 which were inhibited fired faster (>4Hz) than most of the other cells (average 1.6Hz). The excitation was dose related in the range 10^{-6} to 10^{-4} (Figure 3).

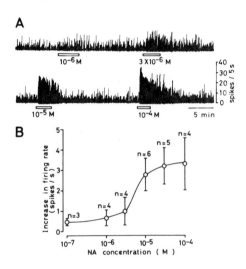

Figure 3. The dose relationship between the firing rate of SON cells and NA concentration; the upper part (A) shows individual ratemeter records and the lower part data from 7 SON cells.

The excitatory effects of NA could be mimicked by the α_1 agonists phenylephrine and methoxamine but the α_2 agonist clonidine and the β agonist isoproterenol had weak and inconsistent effects. The effects of antagonists were consistent with these results since the α_2 antagonist had no consistent effect but the α_1 antagonist prazosin blocked or reversed the effects of NA (see Figure 4). Inhibition of the illustrated cell by NA while it was still influenced by prazosin may indicate that the cell also had other receptors (α_2 or β) for NA.

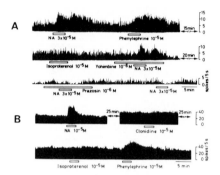

Figure 4. Ratemeter records to illustrate the effects of different NA agonists and antagonists on cells in the SON. α_1 agonists excited these cells and α_1 antagonists depressed them but other agonists and antagonists had little effect on their activity (from Inenaga et al. 1986).

Not all hypothalamic cells behaved in the same way as the magnocellular cells. When cells in the periventricular region were tested, the effects were much less homogeneous. Their responses seemed to fall broadly into 2 categories, those which were excited by NA and behaved in some respects like cells in the magnocellular nuclei and those which were inhibited by NA.

Those cells which were excited by NA, like the magnocellular cells showed a graded response as concentration was increased and the excitatory effects were antagonized by prazosin. The situation was slightly more complex however because the excitation could, in some cases, be partly antagonized by the β antagonist propranolol. This indicates the probable presence of β as well as α_1 receptors.

The responses of those cells which were inhibited by NA also indicated that there was more than 1 type of receptor on their cell surface (Figure 5). Some cells were inhibited by relatively high concentrations of NA but excited by lower concentrations. Methoxamine (α_1 agonist) and isoproterenol (β agonist) slightly increased but clonidine (α_2 agonist) strongly inhibited such a cell (Figure 5). Another cell was inhibited by NA initially but yohimbine (α_2 antagonist) reversed the inhibition.

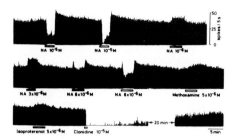

Figure 5. Representative responses of periventricular cells which were inhibited by NA. The activity of the cell was inhibited by high concentrations of NA but excited by lower concentrations and by methoxamine (α_1 agonist); with intermediate concentrations there was a reproducible "on" and "off" excitation which probably occurred as the concentration changed. The β agonist isoproterenol also slightly excited it but the α_2 agonist clonidine caused prolonged inhibition.

All the effects described above appear to be the result of a direct action of the different agonists and antagonists on the cells from which the recordings were made. Both inhibitory and excitatory responses were seen in medium with a lowered calcium concentration and a raised magnesium concentration which blocks synaptic transmission under the conditions used. The effects were thus direct and not the result of an action on other cells with an input to the recorded cells.

DISCUSSION

The majority (91%) of cells recorded from the SON of mice which included both phasic firing (putative vasopressin) and continuously firing (putative oxytocin) cells were excited by NA. Since the proportion of excited cells was so high and because cells with both types of firing pattern were excited it is likely that both oxytocin and vasopressin cells in the SON are excited by an ascending noradrenergic input. While there is evidence that noradrenergic fibres predominate in the ventral part of the nucleus which contains a majority of vasopressin cell bodies (Swanson et al. 1981), it is quite possible that oxytocin cells receive noradrenergic input through ventrally projecting dendrites.

Our results also indicate that the majority of SON cells are excited by α_1 receptors. Furthermore the responses appear to be direct and not to be mediated via interneurones since they persist after synaptic blockade with lowered calcium and raised magnesium concentrations. Since the responses differ from at least one population of other hypothalamic cells it is also probable that they are specific to the particular cell type and not a feature of all hypothalamic cells. There is however some evidence that there is more than 1 receptor type on the surface of the SON cells since, after α_1 blockade with prazosin, NA inhibited rather than excited SON cells. The differences between the effects of iontophoretically applied NA *in vivo* and bath applied NA *in vitro* may be explained if the different techniques expose different populations of receptors to NA.

We are grateful for support from the Ministry of Education, Japan, the British Council and the Japan Society for the Promotion of Science.

REFERENCES

Barker JL, Crayton JW, Nicholl RA (1971). Noradrenaline and acetylcholine responses of supraoptic neurosecretory cells. J Physiol (London) 281:19-32.

Day TA, Ferguson AV, Renaud LP (1984). Facilitatory influence of noradrenergic afferents on the excitability of rat paraventricular nucleus neurosecretory cells. J Physiol (London) 355:237-249.

Day TA, Renaud LP (1984). Electrophysiological evidence that noradrenergic afferents selectively facilitate the activity of supraoptic vasopressin neurons. Brain Research 303:233-240.

Inenaga K, Dyball REJ, Okuya S, Yamashita H (1986). Characterization of hypothalamic noradrenaline receptors in the supraoptic nucleus and periventricular region of the paraventricular nucleus of mice *in vitro*. Brain Research 369:37-47.

Kannan H, Yamashita H, Osaka T (1984). Paraventricular neurosecretory neurons: synaptic inputs from the ventrolateral medulla in rats. Neurosci Lett 51:183-188.

Moss RL, Urban I, Cross BA (1972). Microelectrophoresis of cholinergic and aminergic drugs on paraventricular neurons. Am J Physiol 223:310-318.

Swanson LW, Sawchenko PE (1981). Hypothalamic integration: organization of the paraventricular and supraoptic nuclei. Ann Rev Neurosci 6:269-324.
Swanson LW, Sawchenko PE, Berod A, Hartman BK, Helle KB, Van Orden DE (1981). An immunohistochemical study of the organization of catecholaminergic cells and terminal fields in the paraventricular and supraoptic nuclei of the hypothalamus. J Comp Neurol 196:271-285.

**Organization of the Autonomic Nervous System:
Central and Peripheral Mechanisms, pages 425–434**
© **1987 Alan R. Liss, Inc.**

ROLE OF A1 NORADRENERGIC AFFERENTS IN THE CONTROL OF
VASOPRESSIN SECRETION : *IN VIVO* ELECTROPHYSIOLOGICAL
STUDIES

Trevor A. Day

Department of Physiology and Centre for
Neuroscience,
University of Otago Medical School,
Dunedin, New Zealand.

The release of arginine vasopressin (AVP) from the
neurohypophysis is governed in large part by inputs arising
from sensory receptors located in the periphery. The pathways by which this sensory information reaches the
hypothalamus are unknown. In this regard, however, there
has for some time been considerable interest in the fact
that AVP neurosecretory cells, which are located in the
supraoptic (SON) and paraventricular (PVN) nuclei, receive
a significant projection from noradrenaline (NA) containing
neurons of the brainstem (Fuxe, 1965). Although pharmacological studies directed at elucidating the effect of NA on
AVP secretion have yielded contradictory findings (cf Day
et al., 1985b for refs.), it has generally been held that
NA, and therefore NA-containing afferents, are inhibitory to
AVP release. This view initially stemmed from the observation
that iontophoretically-applied NA commonly inhibits neurosecretory cell discharge *in vivo* (Barker *et al.*, 1971; Moss
et al., 1971, 1972).

In 1981 Sawchenko and Swanson demonstrated that NA
terminal fibers which surround the perikarya of neurosecretory cells originate primarily from neurons located in
the caudal ventrolateral medulla (A1 group of Dahlstrom and
Fuxe, 1964). Moreover, their data indicated that there were
extremely few non-NA cells in that region which projected to
either SON or PVN. Consequently, it was apparent that one
could examine the effects of selectively activating a
population of NA afferents which project directly to AVP
neurosecretory cells. The results which this approach

yielded contradict the view that NA afferents are inhibitory
to AVP release, and have led to a wider re-examination of
the neuropharmacological actions of NA on AVP cells, as will
be described.

The data presented here are taken from studies
conducted in collaboration with L.P. Renaud, A.V. Ferguson,
J.H. Jhamandas and J.C.R. Randle (Day and Renaud, 1984;
Day et al., 1984; Day et al., 1985a; Day et al., 1985b),
and from unpublished experiments by the author.

IN VIVO IDENTIFICATION OF NEUROSECRETORY AVP CELLS

When recording unit activity in the SON or PVN, neurosecretory cells may readily be identified by antidromic
invasion from the neurohypophysis. Furthermore, in the
anaesthetized rat it is also considered possible to
differentiate between AVP and oxytocinergic neurosecretory
cells. In the rat, active neurosecretory cells generally
exhibit either a continuous or a distinctive phasic pattern
of discharge. Stimuli which alter AVP release elicit
corresponding changes in the activity of phasic cells,
whereas stimuli which alter oxytocin release affect the
discharge of most continuous but not phasic units (cf.
Banks and Harris, 1984 and Day et al., 1984 for refs.).
The suggestion that AVP and oxytocinergic cells may be
differentiated on the basis of firing pattern is supported
by in vitro studies in which phasic SON and PVN neurons
have been immunohistochemically identified as AVP-containing
(Cobbett et al., 1986; Yamashita et al., 1983). However,
some continuously discharging neurosecretory cells develop
phasic firing patterns when in a more active state; thus,
it has proven useful to also examine cell responses to
baroreceptor activation, a stimulus thought to inhibit AVP
but not oxytocinergic neurons. In the present studies,
neurosecretory cells which were phasically active, or continuously active but inhibited by baroreceptor activation
(cf. Fig. 1), were classified as AVP-secreting.

FACILITATORY EFFECTS OF A1 STIMULATION

The effect of electrical stimulation of the A1 cell
group area on AVP cell activity was examined in pentobarbital
anaesthetized male Sprague Dawley rats. Cathodal pulses

(0.1 ms, 25-200 µA) delivered within 200-300 µm of the
centre of the A1 cell group enhanced the activity of all SON
(37/37;   Fig. 1) and 78% of PVN (14/18) putative AVP cells
tested.   For PVN responses the mean onset latency was 39.4 ms
(± 1.8 ms SE), which is in good agreement with the low
conduction velocities reported for NA fibres in rat CNS
(Moore and Guyenet, 1983).   Further evidence that A1
stimulation effects were mediated via NA afferents was
provided in the observation that NA terminal plexus
destruction, by microinjection of the neurotoxin 6-hydroxy-
dopamine (6.8 µg in 0.25 µl saline), abolished AVP cell
responses.

These data indicate that A1 NA afferents are likely to
play a facilitatory role in the regulation of AVP secretion.
This suggestion is supported by the recent findings of other
groups who have confirmed that A1 stimulation excites
putative AVP cells in the PVN (Kannan *et al.*, 1984;   Tanaka
et al., 1985), and have demonstrated that chemical

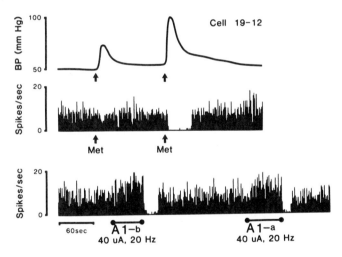

Fig. 1:   Ratemeter and blood pressure records showing effects
of baroreceptor activation (iv bolus of vasoconstrictor
metaraminol) and repetitive A1 stimulation on activity of
putative AVP cell in SON.   Record obtained from animal with
C7 cord transection (cf. Day and Renaud, 1984).   Note the
suppressant effect of baroreceptor activation and the
excitation elicited by A1 stimulation at 2 rostro-caudal
levels.

stimulation of the A1 group increases plasma levels of AVP, as determined by RIA (Blessing and Willoughby, 1985a).

DOSE-DEPENDENT ACTIONS OF NA

The finding that activation of NA afferents excited AVP cells brought into question the effects of NA itself. While previous *in vivo* studies had shown that iontophoretically applied NA generally inhibited neurosecretory neurons, recent *in vitro* work suggested that NA could also exert excitatory effects (Randle *et al.*, 1984; Wakerley *et al.*, 1983). Because of evidence that iontophoretic application procedures produce variable and often surprisingly high local drug concentrations (Armstrong-James *et al.*, 1981), it was decided to re-examine the actions of NA when applied by pressure from micropipettes positioned adjacent to the recording electrode tip. This approach revealed that the *in vivo* effects of exogenously applied NA were dose-dependent. When applied at intra-barrel concentrations of 50-500 µM, NA excited 71% (62/87) of SON putative AVP cells tested. As the concentration of NA applied was increased, however, so was the frequency with which inhibitory responses were elicited: 50-150 µM, 2% (1/45); 200-500µM, 17% (7/42); 1-100 mM, 79% (11/14). These contrasting actions were found to be receptor specific (Fig. 2). The excitatory effects of low concentrations of NA were blocked by the α_1-antagonist prazosin but unaltered by application of the α_2-antagonist yohimbine or the β-antagonist timolol. The depressant actions of high doses of NA, however, were readily blocked by timolol, suggesting that NA-induced inhibitions were β-adrenoreceptor mediated, as has been reported in the earlier iontophoretic studies (Barker *et al.*, 1971).

That NA is capable of exciting neurosecretory AVP cells is in keeping with numerous earlier reports, hitherto largely ignored, that AVP secretion is enhanced following central administration of NA (cf. Day, 1985b for refs.). Additionally, 2 recent studies have now demonstrated that NA and the α_1-agonist phenylephrine stimulate AVP release from hypo-thalamoneurohypophysial explants (Armstrong *et al.*, 1986; Randle *et al.*, 1986).

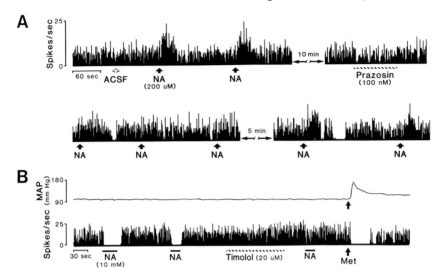

Fig. 2: Ratemeter records from 2 putative AVP neurosecretory cells in SON. A: Excitation produced by brief
pressure application of 200 μM NA was reversibly blocked
by local application of the α_1-antagonist prazosin.
B: Inhibitory actions of a high concentration of NA (10mM)
were blocked by the β-antagonist timolol. Note that
baroreceptor-induced inhibition was unaffected.

IDENTITY OF THE A1 NA AFFERENT NEUROTRANSMITTER

The data summarized thus far suggest that A1 NA
afferents facilitate neurosecretory AVP cell activity via
the interaction of locally released NA with α_1-adreno-
receptors. It was of considerable interest, therefore, to
find that the effects of A1 stimulation on SON AVP cell
activity were not blocked by the α-adrenoreceptor antagonists
prazosin (300 μg -30 mg/kg, n = 6) or phentolamine (10-20
mg/kg, n = 8). This is well illustrated in Fig. 3, where we
see that i.v. prazosin blocked the effect of pressure-
applied NA but not the effect of A1 stimulation. It is
plausible that exogenously applied NA acts at extra-junctional
receptors and that only these were effectively blocked by
prazosin; however, the dose of prazosin given was 50 times
that found sufficient to block the effects of A6 NA cell
group stimulation on lateral geniculate neurons (Rogawski
and Aghajanian, 1982). An alternative explanation is that

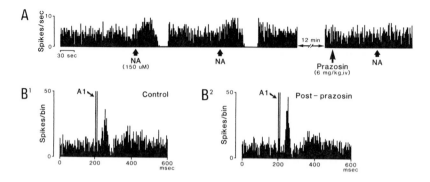

Fig. 3 A: NA-induced excitation of this SON AVP cell was blocked by systemic administration of prazosin. B1: A peristimulus histogram collected before the sequence illustrated in A shows that this cell responded to A1 stimulation (0.5 msec pulses, 100 µA). B2: A peristimulus histogram collected after the sequence illustrated in A; prazosin had not altered the response to A1 stimulation.

A1 NA afferents do not exclusively utilize NA as a neuro-transmitter.

Immunocytochemical studies have demonstrated that, like sympathetic post-ganglionic neurons, A1 neurons contain a peptide similar in structure to members of the pancreatic polypeptide (PP) family (cf. Day *et al.*, 1985a for refs.). In the case of the autonomic nervous system there is increasing evidence that this peptide acts as a neurotrans-mitter (cf. Emson and De Quidt, 1984). Consequently, it was decided to examine the effects on SON AVP cells of 2 PP family members : avian pancreatic polypeptide (APP) and neuropeptide-Y (NPY). Pressure-applied APP (17-170 µM) excited 80% (20/25) of cells tested. Like NA, APP was capable of both initiating bursts and of increasing intra-burst firing rates (Fig. 4). In contrast to APP, NPY at similar concentrations (20-200 µM) excited only 19% (3/16) of units tested; application at a considerably higher concentration (2 mM) excited 30% (3/10). Neither APP nor NPY had any direct depressant effects on AVP cell activity, but it was noted in 4 instances that prolonged exposure to APP reduced the normal excitatory effects of NA. Thus, it would appear that the relationship between PP-related

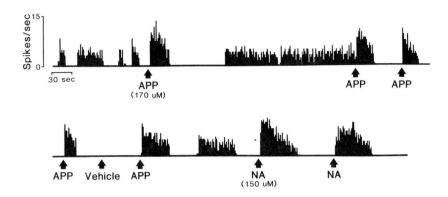

Fig. 4: Both APP (170 μM) and NA (150 μM) excited this putative AVP SON unit. Pressure application of vehicle (5 mM HCl, 1% BSA, 0.9% NaCl) had no effect.

peptides and NA differs from system to system. In the periphery there is evidence that NPY, or an NPY-like peptide, acts post-synaptically to mimic and potentiate the actions of NA on blood vessels, but acts pre-synaptically to inhibit NA release in vas deferens (cf. Emson and De Quidt, 1984). Regardless, the present data are consistent with the possibility that the excitatory effects of A1 NA afferents on AVP secretion may be mediated, at least to some degree and in some circumstances, by a PP-like peptide.

PHYSIOLOGICAL ROLE OF THE A1 PROJECTION TO AVP CELLS

The A1 projection may serve as a pathway for the conveyance of sensory information from the periphery to neurosecretory AVP cells. Accordingly it has recently been shown that blockade of A1 area neuronal function abolishes haemorrhage-induced AVP secretion (Blessing and Willoughby, 1985b). The identity of the sensory receptors involved is uncertain, however. Baroreceptor-unloading may contribute, but it was noted that haemorrhage elicited a metabolic acidosis which was balanced by a reflex alkalosis. This observation strongly suggests some degree of chemoreceptor activation. Banks and Harris (1984) have reported that A1 area lesions block the effect of carotid chemoreceptor

activation on AVP cell discharge. A1 lesions also abolished
baroreceptor-induced depression of AVP cell activity but it
is likely that this involves a pathway through the locus
coeruleus, rather than a direct projection from A1 to hypothalamus (see also Jhamandas and Renaud, 1986).

Attention has thus far focussed on chemoreceptor and
baroreceptor inputs, but the A1 projection may well convey
information related to other sensory modalities also.
Noxious stimuli enhance AVP release (Tata and Buzalkov,
1966) and, as has previously been noted, the A1 cell group
is ideally located for the receipt of nociceptive inputs
from all levels of the spinal cord (Grzanna and Molliver,
1980). Consistent with this possibility, it has recently
been observed (Day, unpublished findings) that blockade of
A1 area neuronal function abolishes the excitation of AVP
cells produced by injection of the algogenic substance
capsaicin into the vascular supply of the hindlimb.

CONCLUDING REMARKS

The data presented here, in combination with the
findings of other workers, suggest that afferents originating
from the A1 NA cell group stimulate the secretion of AVP.
This action may involve the release of both NA and a PP-like
neuropeptide. It appears that the A1 NA projection may
integrate inputs from diverse populations of peripheral
sensory receptors and convey the sum of this information to
hypothalamic neurosecretory AVP cells.

REFERENCES

Armstrong WE, Gallagher MJ, Sladek CD (1986). Noradrenergic
    stimulation of supraoptic neuronal activity and vaso-
    pressin release *in vitro* : mediation by an α_1-receptor.
    Brain Res 365: 192.
Armstrong-James M, Fox K, Kruk ZL, Millar J (1981).
    Quantitative ionophoresis of catecholamines using multi-
    barrel carbon fibre electrodes. J Neurosci Meth 4: 385.
Banks D, Harris MC (1984). Lesions of the locus coeruleus
    abolish baroreceptor-induced depression of supraoptic
    neurones in the rat. J Physiol (Lond) 355: 383.

Barker JL, Crayton JW, Nicoll RA (1971). Supraoptic neurosecretory cells: adrenergic and cholinergic sensitivity.
Science 171: 208.

Blessing WW, Willoughby JO (1985a). Excitation of neuronal
function in rabbit caudal ventrolateral medulla elevates
plasma vasopressin. Neurosci Lett 58: 189.

Blessing WW, Willoughby JO (1985b). Inhibiting the rabbit
caudal ventrolateral medulla prevents baroreceptor-
initiated secretion of vasopressin. J Physiol (Lond) 367:
253.

Cobbett P, Smithson KG, Hatton GI (1986). Immunoreactivity
to vasopressin- but not oxytocin-associated neurophysin
antiserum in phasic neurons of rat hypothalamic paraventricular nucleus. Brain Res 362: 7.

Dahlstrom A, Fuxe K (1964). Evidence for the existence of
monoamine-containing neurons in the central nervous
system. I. Demonstration of monoamines in the cell bodies
of brainstem neurons. Acta Physiol Scand, Suppl 232: 1.

Day TA, Ferguson AV, Renaud LP (1984). Facilitatory
influence of noradrenergic afferents on the excitability
of rat paraventricular nucleus neurosecretory cells.
J Physiol (Lond) 355: 237.

Day TA, Renaud LP (1984). Electrophysiological evidence
that noradrenergic afferents selectively facilitate the
activity of supraoptic vasopressin neurons. Brain Res
303: 233.

Day TA, Jhamandas JH, Renaud LP (1985a). Comparison between
the actions of avian pancreatic polypeptide, neuropeptide
Y and noradrenaline on rat supraoptic vasopressin neurons.
Neurosci Lett 62: 181.

Day TA, Randle JCR, Renaud LP (1985b). Opposing α- and
β-adrenergic mechanisms mediate dose-dependent actions of
noradrenaline on supraoptic vasopressin neurones *in vivo*.
Brain Res 358: 171.

Emson PC, De Quidt ME (1984). NPY - a new member of the
pancreatic polypeptide family. Trends Neurosci 7: 31.

Fuxe K (1965). Evidence for the existence of monoamine
neurons in the central nervous system. IV. The distribution of monoamine nerve terminals in the central nervous
system. Acta Physiol Scand 64, Suppl 247: 37.

Grzanna R, Molliver ME (1980). Cytoarchitecture and
dendritic morphology of central noradrenergic neurons.
In Hobson JA, Brazier MAB (eds): "The Reticular Formation
Revisited" New York: Raven Press, p 83.

Jhamandas JH, Renaud LP (1986). Diagonal band neurons may
mediate arterial baroreceptor input to hypothalamic vasopressin-secreting neurons. Neurosci Lett 65: 214.

Kannan H, Yamashita H, Osaka T (1984). Paraventricular
neurosecretory neurons: synaptic inputs from the ventrolateral medulla in rats. Neurosci Lett 51: 183.

Moore SD, Guyenet PG (1983). Alpha-receptor mediated
inhibition of A2 noradrenergic neurons. Brain Res 276:
188.

Moss RL, Dyball REJ Cross BA (1971). Responses of antidromically identified supraoptic and paraventricular
units to acetylcholine, noradrenaline and glutamate
applied iontophoretically. Brain Res 35: 573.

Randle JCR, Borque CW, Renaud LP (1984). α-adrenergic
activation of rat hypothalamic supraoptic neurons maintained
in vitro. Brain Res 307: 374.

Randle JCR, Mazurek M, Kneifel D, Dufresne J, Renaud LP
(1986). α_1-adrenergic receptor activation releases vasopressin and oxytocin from perfused rat hypothalamic
explants. Neurosci Lett 65: 219.

Rogawski MA, Aghajanian GK (1982). Activation of lateral
geniculate neurons by locus coeruleus or dorsal
noradrenergic bundle stimulation: selective blockade by
the $alpha_1$-adrenoreceptor antagonist prazosin. Brain Res
250: 31.

Sawchenko PE, Swanson LW (1981). Central noradrenergic
pathways for the integration of hypothalamic neuroendocrine
and autonomic responses. Science 214: 685.

Tanaka J, Kaba H, Saito H, Seto K (1985). Inputs from the
A1 noradrenergic region to hypothalamic paraventricular
neurons in the rat. Brain Res 335: 368.

Tata PS, Buzalkov R (1966). Vasopressin studies in the rat.
III. Inability of ethanol anaesthesia to prevent ADH
secretion due to pain and haemorrhage. Pflug Arch ges
Physiol 290: 294.

Wakerley JB, Noble R, Clarke G (1983). *In vitro* studies of
the control of phasic discharges in neurosecretory cells
of the supraoptic nucleus. Prog Brain Res 60: 53.

Yamashita H, Inenaga K, Kawata M, Sato Y (1983). Phasically
firing neurons in the supraoptic nucleus of the rat
hypothalamus: immunocytochemical and electrophysiological
studies. Neurosci Lett 37: 87.

Organization of the Autonomic Nervous System:
Central and Peripheral Mechanisms, pages 435–445
© 1987 Alan R. Liss, Inc.

THE SUBFORNICAL ORGAN: A CENTRAL INTEGRATOR IN THE
CONTROL OF NEUROHYPOPHYSIAL HORMONE SECRETION

Alastair V. Ferguson

Department of Physiology
Queen's University
Kingston, Ontario
CANADA K7L 3N6

INTRODUCTION

Blood borne hormones are known to influence many
physiological functions by actions within the central
nervous system (CNS). However the mechanisms through
which such substances gain access to the brain, and
influence neuronal excitability remain poorly understood.
Although the blood-brain barrier is relatively impermeable
to peptide hormones these substances are known to play
major roles in the feedback control loops through which
many homeostatic functions are controlled. Recent studies
suggest that specific windows exist in the CNS, known as
circumventricular structures, which lack the normal
blood-brain barrier (Dellman and Simpson, 1979), and
contain high densities of specific peptidergic receptors.
One such structure the subfornical organ (SFO) has been
implicated as a CNS structure at which circulating
angiotensin II (AII) acts to modify the secretion of
vasopressin from the posterior pituitary (Iovino and
Steardo, 1985; Knepel et al., 1981). Systemic AII has
been shown to reach the SFO and bind to specific AII
receptors within this structure (Mendelsohn et al., 1984).
It has been demonstrated also, that destruction of the SFO
abolishes the increases in arterial blood pressure
(Mangiapane and Simpson, 1980), drinking behaviour
(Simpson et al., 1978) and secretion of vasopressin
(Knepel et al., 1981) normally observed in response to
systemic AII.

Anatomical studies describing efferent projections from the SFO to the hypothalamic supraoptic (SON) and paraventricular (PVN) nuclei (Lind et al., 1982; Miselis, 1981) demonstrate pathways through which the SFO may influence neurohypophysial hormone secretion. This chapter will review recent studies which provide new information as to the cellular mechanisms through which neural elements of the SFO may play a role in the control of pituitary hormone secretion by influencing the excitability of hypothalamic oxytocin and vasopressin secreting neurons. These studies fall into one of two complimentory areas investigating the role of either systemic AII or electrical activation of SFO efferents in the control of oxytocin and vasopressin secretion.

SYSTEMIC ANGIOTENSIN II

Vasopressin Secretion

Systemic AII stimulates the release of vasopressin from the posterior pituitary although until recently the mechanisms underlying this effect were poorly understood. It has now been reported that lesions of the SFO abolish these effects of AII on the release of vasopressin (Iovino and Steardo, 1985; Knepel et al., 1981) indicating this to be the CNS site of action for the former peptide. In agreement with such a conclusion is the observation that systemically administered AII binds to specific receptors within the SFO (Van Houten et al., 1983; Mendelsohn et al., 1984). Other forebrain regions including the organum vasculosum of the lamina terminalis (OVLT), AV3V (Lind et al., 1984) and nucleus medianus (Mangiapane et al., 1983) may play a role in these responses, although metabolic studies demonstrating selective stimulation of the SFO following AII (Gross et al., 1985) suggest this structure to be of primary importance. Another question which deserves attention is the role of AII in controlling the secretion of oxytocin specifically in view of recent electrophysiological and endocrine studies (see Electrical Stimulation of SFO) indicating a facilitatory role.

SFO Neurons

Extracellular single unit recordings from SFO neurons both in vivo and in vitro report a relatively slow ($<$ 5 Hz) spontaneous firing frequency (Buranarugsa and Hubbard, 1979; Felix and Akert, 1975; Ishibashi et al., 1985). These studies also report that SFO neurons increase their firing rate in response to both systemic and iontophoretic administration of AII, establishing at the cellular level the responsiveness of SFO neural elements to this peptide. Recent studies demonstrating that a population of these SFO neurons which respond to systemic AII may be antidromically activated by electrical stimulation in the PVN (Tanaka et al., 1985) support the hypothesis that these are primary CNS pathways through which this peptide influences neurohypophysial hormone secretion.

Oxytocin and Vasopressin Secreting Neurons

Considerable information therefore indicates that circulating AII influences the secretion of vasopressin through an action within the SFO. We have now addressed this question at the cellular level by examining the effects of systemic AII on the excitability of identified oxytocin and vasopressin secreting neurons in the hypothalamic SON and PVN (Ferguson and Renaud, in press). In agreement with previous (Mitchell et al., 1982) studies it was found that putative vasopressin secreting neurons showed increases in excitability following AII administration. A more novel and surprising finding of these studies was the similar demonstration of a facilitatory influence of AII on the activity of putative oxytocin secreting neurons. A third group of identified neurons within the PVN, those projecting to the nucleus tractus solitarius, were unaffected by AII (Ferguson, 1986) indicating the effects of AII to be specific to the neurohypophysial oxytocin and vasopressin secreting neurons. Also these studies demonstrated, that following destruction of the SFO by electrolytic lesions, these effects of systemic AII on neurohypophysial cell excitability were abolished (Table 1).

TABLE 1. Effects of systemic AII on the excitability of oxytocin and vasopressin secreting neurons in intact and SFO lesioned rats. N = number of cells tested. Other columns represent % of cells tested in which activity was enhanced (↑) inhibited (↓) or unaffected (→) by systemic AII.

	PHASIC/BP SENSITIVE (putative vasopressin)				CONTINUOUS/BP INSENS. (putative oxytocin)			
	N	↑	↓	→	N	↑	↓	→
INTACT	12	83	17	0	32	75	0	25
LESIONED	5	0	100	0	10	0	0	100

ELECTRICAL STIMULATION OF SFO

Oxytocin and Vasopressin Secretion

As outlined in the preceeding section considerable circumstantial evidence suggests that systemic AII acts at the SFO to stimulate the release of vasopressin and possibly oxytocin from the posterior pituitary. However until recently no direct evidence was available as to the effects of activation of SFO efferents on the circulating concentrations of these peptide hormones in conscious animals. Studies in my laboratory have now shown that discrete electrical stimulation in the SFO, but not in immediately adjacent regions such as the hippocampal commissure or medial septum , results in significant increases in the circulating concentrations of not only vasopressin but also oxytocin (Fig. 1) in freely moving rats (Ferguson and Kasting, 1986). These data support the view that activation of SFO efferents facilitates the activity of hypothalamic neurohypophysial neurons.

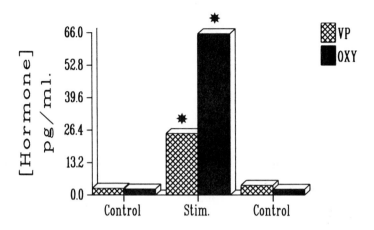

Figure 1. Histogram illustrating plasma oxytocin (N=4) and vasopressin (N=5) concentrations 60 min before (Control), immediately following (Stim.) and 60 min after (Control) electrical stimulation (200 µA, 10 Hz, 30 sec On-Off, 3 min) in the subfornical organ of conscious freely moving rats. * p < 0.01.

Effects on Neurohypophysial Cell Excitability

The anatomical demonstration of dense efferent projections from the SFO to the hypothalamic SON and PVN (Lind et al., 1982; Miselis, 1981) showed direct CNS pathways through which activation of SFO neurons could influence the excitability of oxytocin and vasopressin secreting neurons located within these two nuclei (Swaab et al., 1975; Vandesande and Dierickx, 1975). Studies at the ultrastructural level have confirmed that at least a portion of these SFO efferents synapse directly on the oxytocin and vasopressin containing neurosecretory cells (Renaud et al., 1983).

Electrophysiological studies have now examined the functional nature of these SFO connections with neurohypophysial neurons. It has been reported that electrical stimulation in the SFO has predominantly excitatory effects on antidromically identified neurohypophysial neurons (Fig. 2a, b, d) in both the SON and PVN (Ferguson et al., 1984; Sgro et al., 1984; Tanaka et al., 1985), although inhibitory responses were observed in a small proportion of these neurosecretory cells (Fig. 2b, c). These excitatory responses were either of

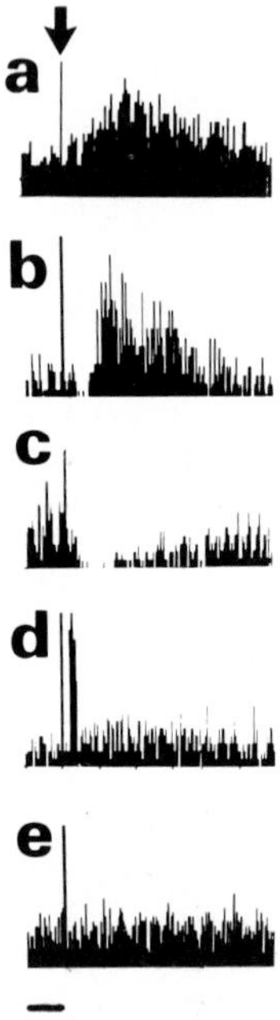

	VP NEURONS	OXY NEURONS
	(phasic : n=38)	(contin : n=116)
a	45	43
b	24	15
c	13	3
d	5	18
e	13	21

Figure 2. Summary of data comparing the effects of electrical stimulation in the subfornical organ (↓) on the excitability of putative vasopressin (VP) and oxytocin (OXY) neurons in the hypothalamic supraoptic and paraventricular nuclei. Peristimulus histograms (a-e, bar = 100 ms) represent the five response profiles observed, while figures indicate the % of neurons tested showing that response.

short latency and short duration (Fig. 2d), or were in the form of a longer latency prolonged response lasting up to 500 ms (Fig. 2a). The observed inhibitory effects suggest some degree of functional heterogeneity in these SFO projections to the hypothalamus, specifically as in some cases mixed effects were observed (Fig. 2b). Preliminary information suggests that such heterogeneity may result from the involvement of secondary polysynaptic connections between these two structures (see Medial Septum/Diagonal Band Neurons). Also we find that cells demonstrating long duration excitatory effects following SFO stimulation show enhanced excitability in response to systemic AII (Ferguson and Renaud, 1986), indicating that this functional pathway may be specifically activated by AII.

A second important question addressed by the above electrophysiological studies related to whether SFO efferents were preferentially distributed to the vasopressin secreting neurons, as had been suggested by anatomical studies at the light microscopic level (Sawchenko and Swanson, 1983). However similar effects of SFO stimulation were observed on both putatively identified oxytocin and vasopressin secreting neurons (Fig. 2). This finding draws strong support from the endocrine studies outlined above reporting increased plasma concentrations of both of these peptide hormones in response to electrical stimulation in the SFO (Ferguson and Kasting, 1986).

Medial Septum/Diagonal Band Neurons

It has already been suggested that SFO effects on hypothalamic neurosecretory cells may result from the activation of polysynaptic as well as monosynaptic pathways. Anatomical studies have reported that SFO sends efferent projections to the medial septum (Miselis, 1981; Lind et al. 1982), a region known to project to the SON (Zaborsky et al, 1975), while electrophysiological studies have reported that electrical stimulation in the medial septum has primarily inhibitory effects on neurohypophysial neurons (Cirino and Renaud, 1985; Negoro et al., 1973; Poulain et al., 1980). Recent studies have demonstrated that some 60% of neurons in the medial septum/diagonal band region antidromically identified as projecting to the region of the SON are orthodromically activated by electrical stimulation in the SFO (Ferguson et al., 1985). It is therefore possible that these polysynaptic connections may mediate the inhibitory effects of SFO stimulation on oxytocin and vasopressin secreting neurons.

CONCLUSIONS

Evidence now suggests that the SFO may act as a window through which circulating peptide hormones gain access to the nervous system and thus influence further hormone secretion. It has been demonstrated that systemically administered AII binds to specific receptors within the SFO causing the activation of both oxytocin and vasopressin secreting neurohypophysial neurons and, increased plasma concentrations of the latter peptide. Other studies report that electrical stimulation in the SFO causes increased plasma concentrations of oxytocin and vasopressin, as well as facilitating the excitability of the majority of neurohypophysial neurons tested. In conclusion it would appear that the SFO may act as a sensory structure within the CNS responding to changes in peripheral hormone concentrations and modifying the secretion of oxytocin and vasopressin from the posterior pituitary in response to such changes.

Acknowledgments: Research supported by MRC of Canada. Thanks to Wendy Brown and Dorothy Robichaud for secretarial and technical assistance.

REFERENCES

Buranarugsa P, Hubbard JI (1979). The neuronal organization of the rat subfornical organ in vitro and a test of the osmo- and morphine- receptor hypothesis. Journal of Physiology 291:101-116.
Cirino M, Renaud LP (1985). Influence of lateral septum and amygdala stimulation on the excitability of hypothalamic supraoptic neurons. An electrophysiological study in the rat. Brain Res 326:357-361.
Dellman HD, Simpson JB (1979). The subfornical organ. Int Rev Cytol 58:333-421.

Felix D, Akert K (1974). The effect of angiotensin II on neurones of the cat subfornical organ. Brain Res 76:350-353.

Ferguson AV (1986). Lesions of the subfornical organ abolish activation of hypothalamic oxytocin and vasopressin neurons in response to systemic angiotensin II. Canadian Journal of Physiology and Pharmacology 64(4):Aix-Ax.

Ferguson AV, Kasting NW (1986). Electrical stimulation in subfornical organ increases plasma vasopressin concentrations in the conscious rat. American Journal of Physiology 251:(in press).

Ferguson AV, Renaud LP (1986). Systemic angiotensin II acts at the subfornical organ to facilitate the activity of neurohypophysial neurons in the rat. Ameri-Journal of Physiology (in press).

Ferguson AV, Day TA Renaud LP (1984b). Subfornical organ afferents influence the excitability of neurohypophysial and tuberoinfundibular paraventricular nucleus neurons in the rat. Neuroendocrinology 39:423-428.

Ferguson AV, Bourque CW, Renaud LP (1985). Subfornical organ and supraoptic nucleus connections with septal neurons in rats. American Journal of Physiology 249:R214-R218.

Gross PM, Kadekaro M, Andrews DW, Sokoloff L, Saavedra JM (1985). Selective metabolic stimulation of the subfornical organ and pituitary neural lobe by peripheral angiotensin II. Peptides 6(1):145-152.

Iovino M, Steardo L (1984). Vasopressin release to central and peripheral angiotensin II in rats with lesions of the subfornical organ. Brain Res 322:365-368.

Ishibashi S, Oomura Y, Gueguen B, Nicolaidis S (1985). Neuronal responses in subfornical organ and other regions to angiotensin II applied by various routes. Brain Res Bull 14:307-314.

Knepel W, Nutto D, Meyer DK (1982). Effect of transection of subfornical organ efferent projections on vasopressin release induced by angiotensin or isoprenaline in the rat. Brain Res 248:180-184.

Lind RW, Van Hoesen GW, Johnson AK (1982). An HRP study of the connections of the subfornical organ of the rat. J Comp Neurol 210:265-277.

Lind RW, Thunhorst RL, Johnson AK (1984). The subfornical organ and the integration of multiple factors in thirst. Physiology and Behaviour 32:69-74.

Mangiapane ML, Simpson JB (1980). Subfornical organ lesions reduce the pressor effect of systemic angiotensin II. Neuroendocrinol 31:380-384.

Mangiapane ML, Thrasher TN, Keil LC, Simpson JB, Ganong WF (1983). Deficits in drinking and vasopressin secretion after lesions of the nucleus medianus. Neuroendocrinology 37:73-77.

Mendelsohn FAO, Quirion R, Saavedra JM, Aguilera G, Catt KJ (1984). Autoradiographic localization of angiotensin II receptors in rat brain. PNAS, USA 81:1575-1579.

Miselis R (1981). The efferent projections of the subfornical organ of the rat: a circumventricular organ with a neural network subserving water balance. Brain Res 230:1-23.

Mitchell LD, Barron K, Brody MJ, Johnson AK (1982). Two possible actions for circulating angiotensin II in the control of vasopressin release. Peptides 3:503-507.

Negoro H, Visessuwan S, Holland RC (1973). Inhibition and excitation of units in paraventricular nucleus after stimulation of the septum, amygdala and neurohypophysis. Brain Res 57:479-483.

Poulain DA, Ellendorff F, Vincent JD (1980). Septal connections with identified oxytocin and vasopressin neurones in the supraoptic nucleus of the rat. An electrophysiological investigation. Neuroscience 5:379-387.

Renaud LP, Rogers J, Sgro S (1983). Terminal degeneration in supraoptic nucleus following subfornical organ lesions: ultrastructural observations in the rat. Brain Res 275:365-368.

Sawchenko PE, Swanson LW (1983). The organization of forebrain afferents to the paraventricular and supraoptic nuclei of the rat. J Comp Neurol 218:121-144.

Sgro S, Ferguson AV, Renaud LP (1984). Subfornical organ - supraoptic nucleus connections: an electrophysiological study in the rat. Brain Res 303:7-13.

Simpson JB, Epstein AN, Komado JS (1978). Localization of dipsogenic receptors for angiotensin II in the subfornical organ. J Comp Physiol Psychol 92:581-608.

Swaab DF, Pool CW, Nijveldt F (1975). Immunofluorescence of vasopressin and oxytocin in the rat hypothalamo-neurohypophyseal system. J Neural Trans 36:195-215.
Tanaka J, Kaba H, Saito H, Seto K (1985). Subfornical organ neurons with efferent projections to the hypothalamic paraventricular nucleus: an electrophysiological study in the rat. Brain Res 346:151-154.
Vandesande F, Dierickx K (1975). Identification of the vasopressin producing and of the oxytocin producing neurons in the hypothalamic neurosecretory system of the rat. Cell Tiss Res 164:153-162.
VanHouten M, Mangiapane ML, Reid IA, Ganong WF (1983). (Sar^1, Ala^8) angiotensin II in cerebrospinal fluid blocks the binding of blood borne (^{125}I) angiotensin II to the circumventricular organs. Neuroscience 10:1421-1426.
Zaborsky L, Leranth CS, Makara GB, Palkovits M (1975). Quantitative studies on the supraoptic nucleus of the rat. II. Afferent fibre connections. Exp Brain Res 22:525-540.

Organization of the Autonomic Nervous System:
Central and Peripheral Mechanisms, pages 447–456
© 1987 Alan R. Liss, Inc.

THE ROLE OF SUPRAOPTIC NEURONES IN BLOOD PRESSURE
REGULATION

Gareth Leng and Richard E.J. Dyball*

AFRC Institute of Animal Physiology and Genetics
Research, Babraham, Cambridge CB2 4AT and*
Department of Anatomy, University of Cambridge,
Cambridge CB2 3DY, UK.

INTRODUCTION

The vasopressin secreting cells of the magnocellular
hypothalamic neurosecretory nuclei fire in bursts
(phasically) when stimulated by either a rise in plasma
osmotic pressure, or following severe haemorrhage. However,
the bursts of the different cells are not synchronised (Leng
and Dyball, 1983), so this patterning does not result in
pulsatile changes in plasma concentration of the hormone.
The effect of the phasic firing is rather to enhance the
secretion of vasopressin (Dutton and Dyball, 1977) by
facilitating stimulus-secretion coupling at the level of the
neurosecretory terminals in the neurohypophysis. About half
of the cells in the supraoptic nucleus of the vasopressin
deficient Brattleboro rat (DI rat) also display a phasic
pattern of firing, and these cells are believed to be the
defective vasopressin cells. Despite their inability to
synthesize vasopressin normally, these phasic cells respond
to osmotic stimulation like phasic cells in normal animals
(Dyball and Leng, 1985).

Supraoptic neurones in both normal rats (Wakerley et
al., 1975) and DI rats (Figure 1) respond to haemorrhage
with excitation and some respond to a large and rapid
increase in blood pressure (baroreceptor stimulation) with
inhibition. These effects appear to be mediated mainly by
chemoreceptors and baroreceptors in the carotid sinus and
aortic arch, and probably reach the supraoptic nucleus by a
mainly noradrenergic projection arising from the areas of
the A1 and A6 cell groups in the brainstem (Banks and

Harris, 1984). The baroreceptor effects are restricted to vasopressin cells in normal rats: oxytocin cells are not affected, neither are most of the non-neurosecretory cells immediately dorsal to the supraoptic nucleus (Dyball and Leng, 1986). However, in DI rats many oxytocin cells are also affected by baroreceptor stimulation (Leng and Dyball, 1984).

By comparison, haemorrhage, although potent, is likely to be a highly non-specific stimulus. Selective chemoreceptor stimulation is experimentally more elegant than haemorrhage, but also leads to neuronal activation throughout large areas of the brain (Banks, Harris and Stokes, 1985) and may thus be no more specific. Nevertheless, these results suggest that vasopressin may be involved in blood pressure regulation but what precise role does vasopressin play? Vasopressin is of course a very potent vasopressor agent, and there is excellent evidence that its presence in the circulation has a physiologically significant influence on blood pressure regulation under certain circumstances (e.g. Cowley and Barber, 1983; Chapman et al., 1986): we are not questioning the significance of this influence, but rather are asking the converse question, whether there is any real evidence in the rat that the activity of vasopressin cells is influenced by maintained changes in blood pressure within the physiological range.

METHODS

Conventional recording techniques were used to monitor the activity of magnocellular neurosecretory cells in the hypothalamus of rats anaesthetized with urethane (1.25 g/kg; i.p.). Recordings were made extracellularly using glass microlectrodes filled with 0.15M NaCl solution with a tip resistance of 20-30 megohms. The supraoptic nucleus was exposed from the ventral side and the cells identified as neurosecretory if they could be antidromically excited by electrical stimulation of the neural stalk (1 mA biphasic pulses; 1 ms pulse width). Blood pressure was monitored from a femoral artery, and a right atrial catheter was inserted for injection of pressor agents or removal of blood. Recordings from Brattleboro rats homozygous for diabetes insipidus (DI rats) from the AFRC Babraham colony were compared with recordings from a homozygous normal "wild-type" strain derived from the same Brattleboro rat colony.

RESULTS

In DI rats after surgery to expose the supraptic
nucleus from the ventral side the blood pressure was low
(30-60 mm Hg) compared with that in control rats following
the same surgery (50-100 mm Hg) but continuous infusions of
arginine vasopressin (1-10 mU/min as a solution of 400 mU/ml
in 0.9% saline) raised blood pressure to control values or
above. It thus appears that following urethane anaesthesia
and the severe stress of ventral surgery, vasopressin may be
an important factor in blood pressure maintenance, but is
the firing of phasic cells affected by changes in blood
pressure within the normal range in these rats?
Baroreceptor stimulation by i.v. injection of phenylephrine
can inhibit phasic cells (Harris, 1979), but in experiments
on both DI rats and on normal controls we consistently
observed that the action depends upon the precise timing of
the increase in blood pressure (Figures 2,3). When blood
pressure was increased by injection of phenylephrine shortly
after a burst started in the recorded cell (0-5 s after the
start of the burst, depending upon the firing pattern of the
particular cell), bursts were either unaffected, or were
lengthened by comparison with preceding and succeeding
bursts. Only if the stimulus was applied after the middle
of the burst was inhibition consistently observed.
Remembering that bursts in vasopressin cells do not occur
synchronously, it follows that baroreceptor stimulation
following phenylephrine injection will have mixed effects
upon vasopressin cells, that the effect is little more than
a re-setting of the phase of the burst, and that the effect
on vasopressin release, although not directly measurable, is
likely to be slight. It should also be stressed that, in
both normal and DI rats, the cells are rather insensitive
and that blood pressure must be raised by 50 mm Hg or more
before inhibition occurs reliably, even when the stimulus is
applied at an appropriate point in the burst.

We therefore attempted to examine the influence of
sustained changes in blood pressure upon the activity of
vasopressin cells. It is well established (Poulain,
Wakerley and Dyball, 1977) that haemorrhage excites
vasopressin cells in normal rats: however a severe decrease
in blood pressure (to 30-40 mm Hg) is required to activate

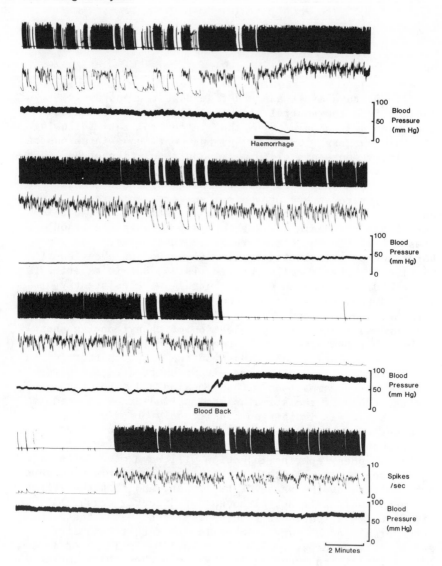

Figure 1. Response of a phasic supraoptic neurone from a DI
rat to withdrawal of 4 ml blood. The top trace marks
individual spikes; the middle trace is a ratemeter record of
the neuronal activity, and the lower trace shows blood
pressure. The haemorrhage caused a large fall in blood
pressure and neuronal excitation: return of the blood
restored blood pressure and transiently inhibited the cell.

the cells reliably. This is consistent with evidence in the cat that vasopressin release does not increase following haemorrhage until blood pressure has fallen by 80 mm Hg or more from control values of greater than 100 mm Hg (Beleslin et al., 1967). In DI rats, phasic cells appear to respond reversibly to haemorrhage like those in normal rats, and require a proportionately similar fall in blood pressure (Figure 1).

We produced sustained rises in blood pressure in DI rats by continuous i.v. infusion of vasopressin (see above). Such infusions did not produce stable blood pressure changes in normal rats, but in DI rats we could, by adjusting the infusion rate, maintain blood pressure at any predetermined value in the range 40-120 mm Hg for 30 min or more. In experiments on seven DI rats, we recorded from eight phasic cells during vasopressin infusions for periods of 1 h or more, and correlated their firing rate with blood pressure during periods when the blood pressure was stable.

It became clear that the rate at which blood pressure changes occurred was important. If the changes occur sufficiently slowly (less than 10 mm Hg/ min) the firing rate of the cells was not substantially affected (Figure 4). Transient excitation or inhibition occurred if blood pressure was changed more rapidly, but these changes in firing rate were not sustained when blood pressure was stabilised within the range 40-120 mm Hg. For each cell, mean firing rate was measured over a period of 8-15 min when blood pressure was stable, and calculated as mean $\pm$ standard error of spikes/10 s segment. The rate of vasopressin infusion was then altered, and firing rate measured again when blood pressure was stable at a new level. Each cell was studied through between four and ten such changes, and no cell showed any significant change in firing rate with blood pressure. Each of these cells responded normally to baroreceptor inhibition: bursts were terminated if 10-20 ug phenylephrine was injected i.v.

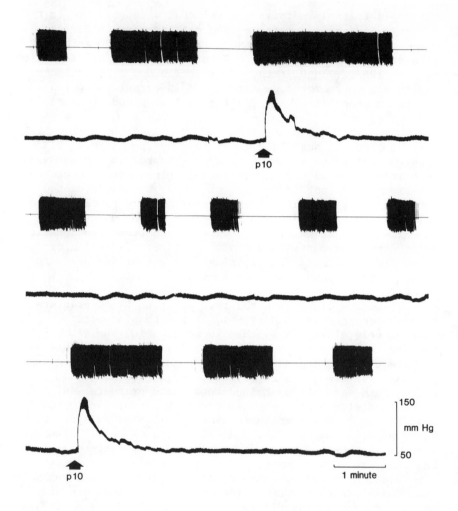

Figure 2. Response of a phasic cell from a normal rat to
i.v. phenylephrine (10 ug, P10). Injections given at the
beginning of a burst prolonged the burst.

Figure 3 (next page). Response of a phasic cell from a
normal rat to i.v. phenylephrine. Injections of 20 ug
(P20), but not of 10 ug (P10) truncated bursts of activity
when given in the middle of the burst. Injections given
between bursts delayed the next burst, and injections given
at the beginning of a burst prolonged it.

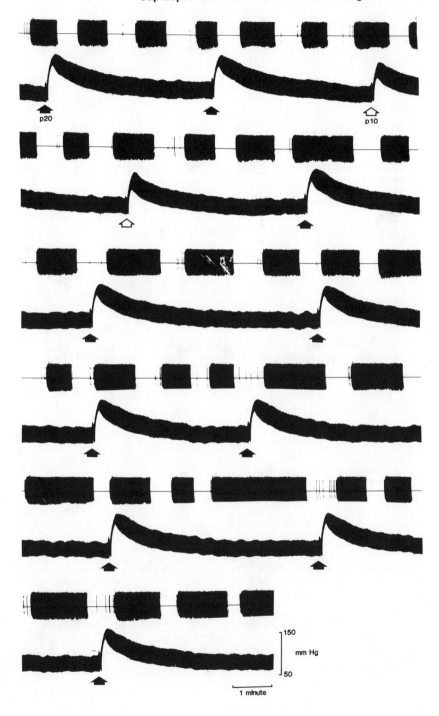

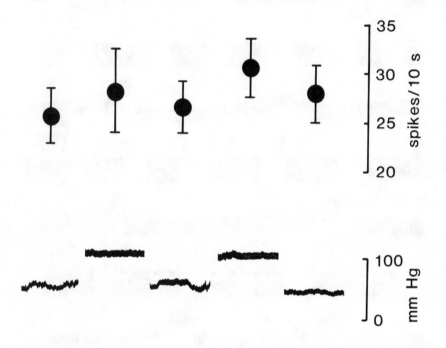

Figure 4. Response of a phasic cell from a DI rat to blood pressure changes produced by i.v. infusion of vasopressin. The symbols show mean number of spikes per 10 s (+ standard error) from 8–15 min of recording when the blood pressure was stable. Below each point is a portion of the blood pressure record from the period over which mean firing rate was calculated. No correlation was found between firing rate and blood pressure in these experiments.

DISCUSSION

It is probable that vasopressin is involved in the maintenance of blood pressure, even though its importance is only clearly apparent under particular experimental conditions, such as following severe haemorrhage or severe surgical trauma. It may be however that what is required under normal circumstances is the presence of sufficient vasopressin to sustain other blood pressure regulating mechanisms rather than that vasopressin secretion is directly related to blood pressure.

What evidence makes us suspect that this is the case? It is clear that the activity of rat vasopressin cells is transiently inhibited by very large rises in blood pressure, and transiently excited by very large drops in blood pressure, but over a very wide range of blood pressure, the firing of vasopressin cells may be independent of blood pressure. The data presented in this paper derive mainly from a study of phasic neurones in DI rats, and what is true for these cells may not be true for normal vasopressin cells. However, phasic cells in DI rats respond as normal vasopressin cells to osmotic stimuli, to baroreceptor stimulation and to haemorrhage. What we believe these results really indicate is the lack of any evidence in normal rats that vasopressin release is related to sustained changes in blood pressure in the range 40-120 mm Hg. Direct evidence is difficult to obtain because the removal of sufficient blood for measurement of plasma vasopressin concentration will in itself constitute a haemorrhage stimulus in rats. However, if vasopressin release in the rat is indeed stimulated only by a virtual collapse of blood pressure, this response may be of little physiological significance. This is not of course to suggest that vasopressin is not important in blood pressure homeostasis: normal vasopressin levels may have a "permissive" effect on other cardiovascular regulatory mechanisms by their tonic effect on the vascular system.

REFERENCES

Banks D, Harris MC (1984). Lesions of the locus coeruleus abolish baroreceptor-induced depression of supraoptic neurones in the rat. J Physiol (Lond) 355: 383–398.
Banks D, Harris MC, Stokes WN (1986). Carotid body chemoreceptor stimulation in rats activates large areas of the forebrain but not the hypothalamus. J Physiol (Lond) 371: 114P.
Beleslin D, Bisset GW, Haldar J, Polak RL (1967). The release of vasopressin without oxytocin in response to haemorrhage. Proc R Soc Lond B 166: 443–458.
Chapman JT, Hreash F, Laycock JF, Walter SJ (1986). The cardiovascular effects of vasopressin after haemorrhage in anaesthetized rats. J Physiol (Lond) 375: 421–434.
Cowley AW, Barber BJ (1983). Vasopressin vascular and reflex effects – a theoretical analysis. Progr Brain Res 60: 415–424.
Dutton A, Dyball REJ (1979). Phasic firing enhances vasopressin release from the rat neurohypophysis. J Physiol (Lond) 290: 433–440
Dyball REJ, Leng G (1985). Supraoptic neurones in Brattleboro rats respond normally to changes in plasma osmotic pressure. J Endocr 105: 87–90.
Dyball REJ, Leng, G (1986). Regulation of the milk-ejection reflex in the rat. J Physiol (Lond) in press
Harris MC (1979). Effects of chemoreceptor and baroreceptor stimulation on the discharge of hypothalamic supraoptic neurones in the rat. J Endocr 82: 115–125.
Leng G, Dyball REJ (1983). Intercommunication in the rat supraoptic nucleus. Q J Exp Physiol 68: 493–504.
Leng G, Dyball REJ (1984). Altered baroreceptor inputs to the supraoptic nucleus of the Brattleboro rat. Exp Brain Res 54: 571–574.
Poulain DA, Wakerley JB, Dyball REJ (1977). Electrophysiological differentiation of oxytocin- and vasopressin-secreting neurones. Proc R Soc Lond B 196:367–384.
Wakerley JB, Poulain DA, Dyball REJ, Cross BA (1975). Activity of phasic neurosecretory cells during haemorrhage. Nature 258: 82–84.

Postscript

Organization of the Autonomic Nervous System:
Central and Peripheral Mechanisms, pages 459–463
© 1987 Alan R. Liss, Inc.

THE AUTONOMIC NERVOUS SYSTEM AND RECENTLY ACQUIRED UNDER-
STANDING OF ITS FUNCTION AND ORGANIZATION

Chandler McCuskey Brooks,
Distinguished Professor of State Univ. of N.Y.

Department of Physiology, SUNY, Health Science
Center at Brooklyn, 450 Clarkson Ave., Brooklyn,
New York 11203, USA

During this symposium many of the major figures who,
during the past 20 years have supported a new surge of
interest in the autonomic system complex, have reported
their recent findings and conclusions relative to this
component of the nervous system. I have watched and considered what I have heard.

Time and circumstance determine one's role in life
and I assume that my present commission in the concluding
of this meeting should be different from the common analytical approach. No longer swimming in the river of
"hands-on-research" I have been standing on the shore watch-
ing what is passing, what has passed and what is approaching.
It is appropriate that I express a somewhat different view.

I offer no criticism but recognize the present emphasis
and appropriateness of reductionist thought. Of the 45
papers presented by title at least 30 dealt with very
specific matters such as properties of various neuron types,
transmitters, the pathways of reflex actions. The word
organization was used frequently but relative only to restricted performances of parts. Approximately 10 dealt
with foci of control or regulation of specific reactions.
There were 4 papers that definitely dealt with integrative
control of behavior and revealed thought concerning the
unity of the totality. It is this type of concept that I
wish to emphasize because I consider "integrative" power
the essence of life and the autonomic system to be the
integrator of body function in its totality.

I agree with those who conceive of the biological world as a totality with each living thing playing its role in support of the whole. There are factors of safety and a few species may die without noticeable consequence but not without effect. The marvel is the integrative power that correlates this diversity to make strong the whole.

Man is a totality, the autonomic system plays a truly major role in the integration maintaining required balances, adaptability, effectiveness of perception and the qualities of behavior. Its study leads to the goals of the future because physiology must become more of a behavioral, sociological and philosophical science. The big problems and the big objectives pertain to totalities and not minutia.

The work reported during this symposium has added to the extent and refinement of our knowledge. Month by month our concept is confirmed that the autonomic system inner- vates all tissues and participates to some degree in all functions even the development of the ovum (11) and ovulation (8), metabolism in all its complexities (6) and in the genesis and expressions of emotions (7). It participates not only in the organization but also the execution of reaction pat- terns. In this symposium there was consideration of the integration of alarm reactions, of homeostatic reflex actions. There was discussion of the role of afferents in triggering integrative reactions. However, reductionist thought is overwhelmingly dominant and on the whole many of our most recent such studies have added to the difficulty of understanding how central control and integration can dominate peripheral reactions to deliver visceral support to somatic system performance. I refer of course to studies of local reactions within ganglia and plexuses (5).

Recent knowledge of neurohumoral relations between the gut, the liver, the hypothalamus and pancreas have advanced integrative thought. Another example of new thought has arisen from studies of cardiac-renal relation- ships. Reflexes originating in the heart affect the kidney. Emissions from the kidney (renin-angiotension) and the heart - the atrial natriuretic peptide -affect the kidney and the hypothalamic - controlled reactions are involved. The point I make is that stimuli reverberate through the body and affect the totality. Our problem now is that of determining whether what can happen does happen normally and that of determining the degree of significance of that which does happen.

Another field of modern thought originated from studies of immunology (Paul Ehrlich 1854-1915) and of the autonomic nervous system (John N. Langley 1852-1925). Walter B. Cannon in his studies of transmitters and their action also used the concept of receptors (2,3). Receptors are now a world unto themselves. There are receptor points on receptors, receptors can be sensitized or chemically obtunded. For a while it was thought that receptors could be the recorders of experience and provide the mysterious power of memory but receptors have various half lives, they degenerate and regenerate (5), they are not the end of the line. Humoral agents and receptors combine and move in cell membranes - "lateralization." They trigger the release of messengers that effect more basic processes. The study of the humors, the receptors is beginning to merge with the chemistry of genetics. If we could just know more, remember more perhaps we could see in the avalanche of facts the beginning of the understanding of the totalities - but I cannot perceive it. However, we are making progress.

Of recent years there has been a greater realization of the role of the autonomic system in disease - in the creation of disease states by its excessive actions and/or its functional failures. Books have recently been published (1) and organizations have been formed and health organizations are attempting to deal with autonomic system disease-causing abnormalities (9).

Men more than any other creatures must learn. What is learned is of vital importance. Since Pavlov's day (3) we have known that the autonomic nervous system is highly involved in conditional learning. Obviously the conditioning of this system plays an important role in the quality and "color" of behavior. Since Galen's day (9) we have had the realization that the autonomic nervous system has a role to play in establishing the emotion of sympathy. Since sympathy even more than reason may tend to prevent man's imbalancing greed, acquisitiveness and destructiveness it seems reasonable that we should study the genesis of sympathy.

There is another attribute of man and society akin to sympathy. I refer to the ability to Hope. This kind of talk is far from the concepts we rely on in science and the purity of our methodology but creeping into our literature

is the evidence of a curative power of sympathy
and of hope (10). This is spiritual but man is both
physical and spiritual. The question arises - how are
the two linked. This is a question I see approaching us
and it probably is already here. Can the autonomic system
and the integrative centers that control it be better
trained to cultivate sympathy and entertain hope? The
diagram below at least expresses to me a concept of where
we are and how we are proceeding.

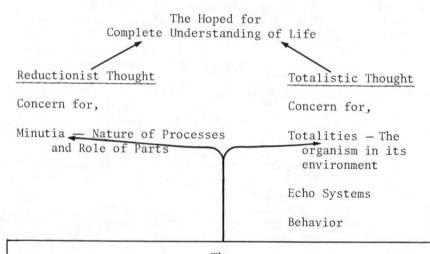

The Hoped for
Complete Understanding of Life

Reductionist Thought   Totalistic Thought

Concern for,   Concern for,

Minutia — Nature of Processes   Totalities — The
    and Role of Parts   organism in its
                                            environment

                                        Echo Systems

                                        Behavior

The
Basic Concepts of Physiological Thought

Functions characterize Life

Irritability: Excitability and Inhibition: Responsiveness

Metabolism: Use of Energy: Anabolism and Catabolism

Adaptation to effect change and maintain essential
constancies

Reproduction: Of parts and totalities, healing,
duplication growth, differentiation

Integrative Control: Of parts to serve the whole

The Parts   ←—┴—→ The Totalities

1. Bannister R (1983). Autonomic Failure: A Textbook of Clinical Disorders of the Autonomic Nervous System. Oxford Univ Press Oxford.
2. Brooks C McC (1983). Newer concepts of the autonomic system's role derived from reductionist and behavioral studies of various animal species. J auton Nerv Syst 7:199-212.
3. Brooks C McC (1985). I P Pavlov and W B Cannon: Founders of modern physiological thought relative to behavior and the autonomic system. Pavlovian J of Biol Sci 20:1-6.
4. Garrison F H (1914 & 1929). History of Medicine. W B Saunders Co Philadelphia.
5. Karczmer A G, Koketsu K and Nishi S (1986). Autonomic and Enteric Ganglia: Transmission and its Pharmacology. Plenum Press New York.
6. Mei N, Niijima A and Brooks C McC (Eds) (1984). General involvement of enteroreceptors in motor, homeostatic and behavioral regulations. J auton Nerv Syst 10:209-392.
7. Oomura Y (Ed) (1986). Emotions: Neuronal and Chemical Control. Japan Scientific Societies Press Tokyo S Karger A G Basle Switzerland.
8. Owman C, Edvinsson L, Sjöberg N-O, Sporrong B, Stefenson A and Walles B (1977). Influence of sympathetic nerves, amine receptors and anti-adrenergic drugs on follicular contractility and ovulation. Proc XVII International Congress of Neurovegetative Research: Homeostasis in the Autonomic Nervous System - Basic and Clinical Research Tokyo.
9. Pamnani G, Mueller G and Hom J (1986). Role of atrial natriuretic factor (ANF) in the development hypertension in reduced renal mass, saline drinking rats. Abstract Federation Proc #4305.
10. Schaefer H (1986). Social factors as causes for the dysfunction of the autonomic system. Proc. XIXth International Congress of Neurovegetative Research J auton Nerv Syst In Press.
11. Trzecrok W H, Ashmed C E, Simpson E R and Ojeda S R (1986). Vasoactive intestinal peptide induces synthesis of the cholesterol side-chain cleavage enzyme complex in cultured rat ovarian granulosa cells. Proc Nat Acad Sci, USA In Press.

Index